HEALTH CARE MARKETING MANAGEMENT

A Case Approach

Philip D. Cooper, Ph.D.
Associate Professor of Marketing
The University of Tulsa
Tulsa, Oklahoma

Larry M. Robinson, Ph.D.
Vice President—Research
Nationwide Insurance Companies
Columbus, Ohio

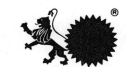

AN ASPEN PUBLICATION®
Aspen Systems Corporation
Rockville, Maryland
London
1982

Library of Congress Cataloging in Publication Data

Cooper, Philip D., 1942-
Health care marketing management.

Includes index.
1. Medical care—Marketing—Case studies.
2. Marketing management—Case studies.   I. Robinson,
Larry M.   II. Title.
RA410.5.C65   362.1′068′8   82-3904
ISBN: 0-89443-394-6   AACR2

Publisher: John Marozsan
Editorial Director: Mike Brown
Managing Editor: Margot Raphael
Editorial Services: M. Eileen Higgins
Printing and Manufacturing: Debbie Swarr

Printed in the United States of America

1 2 3 4 5

Table of Contents

Preface

The late 1970s witnessed a phenomenal surge of interest in the application of marketing to health care. Well over 200 articles were written, at least three books were published, several universities began to offer coursework in health care marketing, and many seminars on the topic were well attended by administrators. The authors were prompted to write this book because many administrators expressed to us their frustration over the lack of published health care situations amenable to the use of marketing concepts and techniques. We undertook to develop visible examples that could provide guidance as they formulate market-based plans and strategies.

This book represents the first collection of cases to examine the application of marketing concepts and strategies to the solution of challenges that health care administrators face. The 22 cases are not written to exemplify effective or ineffective handling of an administrative situation. Rather, they are presented to provide a focus for the reader and student and to develop a dialogue about the differing situations and uses of marketing. The overviews at the end of each case present opinions with which the reader may or may not agree.

Cases are drawn from a variety of health care settings. Nine concern the efforts of hospital administrators to develop market-based strategies. The others center on marketing efforts of primary clinics, health maintenance organizations, nursing homes, hospices, free-standing emergency rooms, multiphasic testing centers, medical associations, well-child clinics, and group practices.

Each case is based on a real situation. Great care has been taken to obtain approval for use of each organization's name. We are indebted to administrators at the following institutions for undisguised use of cases involving their organizations: Grady Memorial Hospital, Georgia Medical Plan, Moody Nursing Home, Minneapolis Hospice, Ohio State Medical Association, Southern Jamaica Plain Health Center, Sunrise Hospital, St. Elizabeth Hospital, Mt. Carmel Mercy Hospital and Medical Center, Toco Hills Medical Emergency Center, Mt. Zion Hospital and Medical Center, and West Oakland Osteopathic Amcare Center. The remaining cases also are about real situations but the sponsoring organizations requested that their identities not be revealed. For those cases, we have changed the setting and, in some instances, the data, to protect anonymity while maintaining the integrity of the situations.

Each case is self-contained in that all information available to the administrator at the time of a decision is provided for the reader. Each case also is followed by an overview of central issues addressing the marketing concepts involved. A variety of practitioners was invited to provide overviews and the reader will note the contrasts in presentation. These overviews remain in as close to original form and content as possible to preserve the different perspectives.

The book is divided into four parts. Part I introduces health care marketing concepts and the marketing process and includes two cases. The first, on the Faculty Medical Practice Corporation, examines the multiple publics, each with its own interests and concerns, that the health administrator must satisfy. The second, Good Samaritan Hospital (A), describes the reasoning and early steps involved in developing a marketing function for such an institution.

The cases in Part II examine efforts to define the market for health services, including marketing research to identify consumers' perceived needs and the steps involved in identifying viable market segments.

Part III addresses the controllable elements of a marketing plan. The cases focus on specific decisions on services to be offered; how the services are to be communicated to market segments; how, when, and where they are to be made available; and what cost considerations are involved in the decision to utilize health care services in general and a specific provider in particular.

The introduction to Part IV addresses questions central to a review of a marketing strategy. The cases are intended to help in reviewing or auditing marketing efforts and in preparing appropriate plans.

A remarkable number of debts are incurred in the process of bringing a book such as this to completion. Perhaps we should acknowledge first the splendid cooperation of the health care providers who permitted analysis of cases involving their organizations. Such involvement requires not only time but also a trust in academic integrity and a belief in the value of dialogue. Furthermore, we are heavily indebted to those who coauthored with or provided early drafts of cases to us. As indicated in the list of credits following the Preface, significant editorial work was contributed by:

Steven F. Ashcraft (Good Samaritan Hospital (A)); James A. Brunner (Northwestern Ohio Health Maintenance Center and Good Samaritan Hospital (A) and (B)); Greg de Lissovoy (Central Alabama Primary Care,

Inc.); Richard W. Maxwell III (University Medical Center); Dan H. Dragalin (Grady Memorial Hospital); Carol Fox (Mount Zion Hospital and Medical Center); Mildred Hedrick (Central Alabama Primary Care, Inc.); Leonard Porter, III (West Oakland Osteopathic Amcare Center); Robert Sweeney (Southland Health Maintenance Organization); Peter Thoreen (Minneapolis Hospice, Inc.); and Myra Tucker (Adamsville Health Center). Equally important and appreciated was the research performed by the following student assistants: Patricia Burkhardt (Good Samaritan Hospital (A)); Arthur Isack (Faculty Medical Practice Corporation); James Hite (Northwestern Ohio Health Maintenance Center); Pat Pons (Moody Nursing Home and Georgia Medical Plan); and Richard Crater (Southern Jamaica Plain Health Center). A special note of thanks to Sam Sharkey, copy editor, for insightful contributions that tied up many loose ends. We are grateful to all of these individuals for their assistance in bringing this volume together.

The authors also are indebted to casewriters who granted permission for use of their cases. The following contributors wrote cases that have appeared elsewhere: David Loudon and Albert Della Bitta (Community Health Plan), Subhash C. Jain and Iqbal Mathur (St. Elizabeth Foundation), C. P. Rao and Gerald Crawford (Colonial Manor Hospital), Roberta N. Clarke (Southern Jamaica Plain Health Center), Jonathon S. Rakich (Mount Carmel Mercy Hospital and Medical Center), and W. Wayne Talarzyk (Ohio State Medical Association). We acknowledge with gratitude the willingness of these casewriters to share their work with a larger audience.

The authors also are grateful to several dedicated health care marketers who provided input for the Overview sections that follow each case: Patrick Mages, vice president, marketing, Methodist Hospitals of Memphis; Patricia Maxwell, then vice president, marketing, St. Francis Hospital, Wichita, Kans.; Jean DeVita, product marketing manager, medical products, Richards Manufacturing Company, Inc., Memphis, Tenn.; Richard Maxwell III, vice president, Lakeview Medical Center, Danville, Ill.; Bob Becker, principal, Hayes/Hill Corporation, Chicago; Cathy Lewis, research analyst, Nationwide Insurance Companies; and Paul Hensler, vice president, program development, O'Connor Hospital, San Jose, Calif. Their help in preparation of the case discussions has been vital.

Finally, Jan Gottemoeller and Sheila Joyner deserve special credit for preparing this manuscript and attending to all the painful details of bringing a book to completion.

Philip D. Cooper, Ph.D.
Larry M. Robinson, Ph.D.

Contributors and Credits

In the following list, contributors cited as "coauthors" worked with Drs. Cooper and Robinson in preparing cases:

Part I

Case 2: James A. Brunner, professor of marketing, Toledo University, Toledo, Ohio, and Steven F. Ashcraft, administrator, Marion General Hospital, Marion, Ohio (coauthors).

Part II

Case 3: W. Wayne Talarzyk, *Contemporary Cases in Marketing* (Hinsdale, Ill.: The Dryden Press, © 1979). Used with permission.
Case 5: James A. Brunner, professor of marketing, Toledo University, Toledo, Ohio (coauthor).
Case 6: Robert Sweeney, director of marketing, Penn Group Health, Pittsburgh (coauthor).
Case 8: Roberta N. Clarke, associate professor of marketing, Boston University. Distributed by the Intercollegiate Case Clearing House, Soldiers Field, Boston, © 1976 by Roberta N. Clarke. All rights reserved.

Part III

Case 9: Myra Tucker, instructor, nursing and community health, Medical College of Georgia (coauthor).
Case 10: Dr. Henry A. Sciullo, Dr. Ed M. Goodin, and Dr. Philip E. Taylor, all of the University of Nevada, Las Vegas. Used with permission.
Case 11: Leonard Porter III, director, public relations, Greenville Hospital System, Greenville, South Carolina (coauthor).

Case 12: Dan H. Dragalin, medical coordinator, Grady Memorial Hospital Satellite System, Atlanta (coauthor).

Case 13: Carol Fox, community relations director, Mount Zion Hospital and Medical Center, San Francisco (coauthor).

Case 14: Subhash C. Jain, professor of marketing, University of Connecticut, and Iqbal Mathur, professor of marketing, Southern Illinois University, *Cases in Marketing Management* (Columbus, Ohio: Grid Publishing, Inc., 1978). Used with permission.

Case 15: Gerald Crawford, associate professor of marketing, University of North Alabama, and C. P. Rao, associate professor of marketing, University of Arkansas at Fayetteville (coauthors). Used with permission.

Case 16: James A. Brunner, professor of marketing, University of Toledo, Toledo, Ohio, and Steven F. Ashcraft, administrator, Marion General Hospital, Marion, Ohio (coauthors).

Case 17: Jonathon S. Rakich, © 1975, by Jonathon S. Rakich. All rights reserved.

Part IV

Case 19: Greg de Lissovoy, executive director, State of Alabama Office of Rural Health Affairs, and Mildred Hedrick, director, Cancer Surveillance Center, Emory University Hospital (coauthors).

Case 20: Richard W. Maxwell III, vice president, Lakeview Medical Center, Danville, Illinois, and Cynthia B. Ligon, administrative assistant, University of Virginia Medical Center (coauthors).

Case 21: Peter Thoreen, resident in health administration, Hennepin County Medical Center, Minneapolis.

Case 22: David Loudon and Albert Della Bitta, professors of marketing, University of Rhode Island. Used with permission.

Part I

Introduction to Health Care Marketing Management

The premise of this book is that marketing is a management tool that can help health administrators to utilize scarce resources more effectively. Marketing focuses on identification and satisfaction of the perceived needs of homogeneous market segments. The underlying logic is applicable to health care providers' relationships with patients, physicians, board members, and other publics with a current or potential interest in their services.

What is health care marketing? Three steps necessary to clarify this question are to:

1. Provide a definition of health care marketing management. Although some key words in that definition are described later, it is important to clarify the concept upon which health care marketing management is based.
2. State the basic concepts from which a health systems management philosophy can be derived. While there may be other concepts upon which such a philosophy might be based, the ones discussed here are service (product), selling, and marketing.
3. Examine decisions made by health care marketers in each of four areas: service, access/availability, promotion, and cost.

HEALTH CARE MARKETING MANAGEMENT

A philosophy of management that coordinates the operation of both profit and nonprofit health delivery systems can be described as follows:

> Health care marketing management is the *process* of understanding the needs and the wants of a *target market*. Its purpose is to provide a viewpoint from which to *integrate* the analysis, planning,

1

implementation (or organization) and control of the health care delivery system.[1]

The output of the health care marketing process is the development of the means to satisfy or facilitate exchange of values between providers and the target market(s). The italicized words (*process, target market,* and *integrate*) are keys to the full understanding of the definition.

Process

Health care marketing management is a process, which implies that it is dynamic, not static. The focal point of the process is the patient/consumer, whose wants and needs are in a constant state of change. Consequently, a process is necessary to keep pace with those changes.

Target Market

While the target market includes a large number of publics (e.g., board of trustees, medical and nonmedical staff, community, etc.), it usually refers to the patient/consumer. The accepted description of a user of a health system is a patient. Unfortunately, that label also suggests the way that an individual is expected to behave once within the system. The more active role that the individual has been taking in speaking out when things are not right, the development of the Patient Bill of Rights, the increase in malpractice suits, etc., suggest that perhaps another label might be more appropriate.

The word consumer is introduced here because commercial organizations use it to describe not only those who have been incorporated into the system (or who have become purchasers of products), but also those the organization hopes to attract. Hence, the word consumer has a much broader meaning than patient.

Integrate

This is a key word in the definition. Activities that can be described as marketing functions already exist in many areas of health delivery systems. Unfortunately, a philosophy or concept has been lacking that could bring these activities into a coordinated process. Health care marketing management, with its focus on patient/consumer satisfaction, can perform this function. One occasional comment is that marketing activities are nothing new and have been carried out for years in the hospital (or other system). What is new is the integrative approach taken to the various activities to provide a common goal.

In the commercial sector, many firms operate as a combination of several insulated units; the production area is the forbidden ground for sales. The production unit provides the product, which then is given to sales to sell (or to get rid of, as the case may be). On the other hand, sales departments do not expect production to tell them how to sell. Many other examples (i.e., public relations, accounting, labor relations, etc.) exist. The same phenomenon is true to a greater or lesser extent in health delivery systems. The patient comes in contact with several groups that are insulated from each other (the office personnel, the bookkeeping department, the provider, the third party payer). Each group has its own objectives.

The marketing concept provides the focus for integrating the organization's efforts. That focus is consumer satisfaction. As health care delivery in the United States moves away from horizontal care (hospital based) toward more vertical care (ambulatory facilities), the patient will become the more predominant focus. It is this focusing function that helps to integrate the previously insulated parts of the system and points up the necessity for organization planning from a marketing management perspective. The basic approaches to health care marketing, as noted, are the service concept, the selling concept, and the marketing concept.

The Service Concept

The first and perhaps the original guiding consideration as health systems began to evolve was the service concept:

> The service concept is the health system's orientation that assumes that the consumer (meaning the physician in many instances) will react favorably to good services and facilities and that very little marketing effort is required to obtain sufficient utilization.

The marketing literature and business publications in general make frequent reference to the aphorism, "Build a better mousetrap and the world will beat a path to your door." The fallacious assumption here is that the product or service stands by itself and is recognized by consumers as being superior. It assumes there is no need to design, package, communicate meaningfully to users, select convenient places to distribute the service (or product), or price (monetary cost as well as other sacrifices) it attractively, etc.

Both profit-making and nonprofit organizations have ascribed to the service concept. The results have been dramatic in some instances. Two classic examples are (1) the railroads' ignoring their competitors' offerings (truckers' ability to pick up and deliver door to door or airlines' ease in saving time) and (2) the performing arts in many cities producing only the old classics and finding audiences and support fading. Health systems are not guaranteed survival by the fact of their existence.

The Selling Concept

This is perhaps more prevalent in the management of profit-making goods than in the health service industry but it still is a major concept that guides management philosophy:

> The selling concept is a management orientation that assumes the system utilizers (physicians or patients) normally will not use the facilities enough unless they are approached with a substantial selling and promotional effort.

The basic tenet behind this concept is that services are sold, not bought. Insurance and encyclopedia salespersons are examples of individuals who feel that the consumer needs to be sought out aggressively. Because of codes of ethics, common sense, and the disdain for making money from the ills of the public, the selling concept is not as prevalent in health systems as in commercial business.

Another tenet is that customers may buy again but even if they don't, there are plenty of other customers out there to be sold. There is no great concern about repeat business. This is not limited to profit-making businesses; nonprofit groups exhibit this concept also. For example, a political party, through the primary election process, has a "product" to sell. Its sales methodology demonstrates another basic tenet underlying this concept: consumers can be convinced to buy through various sales-stimulating devices (e.g., television and radio commercials; billboard, newspaper, and magazine advertisements; personal selling, giveaways, promises, etc.).

The selling of the swine flu program is a good example of this concept in action. The government had a service to perform and concentrated on a series of sales-stimulating devices with little regard to the repeat purchase, i.e., believability in future federal programs. Compliance was far less than expected. Indeed, the insistence on fast action may have prevented careful consideration of the population's needs beyond the predetermined medical issue. Consideration of consumer needs may have resulted in a bit more compliance.

While the selling concept may not be the philosophy behind the operation of health systems, it is introduced here to help clarify the difference between the selling and marketing concepts. While marketing is gaining prominence in the health care system, many confuse marketing with selling. Consequently, they dismiss the marketing concept as inappropriate or unethical.

The Marketing Concept

In the commercial business sector, the marketing concept is only a few decades old, its acceptance beginning in the late 1950s. The concept basically deals with exchange relationships:

> The marketing concept is a health provider's management orientation that accepts that the system's key task is to determine the wants, needs, and values of a target market and to shape the system in such a manner as to deliver the desired level of satisfaction.

This concept is based on several tenets. One is that the system requires an active marketing research plan to determine what these wants, needs, or values might be. Another is that all the activities that relate either directly or indirectly to the target market (the consumer) must be placed under an integrated marketing control. A third is that if the health system is successful in satisfying the consumer, the result will be repeat usage, support for the system (such as volunteer work, referrals, positive word of mouth, etc.), and consumer loyalty. All these results contribute to the satisfaction of the system's goals.

The marketing concept is the antithesis of the selling concept. The latter begins with the system's services and believes that through various sales-stimulating devices an acceptable level of usage can be obtained. The marketing concept begins with existing or potential consumer needs, plans a coordinated set of programs and services to serve them, and in return satisfies its goals through creating consumer satisfaction. As Peter Drucker states, "the aim of marketing is to make selling superfluous. The aim of marketing is to know and understand the consumer so well that the product or service fits him and sells itself."[2]

There is one clear parallel between the focus on consumer needs in the commercial business sector and the health care sector: the difference between true needs and the perception of true needs is the difference between a marketing and a nonmarketing approach. The commercial sector is replete with examples of products that armchair marketers perceived would meet consumer needs. The classic case of the Edsel is perhaps the best known. The introduction of the Mustang is the Edsel's antithesis.

Health professionals have long accepted the responsibility for identifying and responding to consumer needs. The predominant practice, however, has been to define those needs in terms of how the professional felt people should behave rather than in terms of the usages sought or of the motivations that influence human behavior. An argument can be made for the value of experience in the field, yet the Edsel also was designed and sold by professionals. It is precisely this focus on perceived consumer needs that makes marketing so new and different in relation to the predominant mode of patient service planning.

Health care marketing is based on the concept that it is appropriate to manage scarce resources so as to provide quality service to specific population segments. It is not an attempt to stimulate demand for unnecessary or unwanted services. The focus is on demand management to use resources efficiently in meeting perceived needs of target clients. The health care marketer is concerned with management of voluntary exchanges of values; the task is to create, facilitate, and carry out exchanges with specific, carefully defined groups of customers. The measures of marketing success are customer satisfaction, enhanced image, favorable word of mouth, and intentions to return when a need arises.

The health care marketing process can be viewed conceptually in nine discrete steps. The marketer should:

1. Monitor and respond to uncontrollable elements in the external environment. Demographics, social values, government regulations, technology, and competitor actions all must be acknowledged and appropriate responses planned.
2. Identify health care needs perceived by citizens in the service area and offerings to satisfy them. While morbidity and mortality statistics are useful, the approach requires interaction with representative samples of potential clients.
3. Define the total market using secondary data plus projections to determine salient, health-related characteristics of the service area. The definition is future oriented (expected births, predicted cases of byssinosis, and so forth).
4. Define the target market segments because, while the overall objective is to serve all citizens, the reality is that some persons have more acute needs and some groups have a higher probability of utilizing particular services. The health care marketer focuses efforts on clients with the highest potential for service but does not deny care to others.
5. Develop services to meet needs of target markets. Customers buy the results of service usage (continued health, restored health, diminished pain). Services thus should be designed so that care is provided in an efficient manner (from the customer perspective) to maximize the results (also from the patient viewpoint). The customer views the service in terms of total expenditures (time, effort, psychic costs), so that it is essential for the marketer to consider the consumer perspective.

6. Develop access/availability to the services. They must be offered when and where the target customer wants them to minimize inconvenience, pain, and time involved. The brick and mortar orientation that the patient must come to a central, fixed site at rigidly specified times may be counter to providing optimum access and availability. Marketers ask, "How can I maximize access and availability consistent with resource constraints and customer mobility?"

7. Communicate the services and access/availability to target customers. The health care marketer develops objectives for the desired image and awareness with specified groups. All available means of communication (advertising, personal selling, literature, public relations, atmospheres) are planned and executed to meet the objectives. Results are measured and communications altered as necessary to meet the goals.

8. Develop costs to consumers and third parties. The pricing variable generally is recognized as a cost recovery function. It is based on historical data plus projections. However, many costs are sensitive to utilization changes. Therefore, the marketer plans the demand for specific services and prices them based on the plans. Some may be priced below cost to attract trial usage and to enhance utilization in low demand periods.

9. Measure satisfaction of target markets with services offered. The last step in the marketing process is to examine the effectiveness of the organization in meeting the perceived needs of target customers. This step leads back to Steps 1 and 2, the updating of understanding about the market environment and about evolving consumer needs.

NOTES

1. These definitions of the health care environment are adapted from numerous sources. Perhaps the most significant is: Philip Kotler, *Marketing Management* (Englewood Cliffs, N.J.: Prentice-Hall, 4th ed., 1980).

2. Peter F. Drucker, *Management: Tasks, Responsibilities, and Practices* (New York: Harper & Row Publishers Inc., 1973), p. 64.

Chapter 1

Developing a Market Orientation

CASE 1. FACULTY MEDICAL PRACTICE CORPORATION: ENTERING A NEW FIELD

Dr. Crowe, from the small rural community of Wilson, Ark., visited the chief executive officer of the Faculty Medical Practice Corporation (FMPC), K. Casi, to determine whether the corporation would be able to provide some doctors from its staff to serve on a part-time basis where both doctors and medical facilities were nonexistent.

Casi decided the request fit nicely into the kind of objectives and missions that the FMPC was beginning to develop for itself. Specifically, he felt it would help to expand the FMPC operation and perhaps provide a number of referrals for the medical staff. These referrals would benefit the whole corporation because of the broad scope of specialties it offered. At the same time, this breadth of service would reduce Dr. Crowe's efforts to locate the types of specialties needed. Casi placed the announcement in the weekly newsletter (Exhibit 1-1) that went to all the FMPC professional staff.

The day after the newsletter was distributed, Casi received a telephone call from a concerned administrator, Barnes, at the university medical center. Barnes asked, "How would a faculty physician visiting a small rural city serve medical education?" The unstated problem was the medical center's perception that the expansion of the FMPC to more community-centered service would limit the physician/teacher's time devoted to teaching, and research would be limited severely, thus defeating the contribution that the faculty member could make to medical education.

Faculty Medical Practice Corporation

In 1974, the medical school of a prominent university established a Faculty Medical Practice Incorporation (FMPI). Its purpose was to handle

9

Exhibit 1-1 Excerpt from an FMPC Newsletter

Newsletter Memo #2
November 9, 1977

Some of the recent items of interest in FMPC are these:

- The good news is that the number of patient visits in the Pauline Building is increasing rapidly and currently is averaging 130 per day, which is 20 percent more than was the case six months or a year ago. The patient load continues to rise. However, the bad news is that we are overstaffed in certain areas and have begun to make cutbacks. Specifically, we have recently reduced the number of receptionists in the lobby of the Pauline Building.

- We are looking into the possibility of a centralized Management Information System (MIS) for all of FMPC. An MIS Users Committee has been created to assist in determining our computer needs with initial emphasis on financial consideration. On this Committee are several business managers, administrative staff, a physician and myself. The Management Information System is critical for FMPC and I will keep you aware of developments through future Newsletter Memos.

- In the near future we expect to have a cashiering service available in the lobby of the Pauline Building for patients who wish to pay for their services on the day the care is given. This service will apply to Pauline Building ancillary services as well as services from any endeavor unit. In addition, we hope to be able to accept Mastercharge and Visa credit cards for services rendered in FMPC and paid for in the lobby of the Pauline Building. More information will be given in future Newsletter Memos as the plans are finalized.

- I have been contacted by a physician who is organizing a multispecialty clinic in Wilson, Arkansas, which is between West Memphis and Blytheville. He would like to develop a contractual arrangement with FMPC to provide physician services on a part-time basis. We also hope to develop an arrangement by which the Pauline Building will be the site of referral and specialty backup. Physicians interested in learning more about the new clinic in Wilson such as the types of physicians needed, financial arrangements, etc., should get in touch with me for more details.

- The FMPC Accounting Department has now completed the programming necessary for documenting accounts payable so that the vendor and the endeavor units both have sufficient documentation to identify the payment. Prenumbered check requests are now being identified, along with the vendor invoice number, thereby giving the ability for easy identification to both the vendor and the requesting party.

- A number of questions have arisen concerning the use of professional courtesy in charging for physicians' services. It is the physicians' prerogative to decide whether to give a discount on his services and to whom he may wish to give it. It is suggested, however, that in lieu of providing a total discount, the physician may want to charge "insurance only" so that the patient will not receive a bill, but the endeavor unit will receive whatever payment the insurance company makes as payment in full.

Exhibit 1-1 continued

The physician ultimately, however, is the one to decide whether professional courtesy is given, e.g., to other physicians, their families, house staff, medical students, FMPC employees, nurses, etc.

- FMPC has ordered a defibrillator for the Pauline Building. Specifically, it is a Pulsar 4 defibrillator by American Optical. The defibrillator will be located in the area of the Pain Clinic on the third floor of the Pauline Building. A future Newsletter Memo will list the date when the equipment is in place.

- Recently there have been a number of requests for release of medical record information. Often these requests are from lawyers, insurance companies, etc., ...

central billing and collection for the private practice of doctors associated with the medical center. Unfortunately, this became extremely expensive and ineffective and was abandoned in its second year. In 1977, a new organization, the Faculty Medical Practice Corporation, was established. The university's objective was to develop an entity that would allow the medical faculty to be able to carry on private practice that for the most part was independent while also providing the benefits of faculty membership. This would be a selling point for the university in attempting to attract new faculty members.

Current Status

By 1978, the FMPC had 475 employees, of whom 170 were faculty members at the medical center. The others were nonprofessional staff such as billing clerks and secretarial staff. There were 17 departments, referred to as endeavor units to distinguish them from academic departments. However, each endeavor unit corresponded to a similar department in the medical center. They included such areas as nuclear medicine, general surgery, internal medicine, radiology, and so forth. The university had not emphasized primary care[1] until a new faculty member with specialization in that field joined the staff. He attracted two residents in family practice and developed a primary care program.

Organization and Operation

All faculty members automatically were eligible to belong to the FMPC unless their contracts stipulated research or other responsibilities that precluded private practice. While the percentage of the FMPC's income varied from 15 to 85 percent per physician, the average was around 60 percent, with the rest coming from the medical school. All faculty members were entitled to become shareholders in the corporation. As a professional corporation, membership was restricted by state law to members of the medical profession.

The shareholders elected one trustee from each endeavor unit. The trustees in turn elected six directors, who in most instances were not trustees. They basically formed the working group that developed policy and handled day-to-day issues for the corporation. The chief executive officer, Casi, was not a physician, having been hired by the board simply to run the affairs of the corporation. Casi could not be compared to a hospital administrator since the FMPC and its facility was not a hospital. However, its function was similar to a large clinic.

Publics

Five publics were recognized as affecting the FMPC: (1) the university medical center (the most influential); (2) the university itself; (3) the state legislature because the medical center was associated with the state university; (4) physicians in the community; and (5) the patients.

The Missions of the FMPC

Casi felt there were six principal missions that were important for the FMPC:

1. to provide quality medical care
2. to develop a well-managed organization that included economic incentives that would act as a drawing card to attract full-time faculty
3. to establish innovative programs for the community and to work with those being developed there. The FMPC would be able to provide the medical school residents with a hands-on experience in those programs
4. to develop community-centered, coordinated health care programs— basically one-stop shopping centers for health care—an increasingly important factor
5. to provide medical care that was both convenient and cost effective
6. to meet the community's unmet health care needs, specifically in the underprivileged sector

Perceived Problems

The telephone call from the medical center underscored one of the major problems that Casi perceived for the FMPC: the conflict between medical education and the development of a community-centered approach. The question was, "Is the best interest of medical education served by the FMPC's becoming more community centered?" The concern was the amount of time a faculty member would be spending with the community as opposed to the physician's educational responsibilities. The university had no written policy statement on this issue.

A second major problem was the FMPC's high level of dependence on community physicians for referrals. A related problem was the fact that FMPC lacked an emphasis on primary care. If this could be improved, referrals could be developed internally. A related consideration was the existing facility—a single building that was suitable as long as only secondary or tertiary care was provided. Expansion to encompass primary care would necessitate expensive changes and possibly a more convenient location for these services.

Another difficulty was that the 17 endeavor units had coordination problems. The failure of the 1974 Faculty Medical Practice Incorporation made it difficult to convince endeavor units that it would be advantageous for them to consider a centralized billing and collection function again. A subset of that problem was that each endeavor unit collected its own patient data rather than using a central information source.

Current Action and Planning

In an effort to develop quality medical care, Casi had initiated a program for evaluating the quality of the physicians' records. Training sessions were held to demonstrate the specific requirements for record content. To ensure that the professional staff provided consistently good medical records, the board of directors established a program of sanctions against those who failed to comply, including economic sanctions as well as the possibility of restricting the practice of the physician.

In an effort to develop an emphasis on primary care, the FMPC, as noted, added a local physician with a large practice in internal medicine who was in the process of developing a primary care program. There also was a possibility that the medical school's family practice department, not then participating in the FMPC, might join in the next year. Consideration had been given to the development of satellite centers around the city within the next five years. However, these plans were in only the initial stage. A physical fitness program for executives for a number of large corporations in the city also was in the planning stages.

The question still bothering Casi was whether the missions of the FMPC involving a higher level of community orientation and the medical education objective of the university were consistent. If the FMPC continued to develop a higher level of consumer orientation or consumer centeredness, would medical education be hampered? What impact would this have on the plans under consideration?

NOTE

1. Primary care generally is referred to as the initial physician contact with the patient. Secondary care is that provided by a physician to whom the patient has been referred by the primary doctor. The next level of referral is tertiary care. For example, if the general practitioner refers the patient to a surgeon, who in turn refers the person to a neurosurgeon, the last-named provides tertiary care.

OVERVIEW OF CASE 1

Issues to Consider

1. Does a marketing or consumer-centered approach preclude the satisfaction of the university medical center's objectives?
2. What publics should be added to those listed? Are the statements of missions applicable to each public? Should the statements of missions be rewritten in any manner to eliminate any potential conflicts?
3. What should the priority of the various problems be? Which is most important?

Discussion

1. The Objectives and the Faculty

On the surface it would appear as though the FMPC and the medical center are indeed at odds. If faculty members are spending more time in practice, obviously they devote less time to teaching. This needs to be brought into perspective. The case mentions that the university had developed no policy regarding its expectations of its faculty. Before any steps can be taken, this must be done.

The compatibility between a marketing approach and health care is the greatest with primary care and diminishes in its applicability as it moves to the secondary and tertiary levels. The reason primary care is compatible is the consumer perception of health needs. A major part of primary care deals with preventive medicine. Such "purchases" tend to be postponable since the problem often is perceived as minor. In that situation, the individuals are not unlike the consumers of most commercial products: they have the choice to utilize or not to utilize the services being offered. This is unlike secondary or tertiary care where the problem exists and there is no choice or little choice because of the referral process.

As the university increases its emphasis on primary care, the apparent conflict with the FMPC will diminish since the instruction of such physicians must be community oriented. Practice in the community can enhance the FMPC's ability to sense health care needs of families. From the FMPC's perspective, the dependency on referrals from community physicians can be reduced as the organization develops its own referral system through offering primary care services.

2. The Role of the Various Publics

The FMPC has many publics to consider. Most health delivery systems serve multiple publics such as physicians, staff, consumers, board members, regulators, and third party reimbursement organizations. This is one of the challenges that makes marketing in this field so interesting. A marketing program theoretically could be developed for each public.

Under a functional definition of publics, there are four levels that become involved in the resource-conversion machine called a health delivery system: input publics, internal publics, agent publics, and consuming publics. Input publics for hospitals in general include:

- Supporters—those who lend the organization its resources (time, money, encouragement) such as (1) the volunteers who serve a hospital or clinic such as the FMPC, (2) the community physician, and (3) the university medical center.

- Supplier publics—those who sell goods and services to the organization, such as medical supply houses.

- Regulatory publics—the local Health Systems Agency and local, state, and federal governments.

Internal publics process the inputs and include the staff, both professional and nonprofessional (billing clerks, housekeeping, administrators, etc.). Subgroups such as the board of directors and the trustees can take on roles different from just being staff physicians. Internal publics become critically important in this case, especially because of the history of inefficiency and waste in the predecessor organization, the FMPI.

The services of the FMPC may be distributed through agent publics or directly to the consuming public. If the corporation becomes more oriented to primary care, then agent publics will take on a less critical role, but that change is not imminent. Examples of agent publics include the community physician because of the referral process. The mass media also are agents. FMPC physicians, in addition to being internal publics, are agent publics since they can refer patients to other doctors in the group as well as bring patients in from private practice.

Consuming publics are composed of two main groups—client publics and general publics. The main client public includes current and prospective patients and, from a different point of view, business firms whose employees are patients of the FMPC. The general publics include the community at large and relatives of patients. Since the FMPC is a referral center and draws patients from beyond the local community, the mass publics also should be considered.

Some of the FMPC's six missions are established with specific publics in mind. For example, the second mission—economic incentives—is aimed specifically at the university medical center and the faculty physicians. The third, fourth, and sixth missions all deal with community centeredness and seemed to be producing problems for the medical center. However, as the medical center developed its primary care program, these missions became less incompatible. The only major revision to the mission statements is to combine the first (quality care) with the fifth (cost effectiveness of medical care). If treated separately, they could produce conflicting results such as a program that is of top quality but also is ineffective.

3. Priorities

While Casi views the conflict with the medical school as based on major problems, it may be blown out of proportion because of the change in emphasis to include primary care in its medical education program. Perhaps the most important problem that demands attention is the lack of coordination among the endeavor units. This top priority problem should be addressed by the FMPC's administration because it has the broadest impact on most of the missions. It certainly affects the cost and convenience issue and has an impact on quality because of the potential lack of continuity of care. The lack of coordination, if perceived negatively by the community physicians, can lead to reduced referrals. If the consuming publics also perceive that lack, self-referrals also may decline.

Chapter 2

Organizing a Marketing Operation

CASE 2. GOOD SAMARITAN HOSPITAL (A): FEASIBILITY STUDY FOR A HOSPITAL MARKETING DEPARTMENT

"It's happened again," Glen Blackwell complained to his wife. As the assistant administrator of Good Samaritan Hospital responsible for its marketing activities, he had been planning a community awareness campaign centering on its new x-ray equipment.

"Now I find out through the newspaper that our public relations office already has one started," he said. "It didn't even emphasize the important aspects of the new equipment. Lately, it always seems to be the same old story—public relations doubling up on projects that should be left to my office. Well, perhaps at tomorrow's meeting the hospital board will make a final decision concerning the development of the marketing activities."

He explained that he had sent in a report some time ago outlining the marketing function at the hospital and had suggested a format for a plan of action for implementation of the program (Exhibit 2-1).

"For the last three months the board has been going in circles trying to decide how extensive a program to begin and where the marketing department should be positioned in the hospital structure," Blackwell said. "The president even told me a couple of days ago that some résumés already had been received from people who are interested in the marketing manager's position. The board is quite sure that it will be hiring an experienced marketing person to head up the program. But so far, it hasn't decided what the person will be responsible for or to whom."

The Hospital's Background

Good Samaritan Hospital was established in 1874 by a group of church women to minister to the sick and infirm among the newcomers and im-

Exhibit 2-1 Example of Part of a Plan for a Marketing Function

To: Russell Fruth, President, Good Samaritan Hospital

From: Glen Blackwell, Administrative Assistant

Re: Marketing Proposal for Good Samaritan

This report is the result of a project assignment whose purpose was to (1) research the state of the art of marketing and the marketing function as it relates to hospitals and (2) provide recommendations as to the implementation of a marketing function at the Good Samaritan Hospital.

The Marketing Function

This section of the report presents, in general terms, the nature of marketing from an operational perspective. The role of marketing management, marketing activities, and the administration of a marketing program shall be presented.

The mission of a hospital's marketing department is to analyze, plan, implement, and control programs designed to bring about desired exchanges with target medical care markets for the purpose of achieving organizational objectives. A heavy reliance is placed upon designing the organization's offering in terms of the target markets' needs and desires, and using effective pricing, communications, and distribution to inform, motivate, and service the market.

In developing a marketing strategy, the hospital's marketing manager must address his attention to four basic concerns. The first, market segmentation, involves analyzing potential customers by pertinent characteristics such as demographic and psychographic factors. The second, market positioning, involves a decision as to which target markets the firm is to serve. Third, market entry, is a consideration of how the product or service shall be produced. And fourth, market mix, involves a coordination of factors called the 4 Ps, which will produce the desired results.

The 4 Ps are Product, Place, Price, and Promotion. In the hospital setting, we would view the product as the type of service to be offered: preventive, diagnostic, therapeutic, especially viewed in terms of the benefit of the service to the patient—relief of pain and anxiety, longer life, less disability, etc. Place refers to how the service will be delivered to the patient. Such factors as location, hours of service, and referral mechanisms that determine the extent and mode of access to the service are reviewed. Price refers not only to the financial charge for the

Exhibit 2-1 continued

service but also to everything the patient must "endure" to utilize the service. This would include such considerations as waiting time, physical discomfort, emotional upset, and any loss of personal dignity. Promotion deals with how and what the prospective patient learns about the organization and the service it offers. The marketer is interested in how the patient can become aware of the service, develop an interest in it, use the service, use it regularly, and recommend it to others.

Although the patient has been used. as the basis for the preceding illustration, this was not meant to imply that the patient should be the primary or only focus of the marketer. The above considerations apply equally to physicians, other health care institutions, and any other identifiable marketing opportunity.

migrants to Toledo who had neither homes nor families. After 104 years of growth and expansion, Good Samaritan, located in West Toledo, was the largest metropolitan hospital in northwestern Ohio. The institution maintained 732 beds, numerous outpatient clinics and services, and a staff of 620 physicians and 750 nurses to provide medical and health care to the Toledo metropolitan area and surrounding communities.

In early 1978, Blackwell had had no experience in marketing until the hospital president, Russell Fruth, approached him about developing a formalized marketing program.

In the previous two years several hospitals throughout the country had attracted attention by instituting marketing departments. Blackwell could still remember Fruth saying, "It won't take that much of your time and it will be very good experience."

However, it had not taken Blackwell long to recognize that hospital marketing required expertise and time. He had been relying upon the advice of a marketing consultant but felt the time had arrived for the establishment of a formal department. Dr. Stewardson, the consultant, had helped to construct several model marketing departments, which the board now was considering.

Rationale for the Marketing Function Proposal

When the proposal for an expanded marketing function was requested, Blackwell submitted a detailed report on why a larger, more detailed program was necessary. He summarized the needs as follows:

1. To enable Good Samaritan to compete efficiently with the eight other metropolitan hospitals. Today's consumers are able to choose more

than ever before which hospital is to provide the services requested by the patient.

2. To coordinate planning and promotion with public relations to minimize the risk of creating a distorted or perhaps contradictory image of the hospital.
3. To maximize the utilization of services and equipment and to identify services required and those no longer needed.
4. To recognize who constitutes the hospital's prime markets and then determine how to reach those markets effectively.
5. To strengthen ties with physicians since a strong doctor core is essential to a hospital's growth.
6. To maintain or increase the current census level by promoting a strong community commitment and awareness of the hospital's capabilities.
7. To expand the hospital's services into new areas to offset any loss of revenues that might result from the drive for legislation to reduce patient days' reimbursed by third parties.
8. To promote the availability of the hospital's shared services such as the computer-assisted electrocardiograph program and the management assistance that are available to other hospitals desiring to use the expertise of Good Samaritan's staff in any of their departments (pulmonary function, pharmacy, information services, etc.).

It also had been discovered during the research phase of the project that key administrative persons were relatively unfamiliar with some of the fundamental concepts and philosophies of marketing. The hospital essentially was being guided by decisions based on intuition, so the need for education on marketing was apparent.

Good Samaritan had long been involved in activities that might be included in a marketing program. Exhibit 2-2 lists 17 activities that Blackwell considered to be part of marketing. Good Samaritan, and hospitals in general, had participated in marketing decisons but they had been fragmented among various departments, and the top administrators had not provided the extensive information and analysis needed in many instances.

Blackwell knew that many hospitals had public relations departments and various other offices that often led to duplicate efforts. Further, he was aware that many public relations departments did not have the expertise to delve into in-depth projects.

Good Samaritan's marketing efforts, like those of a majority of other hospitals, were focused on the short run. Blackwell recognized, however, that the marketing objective concept should focus on the long run as well as the short run, with a wide spectrum of activities and influence. The primary focus of a marketing program should be the long-term survival of

Exhibit 2-2 Patient Marketing Activities of the Good Samaritan Hospital

1. Public Relations Department (publications, news releases, news coverage)
2. Hospital-sponsored seminars and conferences
3. Certificate-of-need applications
4. "Hospital Week" activities
5. Establishment of referral bases
6. Heart monitor program
7. Expectant parent classes
8. Statistical data gathering
9. C.V. laboratory exhibit
10. Patient representative and patient questionnaires
11. Physicians' office building project
12. Maintenance of pleasant physical facilities
13. Hobby fair
14. "At GSH We Read You Loud and Clear"
15. Long-range plan development
16. Effort against unionization (primary marketing)
17. Physician data stat report

the institution. The program should include searching for new market opportunities; predicting, monitoring, and evaluating levels of service; monitoring the marketing environment; and appraising the hospital's market position.

Blackwell was aware that an essential element of any program is the marketing information system. Its primary components should be: (1) an internal accounting system to provide data for pricing, (2) a marketing intelligence system to monitor developments and changes in the marketing environment, and (3) a marketing research system for conducting specific studies of market opportunities, marketing effectiveness, and the identification of marketing problems.

Good Samaritan's Board Meeting

Before the board meeting, Blackwell met with Dr. Stewardson to review organizational proposals he was planning to present if requested. Figure 2-1 shows part of the organizational structure of Good Samaritan Hospital. Figure 2-2 describes the four alternative marketing department structures he developed.

"The four alternatives proceed from the least to the most complex," Blackwell explained. "They are designed so that if the board should adopt

Figure 2-1 Good Samaritan Hospital Organizational Structure (Partial)

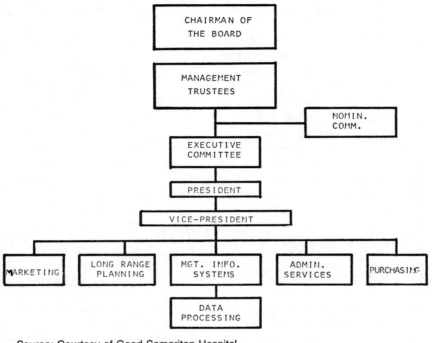

Source: Courtesy of Good Samaritan Hospital.

a less extensive departmental structure, a more sophisticated department could endure. In essence, then, we are offering four alternatives that also can be considered as a single proposal with component steppingstones in the event that the board chooses to develop the department gradually."

"The first alternative is very similar to the present situation," Blackwell said. "It could serve as an intermediate step that could lead into an organizational plan such as either Alternatives 2, 3, or 4. The comparative costs of this proposal are substantially less. Task force members from other areas could be assembled according to the projects under consideration. In addition, under this scheme as well as the others, an outside consultant could continue to be utilized whenever necessary.

"The second proposal would create a marketing department headed by an assistant administrator who would be responsible to the president. As long as access to the president is available, the department would be able to operate in an efficient manner. Even though public relations does not report to the vice president of marketing, coordination would be provided by the president. This plan could allow the marketing department a chance

Figure 2-2 Alternative Marketing Department Structures for Good
Samaritan Hospital

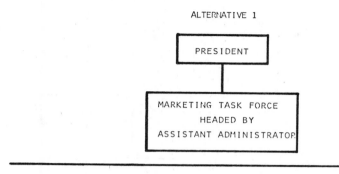

ALTERNATIVE 1

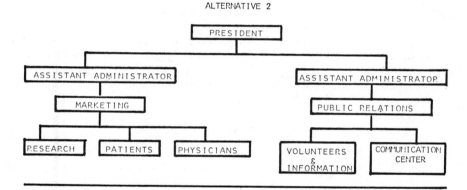

ALTERNATIVE 2

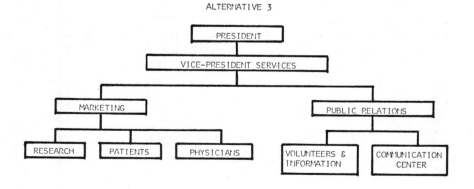

ALTERNATIVE 3

(continued on page 24)

Figure 2-2 continued

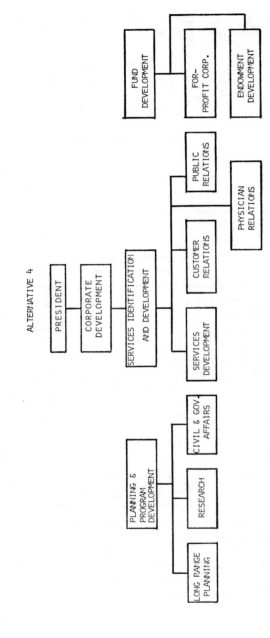

Source: Courtesy of Good Samaritan Hospital.

to develop and prove its expertise and ability to provide the hospital with useful information and planning.

"The third plan overcomes a weakness in the second proposal by placing marketing and public relations under the same vice president (assistant administrator) for marketing. Activities would be more closely coordinated by placing a marketing manager at the level of vice president rather than at the managerial level; the hospital would be assured of the individual's participation at board meetings. It also ensures that the person will be aware of the hospital's mission and its plans for the future. The placement at the departmental head level could also prove effective since the position carries with it sufficient authority to coordinate the marketing function among various departments. This is especially true if the director were allowed to be flexible in maintaining the necessary liaisons as is provided with adequate administrative support."

Blackwell added, however, that "some of the board feel this proposal also involves a large amount of money and staffing. At earlier meetings, many of the board members felt that there were not enough adequate examples of this type of marketing organization at other hospitals. Also, some felt that attempting to establish a department this extensive in a short time could result in confusion. Therefore, some of the members seem to lean toward simpler proposals.

"Finally, there is another proposal I have been developing since we last met. It is probably the most innovative, and I don't know how the board will respond. As you know, there has been some objection to identifying the department as 'marketing' so I am going to suggest that it be designated 'Services,' in the hope that this will overcome the objection to the use of the term 'marketing.' "

"As you know, we have a planning department and I am considering placing research in that department as it is interested in long-range planning as well as civil and governmental activities. The board also has created a new for-profit corporation that it has located under fund development and its function is to take the new activities we plan to market and promote and develop them for profit. My proposal will create a new department that I have designated as Services Identification and Development that will overcome, I hope, the stigma associated with 'marketing.' Under it I plan to place Service Development, Customer Relations, Physician Relations, and Public Relations. Give special consideration to the grouping of responsibilities. This will be an essential element in the determination of the effectiveness of the organizational structure."

"They sound okay to me and spell out the alternatives quite clearly," Dr. Stewardson replied. "Along with your other support, the board should be able to make a decision. I'll back you up if necessary."

The board soon began giving more detailed consideration to the place of marketing within the hospital's organization. Fruth circulated four résumés that had been received in the previous month from persons interested in the marketing position. The board had not been secretive about its plans so the fact that applications were being received already was not surprising. Exhibit 2-3 summarizes the credentials of the four applicants.

"What is your opinion on the applicants' background we have received so far?" Fruth asked. "As far as I am concerned, William Bernard looks like he just could be the type of man we are looking for. He has had a lot of practical marketing experience in industry and is familiar with the Toledo area."

"He might be the man you're looking for," Dr. Stewardson responded, "but then again, he might not be. It all depends on what the board is going to expect out of its services department. Quite honestly, it is pretty hard to fit a man into a position that has not yet been completely formulated. I would suggest the board make its decision regarding the scope of the department's activities in the near future. Then, after the office and its responsibilities have been determined, it will be possible to specify precisely what qualifications would be most advantageous for the position. I urge you not to rush too quickly into the decision on the exact person to hire. I am sure many more applications for this job are yet to be received and it is altogether possible that there will be several who will meet the qualifications you stipulate."

Fruth thanked Dr. Stewardson and asked his assistance in selecting the right person for the position, adding, "You have been most insightful in the past and your experience should be most helpful again."

OVERVIEW OF CASE 2

Issues to Consider

1. How should the marketing function be organized? (The hospital senses that it needs such an operation but does not know where to put it.)
2. What are the functions of a hospital marketing department?
3. What was the board of directors' decision concerning the organization of the marketing program?
4. Who is Good Samaritan's key customer?
5. Is there a process for program and service development?

Discussion

1. Marketing Organization

Is marketing a line or staff function? Who should be in charge of it and where should it report? What organizational structure did Blackwell and the consultant recommend? What would a person in the same job recommend?

Hospital administrators with little marketing training usually see marketing as a staff function. It is in fact a line function. In the final analysis only four functions are necessary in any organization: someone to lead it (the president, chief executive officer, or administrator), someone to keep score (finance), someone to decide what the organization is going to do (marketing), and someone to manufacture the product or service (operations). Finance, marketing, and operations are line functions. It is curious that hospitals often choose to have a financial function and two manufacturing functions—operations and nursing—as their line organization. If marketing exists, they tend to make it a staff function. Who should be in charge of the marketing function?

Ideally the director of marketing should report to the president, chief executive officer, or administrator. Assistant administrators with academic preparation in hospital administration seldom have the background to form or manage a marketing function. Since few academic programs adequately prepare administrators for hospital marketing positions, the M.B.A. or B.A. or someone with proved experience in service marketing would be the logical choice. It was a mistake to saddle Blackwell with the responsiblity for developing a marketing program because he did not have the tools to do the job.

However, he should have had enough management experience to make a recommendation. He developed four alternatives and even had consulting assistance but he committed a fundamental management blunder. As the "expert" in residence on marketing, he did not recommend a course of action. Which organizational alternative should be recommended?

None of the schemes do the job. Alternative 1 is a committee. The result will wind up with a camel instead of a horse. Alternative 2 separates marketing and public relations and suffers from the assistant administrator syndrome, since the two functions probably will work at cross-purposes. Alternative 3 comes close but does not include two critical marketing functions: strategic planning and program development. Alternative 4 is bewildering. Planning and program development are not connected to corporate development and appear to float, without direction. They should be integrated under a box that clearly says "Marketing."

Exhibit 2-3 A Comparison of Résumés Received for Hospital Marketing Manager Position

Element	Candidate			
	William Bernard	Dale Parsons	Michael Green	Earl Williams
Career Objective:	A position that combines marketing, public relations, and advertising.	A position in hospital administration with an expressed interest in feasibility analysis of new projects or departments.	A position that combines a computer and marketing background.	A position that involves salesmanship in a nonprofit organizational environment.
Education:	Graduated from Notre Dame with honors in 1968 with a B.A. in marketing. Earned an M.B.A. from the same institution in 1972 with a specialty in consumer behavior.	Graduated with both a B.S. and an M.B.A. in accounting from the University of Michigan.	Graduated with a B.A. in marketing from the University of Toledo in 1965 and an M.B.A. in 1970, following three years in military service.	Graduated from Bowling Green in 1959 with a B.A. in business. Has taken postgraduate enrichment classes in the field of salesmanship.
Personal Information:	32, married, 2 children.	28, single.	Has lived 35 years in Oregon, Ohio, a suburb of Toledo. Married, with a son and two daughters.	Born and raised in rural northwestern Ohio. Married for 18 years, two daughters, age 42.

Work Experience:	For two years before entering the M.B.A. program, was a salesman for Eaton Products that specialized in artificial surfaces for sports facilities. Since August 1972 employed at Owens-Illinois in a job that entails consumer research prior to marketing new products.	Accountant for Detroit's Riverview Hospital for four years, then for last two years in similar position at Fort Wayne General Hospital.	Worked for eight years as a project head at National Family Opinion, Rossford, Ohio. This provides a wide background in the computer field and market research.	Worked for eight years as a salesman for International Harvestor's Industrial Equipment Division, then for the last ten years as an industrial salesman for Ohio Bell, specializing in business communications networks and development.
Other Activities:	A deacon at St. Paul's Lutheran Church in Toledo. Served on a fund-raising board for the Toledo Zoo. Avid hunter and sportsman.	Served on various hospital boards and community relations activities. Chairman of Fort Wayne Days Summer Festival in 1977. A Red Cross Volunteer.	Troop committee member of Scout Troop 611 in charge of outdoor activities. Teaches junior high Sunday School class. Booster club member at Oregon H.S. United Way volunteer.	Board member at Glendale Baptist Church. Member of Toledo Board of Education 1971–1974.

2. The Basic Functions

The four organizational alternatives do not work because administration is not familiar with the components of a marketing program. Since no tested model for the application of marketing in the hospital exists, there is bound to be confusion.

The four basic functions of a hospital marketing department are marketing research, strategic planning, program and service development, and marketing communications. Public relations functions best as part of the marketing communications group. The model in general terms works this way: research determines the needs of the market segments intended to be served, planning determines what will be done to meet customer need and create long-term customer satisfaction, and program and service development assures that planning priorities are met and developments follow a consistent and orderly process. Marketing communications requires a hospital to tell customers what services are available that will meet their needs. Figure 2-3 shows an organizational scheme for hospital marketing that includes all the key functions.

It is disappointing that the consultant failed to pinpoint the functions of a marketing department or at least suggest that the alternatives were not valid. Surely the consultant should have been pressed for a recommendation.

3. Indecision by Board of Directors

The board adjourned without making a decision on organization. Had Blackwell offered a recommendation, it would have been forced to take some action. Instead, it permitted the horse to push the cart rather than pull it. The members discussed the applicants when they clearly did not have the job defined. The whole issue will continue to drift without a decision on organization.

4. The Wrong Target

Throughout the case study the hospital suggests that the patient, not the physician, is the prime target for the marketing and public relations effort. This is a common error in applied hospital marketing. Yet in about eight out of ten cases, the physician makes the hospital purchase decision. Patients may choose an emergency room and often make a choice for obstetrical services but the majority arrive at the hospital because of a physician's order.

Figure 2-3 A Practical Marketing Organizational Plan

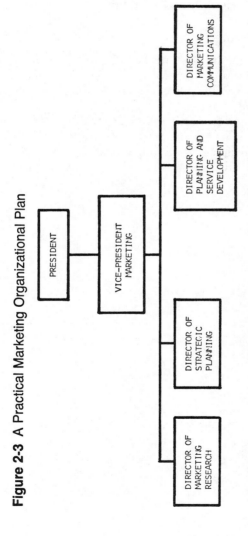

Source: Courtesy of Good Samaritan Hospital.

5. The Need for a Process

Good Samaritan Hospital suffers from a common management deficiency that the marketing process could remedy. It apparently has no process for program and service development. A well-written process could provide answers to all of the questions. It also would require that a new program be developed before personnel selection is even considered. And a program development process would require a financial projection.

Concluding Discussion

Alfred Kahn, when he was President Carter's inflation fighter, was criticized by White House staffers for using the word "inflation." They felt it was negative. So Kahn, with considerable tongue in cheek, decided to substitute the word "banana" for inflation. Absurd? True. And a perfect parallel for the Good Samaritan difficulty with the term "marketing."

Marketing is a management philosophy and process that makes use of sound business principles. Marketing is concerned with meeting needs and creating customer satisfaction. It requires a hospital to perform marketing research and obtain customer input. Marketing requires a hospital to plan, plan, plan.

Market Definition and the Market Environment

A major challenge health care managers face is to define clearly the market and the environment within which health care is to be delivered. Part II focuses on three areas that pertain to market definition and the market environment: consumer behavior, market research and market segmentation.

The cases in the consumer behavior section examine the process by which individuals make health care choices. The study of consumer behavior is an important element in the design of marketing strategy. As illustrated in the first case in this section, an underlying reason for malpractice suits is patients' sense of frustration at not being heard by the medical community. A strategy designed to open communication between physicians and consumers may lead to a reduction in such suits.

Knowing what the consumer thinks is important. It also is essential to understand how the customer uses the facility and what process the person follows in deciding to use a particular service. If the marketing manager understands the consumer decision process, better use can be made of scarce resources to influence or challenge the most important links in the communication channel.

Consumer behavior does not merely mean patient behavior. The "consumer" is a consumer of resources. The physician is a major consumer of resources for a hospital. The government (federal, in many cases) is a consumer of resources of time and money for hospitals, qualified health maintenance organizations, and primary care centers. These also consume organizational resources. Improved understanding of behavior, attitudes, usage criteria, and so forth, can help to meet the perceived needs of key publics in an efficient manner as opposed to a hit-or-miss approach that wastes limited resources.

Market research focuses on development of information to improve decision making. Its objective is to know better and to understand the consumer (i.e., physician, nurse, board member, regulator, etc.). The two cases in the market research section demonstrate the value of information on consumer perceptions, attitudes, opinions, and preferences as input to the formulation of a marketing strategy.

Many health care providers regard the market as an undifferentiated, homogeneous entity. The purpose of market segmentation is to develop a better definition of the most likely prospects for a health care service. The two cases in the final section of Part II suggest that a segmentation strategy can lead to a more efficient use of scarce resources and to the development of strategies that will uniquely satisfy the perceived needs of specific target markets.

The criteria for selection of appropriate segments vary according to the objectives of the health care provider. In a situation similar to the Georgia Medical Plan, where the organization was becoming established, cost effectiveness is of primary concern. On the other hand, while costs certainly are important for the Southern Jamaica Plain Health Center, a need to match the services and skills with specific community market segments also is essential. In both cases, there are many segments with health care needs. The question is: Which segments should be emphasized for resource allocation?

Chapter 3

Consumer Behavior

CASE 3. OHIO STATE MEDICAL ASSOCIATION: A SURVEY OF CONSUMER ATTITUDES TOWARD MEDICAL MALPRACTICE

This case is based on a comprehensive research project designed to measure attitudes toward health care in general and medical malpractice issues in particular. The research involved telephone interviews with 1,500 Ohio residents selected randomly.

Each state's environment for health care is unique in some ways and the results in Ohio are not necessarily applicable to another state. Nevertheless, Ohio is to a degree a microcosm of the entire United States. Thus, it is believed that the findings in this study provide thought-provoking information about the problems of health care and malpractice on a broad geographic scale.

The Changing Environment for Health Care

This report describes a study based on the consumer's right to be heard about a topic of highest concern—medical care. Contemporary consumers want their attitudes and opinions to be heard. Unfortunately, many of their comments and concerns are being presented in the courtroom. Some consumers may feel this is the only way to be heard, to get their questions answered, to finally get someone in society to take them seriously. This study attempts to understand what consumers are saying about their physicians, about health care in general, and especially about malpractice.

The health care environment is characterized by a discontinuity unparalleled in any period of American history. As a consequence of rapid and dislocative change, a different set of planning premises is necessary to provide an acceptable level of health care. This report presents a thorough

35

review of the consumer's viewpoint for all persons who must plan health care programs.

The environment for health care includes four major elements: technological systems; cultural and life style systems; economic and demographic systems; and political, legal, and regulatory systems. Physicians must consider each element of the environment when planning the way a practice should be conducted to maximize consumer satisfaction with health care.

Technological Systems

Technological systems create the potential for satisfying consumers' needs for health care. Interdisciplinary applications of research in areas such as chemistry, electrical engineering, physics, and the behavioral sciences increase the potential of medicine. These advances have a great impact on the practice of medicine and on consumer perceptions of the profession as well.

The American approval of scientific research and technological progress, toward which a great amount of resources is devoted, leads to a faith in medicine and in physicians' capabilities to solve any health problem. Continued improvement in medical technology may result in even higher consumer expectations for physician capabilities. When consumer expectations outpace the ability of medical technology to solve health problems, dissatisfaction is inevitable and malpractice litigation may result.

Cultural and Life Style Systems

Life styles—patterns of activities, interests, and opinions of individuals or groups of individuals in a society—are influenced by demographic and economic influences but basically are a function of the values or cultural norms transmitted to individuals in a society.

Individuals are not born with a set of values about what is right and wrong, good and bad, or desirable and undesirable. Their expectations are learned as the result of interactions with certain institutions—primarily the family, religion, and school—and significant lifetime experiences. Because patients, especially younger ones, have experienced and are experiencing different institutional influences, medicine now is practiced in a changed environment.

New cultural attitudes and life styles of medical service consumers are the understandable and predictable consequences of changes that have occurred in the family, religious groups, and schools. While young consumers probably will grow more conservative as they become older, their values and attitudes about life in general appear likely to remain qualitatively different from those of previous generations. The specific attitudes of this group toward medical services therefore are of particular importance in understanding the future environment for health care.

Economic and Demographic Systems

Economic and demographic influences are critical to understanding or "dimensioning" the environment for any type of consumer product or service, including health care. They may operate either as a positive or negative influence on medical services and may be related in certain segments of the population.

During the 1970s, millions of Americans enjoyed steadily increasing earnings, although there were setbacks in individual years. This increase in affluence resulted in the shift of millions of families from lower earning levels to the middle-income brackets.

Several implications may be drawn from these income changes. One pertains to the social problem created by pockets of poverty in the midst of affluence. When low-income families find themselves the minority rather than the majority, many observers would argue, the frustration of the outnumbered poor is accentuated.

The fastest growing segment of the population during the last decade—the 15-to-24 age group—grew approximately three times faster than the total population. As that group continues to age, however, the fastest expansion among all categories in the decade of the 1980s will be in the 25-to-34 group. More than half the total U.S. population increase between 1970 and 1980 is accounted for by these young people, who are launching employment careers, getting married, setting up households, and having their first child—for whom these are years of intense economic interest.

Another important dimension of the economic and demographic environment is women's greater participation in the labor force. Today, almost 45 percent of wives are employed outside the home. As women attain more employment rights and their wages improve, more economic and political power will shift to them.

Consumers are becoming better educated. In 1960 there were only 8.2 million college graduates in the United States but by 1980 there were more than 19 million. Today more than 60 percent of adults above age 25 are high school graduates whereas in the 1960s the majority were not.

Higher education is likely to mean greater sophistication in a wide range of consumer decisions. Consumers are more demanding in the areas of service, quality, warranties, information, and so forth. Moreover, they are supported in their demands by a multitude of consumer protection agencies that have evolved in recent years and, studies disclose, that proliferate with increasing levels of education.

Political, Legal, and Regulatory Systems

Political, legal, and regulatory systems for both the general and health care environments are proliferating at every level. Increased interest in national health programs has become apparent, although legislation designed to provide national solutions to health care problems failed to be passed. The range of federal and state programs and regulatory forces affecting medical care is nearly limitless, and in recent years some of these have been directed toward the specific problem of malpractice. Several states have enacted malpractice legislation, and the National Conference of Commissioners on Uniform State Laws is working to establish a uniform medical malpractice act for all state governments.

Objectives of the Study

The purpose of the study was to assess attitudes and behavior of consumers concerning health care and physician services, with special attention to consumer support for possible solutions to the medical malpractice problem. Specifically, the objectives were:

1. to describe criteria used by patients to select and evaluate health care by physicians
2. to identify persons likely to bring malpractice suits in specified situations
3. to determine levels of support for alternative approaches for dealing with the malpractice situation

Research Methodology

Telephone Sample

The study used a telephone questionnaire administered to a random sample of 1,500 adult residents in Ohio. The telephone format was selected after consideration of advantages and disadvantages of both mail and personal interviews. The sample was drawn with the assistance of Chicago-based Reuben H. Donnelly Corporation, which maintains telephone directories of all cities of the United States. It provided a computer-generated random sample of telephone numbers in Ohio cities and rural areas.

A sample of 1,500 was considered a reasonable base for making inferences about the Ohio adult population. However, the samples had limitations. For example, persons who were not at home when calls were made or who did not have telephones could be underrepresented. To minimize these problems, three callbacks were attempted at various time periods.

Interviews were conducted by Dwight Spencer Associates from WATS line facilities in Columbus, Ohio, using skilled and continuously monitored interviewers.

Design and Pretest of Questionnaire

The questionnaire was developed from prior studies on medical care and physician services as well as standardized forms used for obtaining demographic and attitudinal data. A preliminary form of the questionnaire was administered by telephone to 20 respondents in the Columbus area; it was tested further through a focus group interview in which male and female consumers discussed each question and possible responses.

After the telephone pretest, the focus group interview, and consultation with the Ohio State Medical Association staff, numerous changes were made to clarify some questions unlikely to provide useful information in their original form. Few difficulties were encountered in the administration of the final questionnaire. Even though it was lengthy—it took an average of 19 minutes for completion—it was of sufficient interest and clarity that few terminations were encountered.

Research Results

This section describes the basic attitudes and behavior of respondents relating to medical care and health issues.

Reasons for Selection of Physician

Respondents were asked to indicate their most important reason for choosing their primary or family doctor. Table 3-1 lists the frequency of various reasons. Recommendation by friends or relatives (40.6 percent) and by other physicians (14.5 percent) are cited as the two most important factors. Convenience of location (6.5 percent) ranks third.

Importance of Physician Characteristics

Respondents were asked to rate 11 physician characteristics on a five-point scale; a 1 indicated that the attribute was very important and a 5 that it was very unimportant. Table 3-2 reports the results, including the mean importance (average rating) for each of the characteristics.

The most important characteristic proved to be the physician's willingness to talk to the patient about the illness. The second most important

Table 3-1 Reasons Cited as Most Important for Having Chosen a Physician*

Reasons for Having Chosen a Physician*	Respondents Citing Reason as Most Important One
Recommended by friend or relative	· 40.6%
Recommended by another physician	14.5
Looked in yellow pages or directory	1.7
Recommended by hospital	1.1
Met the doctor socially or heard of him as a civic leader	3.3
Treated as member of hospital (emergency, etc.)	1.2
Required physician (clinics, insurance, etc.)	.7
Convenient location	6.5
Other reasons	4.5
Can't remember, always been our doctor, etc.	6.1
No response	19.8
	100.0%

*The question asked: Thinking about your primary doctor or family doctor, what was the most important reason for choosing that doctor?

was how long it takes to get an appointment, followed in importance by the doctor's access to the hospital desired by the patient.

The least important characteristic of those listed (all of which are relatively important, however) is the recommendation of friends. This indicates that while friends are the initial source of information, the doctors' actual performance is the key element in continued patient satisfaction. The perception that the doctor has never been sued for malpractice and the fees charged also are of lesser importance.

Quality of Health Care

Ohio residents have a high opinion of the quality of health care provided by their own doctors. Their evaluation of the quality of care by doctors in general, however, is somewhat lower. As shown in Table 3-3, 52.5 percent of the respondents rated their own doctors as providing excellent health care and an additional 34.9 percent as good. Only 12.8 percent ranked care by doctors in general as excellent.

Physician's Charges

The majority of respondents (70.5 percent) feel that the charges they pay their physicians are reasonable for the services provided (Table 3-4).

Table 3-2 Rated Importance of Characteristics of Physicians (Total Sample)

Characteristic	Rated Importance					
	Very Important	Somewhat Important	Neutral Importance	Somewhat Unimportant	Very Unimportant	Mean Importance*
The doctor's office is near you.	40.9%	19.6%	21.7%	9.1%	8.6%	2.25
The doctor has access to the hospital you want.	64.4	19.4	8.9	3.8	3.5	1.63
The doctor has a good personality and appearance.	42.3	27.4	16.5	7.8	6.0	2.08
How much the doctor charges.	33.1	24.6	24.2	10.3	7.7	2.35
The doctor is willing to talk with you about your illness.	93.7	4.9	.8	.3	.2	1.08
The doctor has many years of experience.	38.9	25.9	21.8	8.4	4.9	2.14
The doctor has never been sued for malpractice.	33.5	15.5	24.5	11.7	14.8	2.59
The doctor is recommended by other doctors.	58.2	25.3	10.5	3.9	2.1	1.66
The doctor has evening or weekend office hours.	34.7	24.7	20.9	11.6	8.0	2.33
The doctor is recommended by your friends.	23.9	27.3	23.1	13.1	12.5	2.63
How long it takes to get an appointment.	62.2	27.0	7.3	2.1	1.4	1.54

*The lower the number, the more important the characteristic.

Table 3-3 Evaluation of Quality of Health Care (Total Sample)

Question	Excellent	Good	Average	Poor	Very Poor	No Response
What is your feeling about the quality of health care given by your doctor?	52.5%	34.9%	9.5%	.9%	.4%	1.9%
What is your feeling about the quality of health care given by doctors in general?	12.8	45.9	32.1	4.0	1.2	4.0

Health and Medical Statements

To gain a better understanding of a variety of topics dealing with physicians, personal health and appearance factors, medical communications, and other related subjects, respondents were asked to indicate their agreement or disagreement with a series of Attitude, Interest, Opinion (AIO) statements. The ranges of responses are presented in Table 3-5.

In the AIO statements, physicians again receive high evaluations. More than 90 percent of respondents strongly or somewhat agree that they have a great deal of confidence in their doctors and feel that most physicians are ethical and responsible. Respondents were split in their attitude on the statement "most doctors are overpaid," and almost 20 percent believe most physicians are more concerned about making money than about the welfare of their patients.

Asked if physicians really are to blame in most malpractice suits, a much higher proportion of respondents agree (44.0 percent) that doctors are not to blame than disagree (14.8 percent). However, 40.9 percent are neutral, indicating that a high proportion of the population has little information on which to base a judgment.

In terms of appearance and health activities, almost 40 percent of the respondents said that they generally do exercises at least twice a week, and 37 percent frequently participate in sports where they can get a lot of exercise. Some 68 percent say they are careful about what they eat and 64 percent weigh about what their doctors say they should. About 75 percent generally have a physical checkup at least once a year. Some of the levels

Table 3-4 Evaluation of Charges Patients Pay Their Doctors

Entirely too high for the services provided you	4.5%
Too high for the services provided you	21.7
Reasonable for the services provided you	70.5
Low considering the services provided you	2.2
No opinion	1.1

Table 3-5 Levels of Agreement with Health and Medical Statements (Total Sample)

Statements	Level of Agreement					Mean Agreement*
	Strongly Agree (1)	Somewhat Agree (2)	Neutral (3)	Somewhat Disagree (4)	Strongly Disagree (5)	
Doctor Related Statements						
I have a great deal of confidence in my doctor.	71.5%	19.3%	5.8%	2.1%	.9%	1.41
About half of the physicians in Ohio are not really competent to practice medicine.	4.0	9.2	29.5	26.7	30.3	3.70
Most doctors are overpaid.	16.7	22.9	23.3	22.3	14.5	2.95
In most malpractice suits, the physician is actually negligent or in the wrong.	2.9	7.9	38.0	30.4	20.2	3.57
Most physicians are ethical and responsible persons.	56.5	34.3	6.5	1.7	.7	1.55
Most physicians are more concerned about making money than the welfare of their patients.	5.7	14.1	19.5	33.4	27.1	3.62
Most physicians in Ohio are not very competent.	2.1	4.6	21.2	33.1	38.3	4.02
It is wrong for a doctor to go on strike for any reason.	49.2	13.9	15.3	12.2	8.9	2.17
In most malpractice suits, the physician is not really to blame.	18.1	25.9	40.9	11.2	3.6	2.56
Medical Communications Statements						
I wish there were brochures which explained things to me when a doctor treats me.	52.2%	24.4%	8.9%	8.1%	6.3%	1.92
I often watch TV programs that discuss health problems.	32.7	27.5	10.1	13.2	16.3	2.53
My physician adequately explains my medical problems to me.	61.5	24.6	5.4	5.4	2.8	1.63
If I had a terminal illness, I would not want my physician to tell me.	6.0	3.1	7.9	11.9	71.1	4.39

Table 3-5 continued

Statements	Level of Agreement					Mean Agreement*
	Strongly Agree (1)	Somewhat Agree (2)	Neutral (3)	Somewhat Disagree (4)	Strongly Disagree (5)	
General Statements						
I generally approve of abortion if a woman wants one.	27.4%	14.1%	15.5%	8.6%	34.2%	3.08
I usually read the nutrition information on food packages.	37.3	27.7	8.7	11.1	15.3	2.39
I believe that a very ill person should be allowed to die when there is no chance of recovering again.	54.3	15.7	17.1	4.1	8.7	1.97
Appearance and Health Statements						
I generally have a physical checkup at least once a year.	56.0%	19.7%	4.2%	8.9%	11.2%	2.00
I generally do exercises (like push-ups or sit-ups or jogging) at least twice a week.	21.7	17.4	5.8	14.9	40.1	3.34
I am careful about what I eat.	37.1	31.3	9.9	12.1	9.6	2.26
I usually have a good tan each year.	22.9	19.3	12.9	16.2	28.3	3.08
I frequently play tennis or other sports where I can get a lot of exercise.	19.9	17.1	7.9	16.3	38.7	3.37
I weigh about what my doctor says I should.	39.0	25.4	6.0	15.6	13.8	2.40
I usually go on a weight control diet at least twice a year.	22.7	12.7	5.9	15.5	43.0	3.43
It seems that I am sick a lot more than my friends are.	4.1	5.4	4.1	18.5	67.9	4.41

*The lower the number, the more agreement with the statement.

Table 3-6 Beliefs As to Causes of Increased Costs of Malpractice Insurance

Causes of Increased Costs of Malpractice Insurance*	Percentage of Respondents Believing Each to Be a Cause
Doctors at fault	21.3%†
Lawyers at fault.	19.7
Insurance companies at fault.	11.7
The government or laws are at fault.	8.4
Juries and judges are giving too much.	11.3
People want something for nothing/greedy.	40.7
Other responses.	6.3
No response.	12.7

*The question asked: In recent years, the amount that doctors pay for malpractice insurance has increased drastically. In a few words, what do you personally believe is the cause of increased costs of malpractice insurance?

†Percentages total more than 100 percent because of multiple responses.

of agreement with these statements can be expected to be overstated because of the respondents' desire to give socially acceptable answers; however, it still may be concluded that there is a high degree of involvement and interest in health and appearance activities.

When asked about medical communications, 86 percent agree with the statement, "My physician adequately explains my medical problems to me," while 8 percent disagree. More than 75 percent express agreement with the statement, "I wish there were brochures which explained things to me when a doctor treats me."

Table 3-5 also reports results on medical topics of current interest such as abortion, nutrition information, and euthanasia. There is substantial agreement (70 percent) that a very ill person should be allowed to die when there is no chance of recovery, high interest in nutritional information on food packages, and polarity of opinion about abortion.

General Beliefs about Malpractice

Asked their personal beliefs as to the causes of the increased costs of malpractice insurance, respondents reported a variety of ideas (Table 3-6). Almost 41 percent indicated reasons such as "People want something for nothing" or "People are greedy." About 21 percent felt that doctors were at fault and almost 20 percent blamed lawyers.

Likelihood of Bringing Malpractice Suits

Respondents were presented three scenarios and asked to indicate how likely they would be to bring a malpractice suit under the condition de-

Table 3-7 Stated Likelihood of Bringing Malpractice Suit under Alternative Scenarios (Total Sample)

Alternative Scenarios	Stated Likelihood of Bringing Malpractice Suit					Mean Likelihood*
	Very Likely (1)	Somewhat Likely (2)	Undecided (3)	Somewhat Unlikely (4)	Very Unlikely (5)	
Let's assume that your doctor was unable to determine a cure for you, and you thought your doctor might be at fault. Would you be very likely to bring a malpractice suit, somewhat likely, undecided, somewhat unlikely, or very unlikely to bring a malpractice suit?	1.0%	3.3%	12.6%	16.6%	66.1%	4.44
Let's assume that you developed a serious medical problem in which you thought your physician might be at fault. Would you be very likely to bring a malpractice suit, somewhat likely, undecided, somewhat unlikely, or very unlikely to bring a malpractice suit?	7.1	20.0	29.0	17.0	26.7	3.36
Let's assume that your spouse or your parent died and you thought your physician might be at fault. Would you be very likely to bring a malpractice suit, somewhat likely, undecided, somewhat unlikely, or very unlikely to bring a malpractice suit?	11.2	19.4	29.9	16.3	23.2	3.21

*The lower the number, the greater that stated likelihood of bringing a malpractice suit.

scribed (Table 3-7). Under the scenario of a physician's being at fault in the case of inability to determine a cure, only about 4 percent indicated they would be very likely or somewhat likely to bring a malpractice suit, while almost 83 percent reported they would be unlikely or very unlikely to do so. About 13 percent were undecided.

Some 27 percent said they would be likely to file a malpractice suit if they developed a serious medical problem they thought was the physician's fault. With this scenario, 29 percent were undecided as to their actions and almost 44 percent reported they would be unlikely to sue.

For the scenario involving the death of a spouse or parent, almost 31 percent indicated the likelihood of bringing a malpractice suit, 30 percent were undecided, and almost 40 percent reported they would be unlikely to sue.

Support for Solutions to the Malpractice Problem

The issue of how to handle the malpractice problem was explored by asking respondents to indicate the degree of support they would give to each of nine alternative ways of dealing with the situation (Table 3-8).

Segmentation Analysis of Persons Most Likely to Bring Malpractice Suits

To identify individuals or groups most likely to bring malpractice suits, the dependent variable (likelihood of bringing a suit) was measured with three levels of intensity based upon the three scenarios just described. The overall results for the total sample also are reported in Table 3-9. This section analyzes the likelihood of suing on the basis of three sets of independent variables—patterns of medical treatment, socioeconomic characteristics of patients, and selected attitudinal (AIO) statements.

Medical Treatment Pattern Variables

The importance of the patient-doctor relationship in predicting intentions for malpractice action is demonstrated clearly in this study. Table 3-10 indicates that persons who have a family doctor are far less likely to indicate they would bring a malpractice suit than those who do not. This relationship is true for all three scenarios.

Persons who have not visited a doctor in the last 12 months (for self or a member of the family) also are more likely to state they will sue than are those who have visited a physician. No clear patterns emerge, however, concerning the relationship between malpractice suits and the frequency of visits to a doctor or of days spent in hospitals.

Table 3-8 Levels of Support for Alternative Ways of Handling the Malpractice Problem (Total Sample)

Ways of Handling Malpractice Problem	Levels of Support for Alternative Ways					Mean Support*
	Strongly For (1)	Somewhat For (2)	Neutral (3)	Somewhat Against (4)	Strongly Against (5)	
A law that lowered the proportion of the settlement that lawyers could receive for malpractice suits.	50.8%	20.7%	20.0%	4.6%	3.7%	1.90
A requirement that patients agree to arbitration of malpractice claims (the patient and the doctor would appoint skilled arbitrators to settle malpractice claims).	37.6	29.5	23.5	5.2	4.0	2.08
A state agency, something like the Workmen's Compensation Bureau, which would collect malpractice insurance premiums from all physicians and decide what benefits would be given all patients with malpractice claims.	17.1	21.5	29.5	11.3	20.3	2.96
A state law which limited the amounts that could be collected by patients with malpractice claims.	32.3	21.2	22.6	9.9	13.8	2.52
A peer group review system in which a group of physicians reviewed malpractice claims and decided which ones should be taken to trial.	23.5	21.2	26.8	12.1	16.3	2.76
A release signed before a person is accepted as a patient agreeing not to sue for malpractice.	12.1	10.2	18.1	14.1	45.1	3.70
More time spent by your physician in explaining the risks or potential problems of your operation or medicine even though the charge for the doctor's services would be higher than now.	48.0	21.8	14.7	8.6	6.8	2.04
A state law which requires insurance companies to reduce malpractice rates to doctors in return for correspondingly higher rates on health insurance to the general public.	7.1	9.7	25.7	16.1	41.1	3.75
Countersuits by physicians against patients and their attorneys who sue for malpractice with no basis for the malpractice suit.	47.8	17.5	16.5	8.9	9.1	2.14

* The lower the number, the more support for the way of handling the malpractice problem.

Table 3-9 Likelihood of Bringing Malpractice Suit under Alternative Scenarios by Physician-Hospital Contacts

Classification of Respondents		Likelihood of Bringing Malpractice Suit for		
		Scenario A (64)*	Scenario B (407)	Scenario C (459)
Do you have a family doctor?				
Yes	(1343)†	3.9%‡	26.1%	29.6%
No	(152)	7.2	36.8	40.1
How many times were you, your spouse, and children living at home treated during the past twelve months by a physician?				
1-3	(315)	3.8	27.9	29.5
4-7	(377)	3.7	29.4	31.6
8-11	(234)	2.6	29.9	35.0
12-15	(180)	3.9	17.8	23.3
16 or more	(309)	5.5	23.6	31.7
None or no response	(85)	9.4	38.9	31.8
How many days were you or members of your family in a hospital during the past twelve months?				
1-3	(119)	5.0	30.3	35.3
4-7	(142)	3.5	30.3	37.3
8-11	(66)	4.5	24.2	25.7
12-15	(52)	1.9	28.8	32.7
16 or more	(85)	8.2	22.4	25.9
None or no response	(1036)	4.1	26.8	29.7

*Numbers in parentheses indicate number of respondents stating that they would be "very likely" or "somewhat likely" to bring a malpractice suit under the alternative scenarios.
†Numbers in parentheses indicate number of respondents in each classification.
‡Read: of the respondents in the data base who have a family doctor, 3.9 percent indicated that they would be "very likely" or "somewhat likely" to bring a malpractice suit under the conditions in Scenario A.

Scenario A: Doctor unable to determine a cure for you, and you thought your doctor might be at fault.
Scenario B: You developed a serious medical problem in which you thought your physician might be at fault.
Scenario C: Your spouse or parent died and you thought your physician might be at fault.

Table 3-10 Likelihood of Bringing Malpractice Suit under Alternative Scenarios by Various Classifications of Respondents

Classifications of Respondents		Likelihood of Bringing Malpractice Suit for		
		Scenario A (64)*	Scenario B (407)	Scenario C (459)
Sex:				
Male	(506)†	4.5%‡	32.0%	35.6%
Female	(994)	4.1	24.6	28.0
Age:				
Under 25	(187)	8.0	41.2	52.4
25-34	(362)	3.9	31.8	39.8
35-44	(258)	4.7	23.6	27.1
45-54	(274)	3.6	24.5	24.1
55-64	(227)	3.1	23.8	21.6
65 and over	(185)	3.2	17.8	16.8
Education:				
Elementary/grammar school	(85)	3.5	24.7	21.2
Some high school	(258)	5.4	20.5	25.6
High school graduate	(670)	4.8	28.4	31.8
Some college	(272)	4.0	30.9	34.2
College graduate	(144)	2.1	27.8	31.3
Post graduate studies	(69)	1.4	27.5	34.8
Income:				
Less than $8,000	(257)	3.9	21.8	21.4
$8,000-$14,999	(498)	5.8	32.1	33.1
$15,000-$19,999	(261)	3.1	26.1	35.2
$20,000-$24,999	(128)	3.1	21.1	35.2
$25,000 and over	(143)	4.2	25.9	33.6
Family Size:				
1	(181)	5.0	26.5	25.4
2	(420)	1.7	22.6	25.0
3	(290)	3.8	33.4	37.6
4	(314)	6.1	29.0	36.9
5	(161)	5.0	24.2	30.4
6 or more	(129)	7.0	27.9	25.6
Political Views:				
Very liberal	(85)	7.1	27.1	29.4
Somewhat liberal	(319)	5.6	35.7	37.3
Middle of the road	(665)	3.0	20.8	27.8
Somewhat conservative	(315)	4.1	29.2	29.8
Very conservative	(94)	7.4	34.0	29.8

Table 3-10 continued

Classifications of Respondents		Likelihood of Bringing Malpractice Suit for		
		Scenario A (64)*	Scenario B (407)	Scenario C (459)
Place of Residence:				
Rural area	(253)	4.7	27.3	26.9
Small town	(429)	4.4	24.7	29.1
Urban area	(276)	5.1	30.8	33.7
Suburban area	(540)	3.5	27.2	32.0
Religious Identification:				
Catholic	(364)	4.7	26.4	32.1
Protestant	(972)	3.9	27.5	29.6
Jewish	(16)	0.0	25.0	31.3
Other	(49)	4.1	16.3	24.5
None	(81)	8.6	32.1	40.7

*Numbers in parentheses indicate number of respondents stating that they would be "very likely" or "somewhat likely" to bring a malpractice suit under the alternative scenarios.
†Numbers in parentheses indicate number of respondents in each classification. Numbers may not add to the total sample due to non-response for that classification question.
‡Read: of the males in the data base (506), 4.5 percent indicated they would be "very likely" or "somewhat likely" to bring a malpractice suit under the conditions described in Scenario A.

Scenario A: Doctor unable to determine a cure for you, and you thought your doctor might be at fault.
Scenario B: You developed a serious medical problem in which you thought your physician might be at fault.
Scenario C: Your spouse or parent died and you thought your physician might be at fault.

Socioeconomic Variables

Data on the relationship between likelihood of bringing a malpractice suit and socioeconomic variables (also in Table 3-10) disclose a number of very significant relationships.

Sex

Males are somewhat more likely than females to bring malpractice suits under all three scenarios.

Age

A general trend indicates that as age increases, the likelihood of bringing a malpractice suit decreases. This holds for all three scenarios. A relatively high proportion of young persons (under age 25 and in the 25-to-34 age group) indicate they would be likely to sue. Under Scenario C, for example,

52.4 percent of the respondents under age 25 indicate they would be likely to sue, compared to only 16.8 percent of those age 65 and over. This may signal increased problems for the medical profession in coming years unless these attitudes change. This implication is of special importance since this age group constitutes one of the fastest-growing segments of the population in the near term.

Education

Some variation in malpractice suit attitudes exists among educational groups. Under Scenario A, those most likely to sue have completed some high school or are high school graduates. Under Scenarios B and C, those most likely to bring suits have slightly more education than those likely to sue under Scenario A.

Income

Some variation in attitudes exists among income groups, although the differences are not pronounced. Under Scenario A, the most persons stating that they would be likely to sue are in the $8,000 to $14,999 income group. Under Scenario C, 35.2 percent of those earning $15,000 to $19,999 implied that they would file suit, while only 21.4 percent of the group earning less than $8,000 would.

Family Size

Family size does not appear to be a useful variable in predicting the likelihood of malpractice suits. Under Scenario A, there is no clear pattern. With Scenarios B and C, families with three or four members seem somewhat more likely to bring suits.

Political Views

Under the low-intensity problem (Scenario A), very liberal and very conservative persons are most likely to bring malpractice suits. In the middle-intensity Scenario B, the somewhat liberal and the very conservative are more likely to sue, and under Scenario C, the most likely persons are those who are somewhat liberal. These patterns are somewhat confusing in their complexity but they do imply that persons with middle-of-the-road political views are the least likely to bring a malpractice suit under all three scenarios.

Place of Residence

Only minor variations exist in attitudes toward malpractice suits by place of residence, with the exception that persons in urban areas are the most likely to sue under all three scenarios.

Religious Identification

Minor variations exist among religious groups in their attitudes toward malpractice suits. Once again, such observations must take into consideration the small sample size of some of the religious groups. In general, however, those with no denominational affiliation are the most likely to file under all three scenarios.

Medical and Health Attitude Variables

Segments of the population are increasingly being identified in research studies on the basis of attitudinal (AIO) statements rather than demographic or other variables. These statements may be more valuable in a diagnostic sense because they may indicate more directly the beliefs or feelings associated with certain patterns of behavior and interest. Some of the relationships between selected AIO statements and the stated likelihood of bringing a malpractice suit (Table 3-11) provide revealing insights.

Table 3-11 Likelihood of Bringing Malpractice Suit under Alternative Scenarios by Responses to Selected Health-Medical Statements

Classifications of Respondents		Likelihood of Bringing Malpractice Suit for		
		Scenario A (64)*	Scenario B (407)	Scenario C (459)
I have a great deal of confidence in my doctor.				
Agree	(1363)†	3.7%‡	26.2%	29.3%
Disagree	(46)	10.9	30.4	43.5
About half of the physicians in Ohio are not really competent to practice medicine.				
Agree	(198)	5.6	30.3	33.3
Disagree	(855)	3.5	26.8	27.7
If I had a terminal illness, I would not want my physician to tell me.				
Agree	(136)	6.6	29.4	37.5
Disagree	(1245)	4.4	28.1	31.1
Most doctors are overpaid.				
Agree	(595)	5.9	31.9	37.0
Disagree	(552)	3.1	21.0	26.4
I wish there were brochures which explained things to me when a doctor treats me.				
Agree	(1149)	4.9	29.4	33.5
Disagree	(216)	1.4	19.4	19.9

(continued on page 54)

Table 3-11 continued

Classifications of Respondents		Likelihood of Bringing Malpractice Suit for		
		Scenario A (64)*	Scenario B (407)	Scenario C (459)
In most malpractice suits, the physician is actually negligent or in the wrong.				
Agree	(162)	6.8	37.7	49.4
Disagree	(759)	2.2	22.9	24.4
My physician adequately explains my medical problems to me.				
Agree	(1291)	4.0	26.0	29.4
Disagree	(123)	4.9	31.7	39.0
I generally do exercises (like push-ups or sit-ups or jogging) at least twice a week.				
Agree	(587)	3.9	31.8	33.7
Disagree	(825)	4.2	23.2	27.9
I weigh about what my doctor says I should.				
Agree	(966)	4.0	28.8	32.9
Disagree	(441)	3.9	23.4	24.5
It seems that I am sick a lot more than my friends are.				
Agree	(143)	5.6	24.5	37.1
Disagree	(1296)	4.2	27.2	29.6

*Numbers in parentheses indicate number of respondents stating that they would be "very likely" or "somewhat likely" to bring a malpractice suit under the alternative scenarios.

†Numbers in parentheses indicate number of respondents who "strongly agree" or "agree somewhat" with the statement, followed by the number of respondents who "disagree somewhat" or "strongly disagree" with the statement. The AGREES and DISAGREES do not equal the total respondent base of 1,500 because of neutral answers and non-responses to the statement.

‡Read: of the respondents who "strongly agreed" or "somewhat agreed" with the statement "I have a great deal of confidence in my doctor," 3.7 percent indicated they would be "very likely" or "somewhat likely" to bring a malpractice suit under the conditions described in Scenario A.

Scenario A: Doctor unable to determine a cure for you, and you thought your doctor might be at fault.
Scenario B: You developed a serious medical problem in which you thought your physician might be at fault.
Scenario C: Your spouse or parent died and you thought your physician might be at fault.

As might be expected, respondents who indicated great confidence in their doctors also reported a much lower likelihood of suing under each of the scenarios. Respondents agreeing with the statements "About half of the physicians in Ohio are not really competent to practice medicine" and "In most malpractice suits, the physician is actually negligent or in the wrong" indicated much greater likelihood of filing a suit for each of the scenarios. Those who agree that doctors are overpaid also have a greater likelihood of suing.

Respondents who agree that "My physician adequately explains my medical problems to me" are less likely to sue than those who disagree with the statement. The likelihood of bringing suits was greater for those who agreed with the statement, "I wish there were brochures which explained things to me when a doctor treats me."

In general, those who agree that they exercise and weigh about what their doctors suggest are more likely to bring malpractice suits than those who are overweight and do not exercise. Respondents who agree with the statement "It seems that I am sick a lot more than my friends are" are more likely to sue under Scenarios A and B than those who disagree. Individuals who agree that "If I had a terminal illness, I would not want my physician to tell me," are more likely to file a suit under all three scenarios.

OVERVIEW OF CASE 3

Issues to Consider

1. What is the benefit of gaining information about consumer attitudes about malpractice?
2. What strategic recommendations should be considered for physicians and legislative groups to help reduce the level of unwarranted malpractice suits, based on this research?
3. Could additional analysis be done with the data and/or what further research do the results suggest?

Discussion

1. Attitudes and Behavior

Obtaining information about attitudes is predicated on the assumption that attitudes predict behavior. Knowing the current level of attitudes toward a particular object is believed to assist in determining the level of purchasing of many consumer goods. Conversely, while attitudes may be a precursor to behavior, behavior also may have a similar effect on attitudes. For example, individuals may eat something they did not feel they liked (even though they had not tried it before) only to find out it really was not bad and they did like it. That eating behavior can change an attitude toward food. If the objective is to change attitudes, then allowing behavior to help (in addition to other communications devices) may be useful. However, as the cost of the product or service increases, it is a less practical approach.

In this case, the primary benefits of measuring attitudes are to help determine the potential for malpractice suits under three different scenarios and to segment the population for further study based on feelings of likelihood of initiating malpractice suits. Segmentation is discussed in more detail in following cases.

2. Malpractice Strategies

Not only are malpractice judgments high but the loss of time, court costs, and legal preparations also are costly. If unwarranted malpractice suits could be reduced, savings could be obtained for most parties.

It is apparent from the research, particularly as the scenarios increase in severity of outcome, that those who are more likely to bring malpractice suits are frustrated over a lack of communications. For example, Table 3-11 demonstrates that for such persons the availability of explanatory brochures and literature and the need for adequate explanation by physicians are important issues.

This observation is confirmed by the results shown in Table 3-8, which cites "more time spent explaining . . ." as one of the best ways to handle the malpractice issue. There also was (1) a high level of acceptance for legislation to limit the portion of the settlement obtained by lawyers (the results might be to reduce the encouragement of such suits by the legal profession) and (2) acceptance of arbitration.

One possible strategic recommendation for physicians (particularly if they have practices with a high proportion of the sensitive demographic areas noted in Table 3-10) might be to offer more opportunity to patients to communicate with the doctors or staffs—perhaps develop a "hot line" approach. Another possibility would be to make more literature available to patients. Many medical specialty groups or associations provide such material to their members. Physicians also should be sensitive to and aware of the need to communicate with patients and plan to spend additional time to explain problems in detail.

From a legislative perspective, perhaps the major recommendation is that lawyers' split of settlements be limited. That would attack the problem indirectly by reducing the economic incentive for lawyers to encourage pursuit of questionable cases. Legislation to permit (or even force) arbitration may be of value but its success in discouraging unnecessary suits would be a function of the availability of competent arbitrators.

3. Further Analysis

Additional analysis is possible to gain further insight into possible strategies. For example, the results in Table 3-8 indicate (for the sample population as a whole) which alternatives have the most support. This analysis does not allow for pinpointing methods that could reduce the likelihood of a malpractice suit. Consequently, additional analysis of the table focused on those who would be somewhat or most likely to bring suit under the scenarios would be helpful.

A potential for further research exists based on the results of this study. For example, now that an initial demographic profile has been developed (Table 3-10) for those likely to sue, it may be useful to obtain more information from that segment. This could be done in a variety of ways and on a variety of topics. A focus group of males under 35, with some college education, and living in or around major cities, could be established. Then the development of additional characteristics, alternative communication methods, and variations of malpractice situations could be explored to produce a refined study of the key market segments.

To be sure, other analysis and further research are possible. This material is offered to initiate further discussion.

CASE 4. MOODY NURSING HOME: A CASE STUDY IN BUYER BEHAVIOR

On an early fall morning in 1979, Labe Mell, administrator and corporate president of the Moody Nursing Home, noted that Friday's appointments included an interview with a graduate student who had expressed an interest in following up on a research study conducted at the home five years earlier. Mell mused on the situation then and on events and environmental changes since. He recalled that the study had identified the factors involved in the selection of a nursing home by the patient and family. The results had been useful in his quest to maintain full occupancy for the Moody home. In fact, he had shared the study with the American College of Nursing Home Administrators, which had distributed it to its entire membership. The graduate student's assignment was to write a paper on "Buyer Behavior Research As an Input Into Marketing Strategy."

The Nursing Home Industry

The hospital as a formal, organized, and permanent institution is traceable to the third century. It and more recent institutions (the poor farm, flophouse, almshouse, and sanitorium) all play a part in the history of the nursing home, which finds its roots in the nineteenth century.

In rural areas, the poor farm concept arose when communities began to farm out the responsibility for care of the poor (and usually elderly) to the highest bidder. As a result of the modern trend toward urbanization, the indigent and aged in cities began to settle in hotels, apartments, and multiple-family homes. Care of the sick and aged at first had been provided only by church establishments but gradually had moved into the arena of public responsibility.

Veterans of early American wars fared poorly, too, and tended to turn their hospitals into domiciliary units. Eventually, the government assumed responsibility for providing for them. This concept of caring for the veteran population began to merge with the hospital concept. Eventually, long-term patients were grouped together in locations separate from hospitals. The resultant facility became the immediate forerunner of the modern nursing home. It is only in this century that the licensing of nursing homes is recorded.

The modern nursing home continues to undergo further definition in a struggle to meet changing needs. While it still serves as a place of residence, it now increasingly meets medically oriented needs when its occupants become chronically ill.

The last 40-odd years have seen long-term care develop into a major industry (in 1939, there were 1,200 facilities with a capacity of 25,000 beds;

by 1975, licensed nursing homes numbered 22,000, and about 1,300,000 men and women lived in them.

Factors instrumental in the rapid growth of the industry include: the increasing proportion of the population over age 65, advances in medical technology, changing attitudes of society toward institutionalization of the elderly, the general mobility of the younger generation, the increasing effect of Social Security benefits and private pensions, and the establishment of public programs to pay or share the cost of long-term care.

Because most of the institutions providing services are proprietary, the care of the aged and chronically ill in this country is basically a private industry. However, the industry is governed by local, state, and federal regulations and is generously subsidized by state and federal governments.

Origin and Growth of the Moody Nursing Home and Pavilion

The Moody Nursing Home opened as a privately owned and operated extended care facility in Decatur, Ga., in October 1963, with 104 beds. In July 1967, capacity was increased to 225 beds. Moody was conveniently located near public transportation and shopping centers. It had gardens, terraces, and patios, with bright and cheerful decor and comfortable furnishings indoors. The 70,000-square-foot area of the physical plant provided, in addition to the pleasant and functional residents' rooms, dining rooms, lounges, service offices, inservice classrooms, and a complement of in-house departments that made the home unique.

In-house departments—which proved both convenient and cost effective—included a fully-stocked pharmacy that distributed medications solely on a unit-dose basis, physical and occupational therapy, laboratory, x-ray, EKG, and speech pathology. The special facilities made Moody one of the best-equipped extended-care facilities in the Southeast.

In 1978, the corporation opened a 104-unit facility in Snellville, Ga., offering intermediate care for persons primarily seeking only nursing, housing, and food services. Two blocks from its main building, the corporation also owned Columbia Place, a residential community of 48 units, or flats, for men and women whose condition allowed a greater degree of independence and minimal supervision.

In 1979, the staff for the three facilities consisted of 161 positions:

1 administrator
1 assistant administrator
1 director of nursing services
1 registered nurse, full time
4 registered nurses, part time
1 inservice education director (R.N.)

16 licensed practical nurses (L.P.N.), full time
1 licensed practical nurse, part time
71 nursing aides, full time
1 nursing aide, part time
1 dietitian
1 pharmacist
1 social worker
1 medical records staffer
53 administrative full time (clerks, cooks, custodial, maintenance)
6 administrative assistants part time

The most prevalent rate category for residents living in the Moody Nursing Home ranged from $725 to $795 per month for basic services. Rates were determined by such variables as the degree of medical care needed as well as by Medicare and Medicaid regulations. A computerized billing system was installed in 1972. The 1981 billing was expected to exceed $2 million.

The Meeting

During the long conversation with the visiting graduate student, Mell reviewed aspects of the Moody Nursing Home's marketing strategy. In discussing the earlier marketing study, he commented, "It definitely redirected our marketing efforts. I was amazed to see how little input came from the attending physicians concerning the actual choice of a nursing home facility for their patients."

At that time, radio was the primary advertising medium in what was deemed to be the most cost-effective way of reaching family members who were influential in the decison-making process, characterized by Mell as "40-year-old women."

He noted that Moody rarely had vacancies so radio advertising had been discontinued. The principal promotional activity was word-of-mouth recommendation and an attractive brochure mailed upon request. Mell indicated that he no longer saw any value in traditional marketing efforts for Moody but that if another nursing home was not operating at capacity, promotion based on an understnding of buyer behavior would be essential.

Since the original study, there had been some changes in referral sources. Discharge planners on hospital staffs (sometimes registered nurses, sometimes trained social workers) and Golden Age, a United Way-funded agency, often provided information to prospective residents, although no formal marketing effort was directed to either source.

Perhaps the most fascinating recent development at the Moody home, and the one potentially offering a whole new market segment, was the expansion of the specialized in-house departments to serve off-the-street patients. The same departments—physical therapy, occupational therapy, speech pathology, pharmacy—that had proved complementary to the overall service package and a cost-effective mechanism in terms of financial operation, accepted outpatients on referral from private physicians. Workers in these departments disseminated information on available services in their day-to-day contacts with private physicians. State and federal offices also were alerted to the availability of these services.

The graduate student asked Mell whether the earlier study had been used in formulating the marketing strategy for outpatient care. He said it had been useful but perhaps could be reviewed or followed up by a study focusing specifically on the buying behavior of outpatient clients. Mell provided a copy of the earlier research, which follows.

SUMMARY OF A STUDY OF BUYER BEHAVIOR FOR NURSING HOME SERVICES[1]

The nursing home is a major component in the health delivery system. The elevated status of marketing as a meaningful and acceptable pursuit for any organization, together with the public's accelerated concern for the quality of care provided by all elements of the health delivery system, have drastically altered the nature of marketing efforts in this area.

The very concept of the nursing home itself is changing rapidly: people are living longer; increased urbanization makes caring for the sick and elderly at home less feasible; ever-growing numbers of women who would at one time have been expected to assume these responsibilities are leaving home to return to the work force.

Not to be ignored or minimized, when planning the marketing of nursing homes and their services, are the sensitive and highly personal issues involved—the relocation of a family member out of a home and into an institution, even under optimal circumstances, potentially entails feelings of guilt and anxiety. These factors create a unique purchasing atmosphere.

Given this unique purchasing situation, the marketing mix in the specific case of a nursing home—cost, access, the promotion, and service development—all depend on an understanding of consumer behavior. Here, the critical issue becomes the accurate identification of who makes and/or influences the decision to become a "consumer" or nursing home resident.

Buyer Behavior

First, the institution must understand the buying process of a "customer" in arriving at a purchase decision (in the case of a nursing home, buyer and user are not necessarily the same). Any marketing effort must consider those persons who influence the purchase decision and must begin with an understanding of the entire process, which includes perceived needs, purchase decision, and postpurchase feelings. An awareness of the purchase decision process in selecting a nursing home provides better communications and greater satisfaction to all involved parties: patients, physicians, relatives, third parties (admitting agencies, the clergy, etc.), and the nursing home personnel and administration.

Objective and Methodology

The objective of the project is to study the roles played by patients, physicians, relatives, and third parties as buying participants of nursing home services. It is felt that a marketing effort can be directed more precisely only after identification of these roles. The study was designed to identify and characterize the buying participants. Methodology included a series of interviews with residents (patients), their relatives, the doctors listed as attending physicians at the time of admission, and the nursing home administrator. Twenty-five patients were chosen from the inpatient population of the Moody Nursing Home, according to a random sampling technique.

Findings

The data collected from the patients and their relatives are presented in Tables 3-12 through 3-24, and data from their physicians in Tables 3-25 and 3-26. In Table 3-12, the responses indicate that the family exerts a major initial influence on the patients to enter a nursing home. In 62 percent of the cases in which the relative responded, the family was involved in the decision. The patients acknowledged family participation in only 44 percent of the cases.

Table 3-13 reveals that relatives provide an important source of information to patients in this nursing home. This is an appropriate role in the initial decision. It is worth noting that among the relatives' responses, the largest category (31 percent) was "other." An analysis of this category shows that previous personal knowledge is the most important source of information about nursing homes.

Ninety-four percent of the relatives had knowledge of the nursing home before considering placing the patient there, indicating widespread general knowledge of the particular home (Table 3-14). The fact that so many of the relatives had such prior knowledge, most having received their information from the physician and "other" sources (Table 3-13), suggests that

Table 3-12 Persons or Agencies First Advising Patient to Reside in a Nursing Home

	Patients' Responses	*Relative Responses*
Physician	44%	37%
Family	31%	37%
Physician & Family	13%	25%
Physician & Social Worker	6%	
Friend	6%	

Source: Jac L. Goldstucker, Danny N. Bellenger, and F.D. Miller, "A Case Study of the Buying Participant in the Purchase of Nursing Home Services," *The Journal of Long Term Care Administration* (Summer 1974). Used by permission.

Table 3-13 Source Informing Participant about the Home

	Patients' Responses	*Relative Responses*
Doctor	19%	25%
Relatives	55%	13%
Friend	13%	6%
Church		13%
Advertising		13%
Other	13%	31%

Source: Jac L. Goldstucker, Danny N. Bellenger, and F.D. Miller, "A Case Study of the Buying Participant in the Purchase of Nursing Home Services," *The Journal of Long Term Care Administration* (Summer 1974). Used by permission.

promotional strategies be developed to concentrate on the main decision makers.

Some shopping is involved in selecting a nursing home (Table 3-15). Shopping is much more prevalent for nursing home selection than for other methods of health delivery because the need rarely is as urgent as it is for hospitalization, for example. A high positive response to this question would be expected, as indicated in Table 3-16. People generally are reluctant to admit that the decision they make in any matter is not their first choice. However, the patients are not in accord with their relatives on first choice.

In Table 3-17 the responses of the relatives are aggregated and averaged to arrive at the expense distribution. The patients' knowledge in this area is very poor. The administrator's figures are closer to reality. The relatives' responses may be distorted by a desire to rationalize the placing of loved ones in nursing homes.

Table 3-14 Prior Knowledge of the Home before Decision Made for Patient to Enter Home

	Patients' Responses	Relative Responses
Yes	55%	94%
No	45%	6%

Source: Jac L. Goldstucker, Danny N. Bellenger, and F.D. Miller, "A Case Study of the Buying Participant in the Purchase of Nursing Home Services," The Journal of Long Term Care Administration (Summer 1974). Used by permission.

Table 3-15 Consideration of Other Homes before This Home Was Chosen

	Patients' Responses	Relative Responses
Considered	55%	50%
None Considered	38%	44%
Doesn't Know	6%	6%

Source: Jac L. Goldstucker, Danny N. Bellenger, and F.D. Miller, "A Case Study of the Buying Participant in the Purchase of Nursing Home Services," The Journal of Long Term Care Administration (Summer 1974). Used by permission.

Table 3-16 Nursing Home as First Choice

	Patients' Responses	Relative Responses
Home first choice	69%	87%
Home not first choice	19%	13%
Doesn't know	13%	

Source: Jac L. Goldstucker, Danny N. Bellenger, and F.D. Miller, "A Case Study of the Buying Participant in the Purchase of Nursing Home Services," The Journal of Long Term Care Administration (Summer 1974). Used by permission.

The survey data indicate that relatives chose the home in 69 percent of the cases (Table 3-18). It appears that the opinions of relatives are the most important factor in the selection of the home.

The data in Table 3-19 suggest that the physician either is not involved or, if involved, plays an advisory role in the choice of the home.

In Table 3-20, it is obvious that governmental agencies do not play a large part in the selection process. However, their actual effect on the nursing home's operations is of much greater significance as manifested through federal and state regulations affecting operating standards. The patient's involvement in choosing the home is described in Table 3-21.

The differences in perceptions about who chooses the home may result from several factors: (1) the bias of the interviewer in asking or phrasing

Table 3-17 Perception of Who Pays the Major Portion of Nursing Home Charges

	Relative Response	*Nursing Home Administrator's Response*
Patient	55%	25%
Relative	15%	12%
Medicare/Medicaid	26%	60%
Insurance	4%	3%

Source: Jac L. Goldstucker, Danny N. Bellenger, and F.D. Miller, "A Case Study of the Buying Participant in the Purchase of Nursing Home Services," *The Journal of Long Term Care Administration* (Summer 1974). Used by permission.

Table 3-18 Involvement of Relatives in Choosing the Nursing Home

	Patients' Responses	*Relative Responses*
Relative chose home	69%	69%
Not involved in choice	6%	6%
Advised choice	25%	19%
Gave consent		6%

Source: Jac L. Goldstucker, Danny N. Bellenger, and F.D. Miller, "A Case Study of the Buying Participant in the Purchase of Nursing Home Services," *The Journal of Long Term Care Administration* (Summer 1974). Used by permission.

Table 3-19 Involvement of Physician in Choice of Nursing Home

	Patients' Responses	*Relative Responses*
Gave approval after choice made	31%	19%
Not involved	44%	31%
Suggested several homes	6%	31%
Chose home	19%	13%
Don't know		6%

Source: Jac L. Goldstucker, Danny N. Bellenger, and F.D. Miller, "A Case Study of the Buying Participant in the Purchase of Nursing Home Services," *The Journal of Long Term Care Administration* (Summer 1974). Used by permission.

Table 3-20 Involvement of Medicare/Medicaid Agency in Choice of Home

	Patients' Responses	Relative Responses
Not involved	94%	81%
Provided list from which choice was made		13%
Don't know	6%	6%

Source: Jac L. Goldstucker, Danny N. Bellenger, and F.D. Miller, "A Case Study of the Buying Participant in the Purchase of Nursing Home Services," *The Journal of Long Term Care Administration* (Summer 1974). Used by permission.

Table 3-21 Involvement of Patient in Choosing the Home

	Patients' Responses	Relative Responses
Chose home	25%	6%
Not involved	62%	75%
Indicated preference	6%	6%
Asked someone else to make the choice for them	6%	6%
Joint decision by patient and relative		6%

Source: Jac L. Goldstucker, Danny N. Bellenger, and F.D. Miller, "A Case Study of the Buying Participant in the Purchase of Nursing Home Services," *The Journal of Long Term Care Administration* (Summer 1974). Used by permission.

the question; (2) an attempt by relatives to involve the patients in the decision in a superficial way; and (3) a manifestation by the patients to show that they are involved in decisions regarding their fate. However, it must be noted that 62 percent of the patients indicated they were not involved in the choice.

The administrator listed a tour as a major promotional item. However, the survey sample showed only 44 percent of those making the decision of which nursing home to choose took the tour (Table 3-22).

Indications are that a patient, once admitted, does not often become an influencer to sell others on the home, either directly or indirectly, through communications with relatives (Table 3-23).

Table 3-24 indicates factors considered most important in choosing a nursing home. Other factors of importance not reported were good food, good patient-family communication through staff, good administrative practices, activities, and supervision of employees.

The price of the care being provided and the location of the nursing home are the least important factors of those listed. It often is asserted that, to be successful, a nursing home must be located close to the physician

Table 3-22 Tour Taken before Choice Made to Enter the Home

	Patients' Responses	*Relative Responses*
Tour taken	44%	44%
No tour taken	44%	56%
Doesn't know	13%	

Source: Jac L. Goldstucker, Danny N. Bellenger, and F.D. Miller, "A Case Study of the Buying Participant in the Purchase of Nursing Home Services," *The Journal of Long Term Care Administration* (Summer 1974). Used by permission.

Table 3-23 Acquaintance with a Patient at the Home Prior to Choice of Nursing Home

	Patients' Responses	*Relative Responses*
Prior Acquaintance	31%	25%
No Prior Acquaintance	69%	75%

Source: Jac L. Goldstucker, Danny N. Bellenger, and F.D. Miller, "A Case Study of the Buying Participant in the Purchase of Nursing Home Services," *The Journal of Long Term Care Administration* (Summer 1974). Used by permission.

Table 3-24 Factors Involved in Choice of Home and Importance as Considered by Consumers Making Choice

	Very Important	*Minor Importance*	*No Importance*
Location	58%	37%	5%
Price	48%	52%	
Reputation	89%	11%	
Type of care provided	89%	5%	
Friendliness of nurses & workers	89%	11%	
Cleanliness of facilities	89%	11%	

Source: Jac L. Goldstucker, Danny N. Bellenger, and F.D. Miller, "A Case Study of the Buying Participant in the Purchase of Nursing Home Services," *The Journal of Long Term Care Administration* (Summer 1974). Used by permission.

in order to attract patients. This case study does not support that contention. Of those making 70 percent of the decisions regarding choice of home, almost half felt that location was of minor importance.

Thus, this study indicates that the factors that should be stressed in marketing are type of care provided, quality of the staff, and maintenance of the facility.

Tables 3-25 and 3-26 indicate that physicians are not deeply involved in selecting nursing homes for the patients. The data in these tables are consistent with those in Table 3-20, which suggest that the physician either is not involved or plays only an advisory role.

Table 3-25 Physician Responses

	Yes	*No*	*No Response*
Does the patient normally ask you to choose a nursing home for him?	3	6	3
Is it within medical ethics to recommend a particular nursing home?	7	2	3
Do you require that the nursing home be accredited?	3	2	7
Do you require that the nursing home be near your office?	3	3	6
Do you require that the nursing home be affiliated with a hospital of which you are a staff member?	0	6	6

Source: Jac L. Goldstucker, Danny N. Bellenger, and F.D. Miller, "A Case Study of the Buying Participant in the Purchase of Nursing Home Services," *The Journal of Long Term Care Administration* (Summer 1974). Used by permission.

Table 3-26 How Does the Physician Recommendation Mechanism Operate?

Recommendation is made and then patient chooses the nursing home.	4
Patient chooses home and then approval is given.	4
Recommendation is made and patient is directed in the choice of a nursing home.	3
Don't know.	1

Source: Jac L. Goldstucker, Danny N. Bellenger, and F.D. Miller, "A Case Study of the Buying Participant in the Purchase of Nursing Home Services," *The Journal of Long Term Care Administration* (Summer 1974). Used by permission.

Conclusions

The findings of the random sample indicate that the family exerts the major initial influence on the patient in reaching a decision to enter a nursing home; as such, the family is the most important source of information. Obviously, any promotional strategies should concentrate on the main decision makers. Comparative shopping becomes a real issue in finding a nursing home because, unlike other forms of health care (hospitalization, for example), this form generally is less urgent, as noted earlier.

Another significant finding is that the primary care physician either is not involved in the decision or plays an advisory role only. Government agencies (Medicare/Medicaid) are not involved in the selection process but naturally enter into actual operations through a multitude of federal and state regulations.

Factors indicated by those surveyed as being important in the choice of a nursing home included:

1. reputation of the home
2. type of care provided
3. friendliness of nurses and workers
4. cleanliness
5. price
6. location

The process of choosing begins with advice to the patient to enter a nursing home. This may be initiated by either the physician or the family. Sources of information include relatives, friends, church groups, advertising, other patients, and physicians, with the actual choice most often being made by relatives. After a decision is reached, the attending physician must submit a formal recommendation.

NOTES

1. Jac L. Goldstucker, Danny N. Bellenger, and F. D. Miller, "A Case Study of the Buying Participant in the Purchase of Nursing Home Services," *The Journal of Long Term Care Administration* (Summer 1974), pp. 5–21, adapted with permission.
2. For full discussion, see P. Kotler, *Marketing for Non-Profit Organizations* (Englewood Cliffs, N.J., Prentice-Hall, 1975), pp. 130–141.

OVERVIEW OF CASE 4

Issues to Consider

1. What would be an appropriate marketing strategy for the Moody Nursing Home based on the data from the buyer behavior research?
2. How can the image of the nursing home be measured and, if need be, modified, in light of the four factors rated in the research as influencing selection of a nursing home—(a) the nursing home's reputation, (b) the type of care provided, (c) friendliness of nurses and workers, and (d) cleanliness of facility?
3. What is the difference in buyer behavior for nursing home care and for the outpatient services it offers? How will the two marketing strategies differ?

Discussion

1. Marketing Strategy

The results of the buyer research indicate patient relatives are primary decision makers in the selection of a nursing home. The research also indicates the important factors in the decision process: knowledge of the facility, its reputation, type of care provided, friendliness of the employees, and cleanliness. However, the results must be viewed with caution. It is unclear whether the 25 respondents are representative of the target market. Regardless of the unknowns, this research will assist nursing home management in devising an appropriate marketing strategy.

To follow the market concept, the Moody Nursing Home needs to begin the process by looking outward-in. Consumer input at the outset is the essential component of a marketing strategy. Guidelines suggest a process for development of the marketing strategy. The nursing home should:

1. Identify the target market: the actual market, the potential market, and the nonmarket.
2. Segment the market by demographics, including geography, household size, and income.
3. Identify the perceptions, attitudes, and preferences of the target market by conducting group discussions with prospective patients and family members, followed by quantitative surveys, personal interviews, or telephone interviews.
4. Determine which market segment(s) to target.
5. Define goals and objectives for penetration of chosen market segment(s).

6. Determine how the organization is going to allocate resources to match the needs and desires of the market segment(s).
7. Address the issues of promoting the services to the target market following the determination of location, hours, and price.
8. Implement the program and devise a method of evaluation.
9. Evaluate the program.

2. Analyzing the Image

The image of a health care facility can be measured by using the following techniques: (1) unstructured interviews, (2) judgmental measurement instruments, (3) perceptual and preference mapping, and (4) semantic differential instruments.[2] These tools can provide the data necessary to analyze the perceived image held by the various market segments.

The data must be organized, analyzed, interpreted, and compared with the facility's image of the services it offers, its mission, and its goals. This comparison determines the gap that exists between the image held by the community and that held by the facility. Once the nursing home is aware of how the community views it, it should determine whether a change in image is desired.

That modification can only occur through a full understanding of the factors that have caused its present image. Then the strategies can be developed to influence behavioral changes that will need to occur to bring about the desired image. Not all individuals in the target market will be aware of the revised procedures and practices. Therefore, the nursing home will have to develop a strategy to communicate its efforts. After implementation of the new policies and procedures, management should evaluate the image change by utilizing the measurement tools mentioned earlier.

3. Nursing Home vs. Outpatient Care

The case provides information on buyer behavior for selecting nursing home care but not for the outpatient services the home provides. Obviously, the client populations for the two services are different, although they may utilize both services over time.

The research indicates that the following factors are present in the selection of nursing home care:

1. The decision maker is a relative of the patient rather than the actual consumer of the service.
2. The patient's physician provides information on the facility but does not select it for the patient.

3. The decision maker states that Medicare and Medicaid programs are not involved in the selection process.
4. The decision maker has knowledge of the home before admitting a relative there.

To understand the buyer behavior in the selection of outpatient services, the health care facility should ask the following types of questions:

1. the image of the outpatient clinic
2. the match between services and needs
3. the location, hours, and price
4. the range of facilities utilized for the identical service
5. why (or why not) the home is (or is not) utilized
6. key competitors

The marketing strategies for inpatients and outpatients will be different because of the variances in target markets and market segments as well as in missions, goals, and objectives. Each marketing strategy will differ from the next because of the market mix, the services desired, the programs implemented, and the methods of communicating.

Chapter 4

Market Research

CASE 5. NORTHWESTERN OHIO HEALTH MAINTENANCE CENTER: MARKETING AND PREVENTIVE MEDICINE

Tom McDonald, a CPA and treasurer of the Northwestern Ohio Health Maintenance Center (NOHMC), had suggested to the board of directors that the agency needed to organize its planning more systematically. Harold Meyers, M.D., chairman of the board, could remember thinking, "I only wish that Tom wouldn't keep harping about the need for us to plan more. We are already doing the best we can, considering the circumstances."

He also remembered that McDonald had gone one step further and had made a recommendation: "We just cannot keep operating like this indefinitely. Why don't we admit to ourselves that we could use some expert advice and then try to do a better job of operating the center financially. I am acquainted with Dr. Kevin Randolph, a consultant with Health Care Marketing Services, Inc., and I know he has helped other businesses get on the right track. Maybe he would be willing to help us too."

Dr. Meyers could remember being slightly surprised when the rest of the board had considered this an excellent recommendation and had authorized McDonald to work with Dr. Randolph to discover what possibilities might be open. The two had been working together for several months and now they were to update the board on their progress.

Company Background

The Northwestern Ohio Health Maintenance Center was founded by a group of Toledo area physicians in 1974. The physicians had been in private practice there for an average of ten years. Although the NOHMC was privately owned by the physicians, any Academy of Medicine member was welcome to join on either an owner or nonowner basis. The board felt that the group should be community owned and operated.

The NOHMC was started because the founding physicians saw a need for preventive medicine in Toledo. It was organized in a corporate structure with financing by ten local physicians. A seven-man board of directors— all of them physicians with an average of more than 20 years' medical experience apiece—managed the facility.

The center billed patients separately from the doctor and completed its own insurance forms when appropriate. Preventive medicine, per se, was not covered by health insurance such as Blue Shield.

The founders believed that automated multiphasic health testing services (AMHTS) were a valid answer to the problem of the overworked doctor performing superficial examinations on patients. AMHTS were perceived to fill a void that was plaguing the health care delivery system: regular health checkups for the well person. The time spent with a physician was minimal and often resulted in a less than satisfactory examination. This often was compounded by extended waits to get an appointment and long waits in the doctor's office. The founders felt that people were forced to use less than desirable services because it was difficult or impossible to obtain them in the existing health care framework.

Background of AMHTS

While the concept of AMHTS was new to Northwestern Ohio, more than 130 operations were in existence throughout the country. AMHTS used computers and allied health personnel to provide thorough examinations to both sick and well patients alike. The United States Department of Health, Education, and Welfare best summed up AMHTS as:

> a planned course or series of events or procedures programmed in advance and utilizing allied health personnel and automated instrumentation, through which various categories of persons who may or may not be patients under medical care are processed, in order to accomplish some medical or health related purpose.[1]

AMHTS were used first by health departments to screen for communicable diseases such as syphilis. In time they became multiphasic, that is, more than one test was performed in a single examination. Planned sequences of tests and procedures soon were developed, with analysis performed by a computer. Later it became evident that this approach could be used by physicians to detect many diseases in their early stages. This early detection not only resulted in better treatment but also reduced the total cost to the patient.

There were five discernible uses for AMHTS: (1) health assessment, screening, and disease detection; (2) fitness examination; (3) adjuncts to diagnosis; (4) patient surveillance; and (5) adjuncts to patient management.

Services Offered

The tests performed on an individual ranged from the cardiovascular, such as blood pressure, to chest x-rays, to those for protein levels. Once these tests were performed, the results were entered into the computer to check for abnormalities against the patient's history and physical examination. The tests then could be forwarded to the patient's personal physician. The attending staff of allied health personnel made no assessment of patient well-being. Exhibit 4-1 provides a complete breakdown of services offered.

En route to the board meeting, Dr. Meyers pulled into the parking lot and hurried into the building that housed the NOHMC. The center had rented the rear room of a pathology clinic at a very reasonable rate. "How fortunate," Dr. Meyers thought, "that at least we do not have a lot of. fixed expenses tied up in a building. Our office may be a little bit out of the way, but it is more than adequate for our needs."

The meeting began with the month's financial report (Table 4-1). At its conclusion, McDonald remarked, "It doesn't appear that our financial situation is improving, but at least tonight Dr. Randolph may be able to help us start to realize what we can do to improve the situation." Dr. Randolph then briefed the board on the work he had been conducting.

"Tom McDonald and I have been giving considerable attention to the center's condition in the past few weeks," he began, "to attempt to discover how its operations can be improved. By referring to past records, we have noticed that testing this year is apparently lagging from last year." Dr. Randolph showed the data summarized in Table 4-2. "To be quite honest, the center has never really reached the point of being able to stand on its own feet."

"There are many AMHTS entities throughout the country, however, that seem to be doing a large volume of business on a profitable basis. I hope we will be able to work with them to discover what has made them successful. We first surveyed 57 centers. The clinics were chosen from the (1972) AMHTS Directory."

Their selection depended upon their similarity with NOHMC in terms of sources of testing population. However, he adds, "in order to gain an appropriate perspective of a 'successful clinic,' only those clinics with a monthly testing rate of 400 persons or more were surveyed.

Exhibit 4-1 Tests Performed Routinely by NOHMC on Nonsymptomatic Patients

Anthropometry:		height, weight
Eyes:	vision:	acuity, color and depth perception, muscle balance
	tonometry:	eyeball pressure for detection of glaucoma
	pupillary escape:	diseases of the retina or optic nerve
Audiometry:		hearing at several tonal frequencies
Cardiovascular:		pulse, blood pressure, and electrocardiogram
Spirometry: (lung function)		vital capacity, forced expiratory volume
Chest X-Ray:		abnormalities of heart and lungs
Vibratory Sense:		certain neurological conditions
Women:		breast palpation, instruction in self-examinations
Laboratory:	blood:	glucose, cholesterol, albumin, total protein, urea, uric acid, acid phosphatase in males over 50, alkaline phosphatase, hemoglobin, hematocrit, white cell count, creatinine
	urine:	specific gravity, pH, glucose, ketones, protein, red blood cells, occult blood, casts
	stool:	blood on two specimens taken while patient is on a special diet; designed to reveal bleeding anywhere in the digestive tract
Integrated Report:		data processing printout; abnormalities in both history and physical exam flagged for easy identification

"Concurrently, another survey was prepared to investigate attitudes and acceptance of the NOHMC physicians here in Toledo. This survey was sent to area physicians who were segmented as potential users of this service. The methodology of this study involved the mailing of the survey to a stratified sample of physicians in Northwestern Ohio. Physicians such as psychiatrists, podiatrists, and dermatologists were omitted because it was felt that these categories would have little need for the services of

Table 4-1 Northwestern Ohio Health Maintenance Center

BALANCE SHEET
April 1978

Assets

Cash in bank		$ 5,196.80
Cash on hand		30.00
Leasehold improvements	$ 3,141.12	
Equipment	4,045.59	
	7,186.71	
Less accumulated depreciation	6,606.33	580.38
Deposit—Industrial Commission		12.00
Total Assets		5,099.18

Liabilities

Notes payable—short term	14,220.00	
Payroll taxes withheld	254.00	14,474.00

Net Worth

Capital stock subscribed	50,000.00	
Retained earnings 1/1/78	(56,714.00)	
Net loss for 1978	(2,660.00)	(9,374.82)
Total Liabilities and Net Worth		5,099.18

STATEMENT OF PROFIT AND LOSS

April 1978

	April 1978	Cash Basis Year-to-Date 4/30/78
Income: Regular sources	$ 1,809.12	$ 9,275.55
Expenses:		
Salaries	844.84	3,539.37
Payroll taxes	—	147.50
Rent	600.00	3,000.00
Technical supplies	64.52	382.68
Repairs/maint.—equipment	66.39	66.39
Gas and oil	—	6.66
Office supplies	121.30	411.20
Dues and subscriptions	—	24.00
Professional services—medical	720.27	3,230.06
Professional services—legal, audit	162.00	678.00
Personal property—Ohio franchise tax	—	68.90
Miscellaneous	—	18.04
Total Expenses	2,579.32	11,572.80
Net Profit (Loss) Cy 4/30/78	(770.20)	(2,297.25)

Table 4-2 NOHMC Activity Report by Months and Type of Examinations

	Regular Exams					Preemployment Exams				
	1974	1975	1976	1977	1978	1974	1975	1976	1977	1978
January	10	0	28	48	25	1	17	11	12	17
February	4	17	7	46	19	4	22	0	3	5
March	7	11	12	39	19	0	3	6	3	1
April	6	6	19	31	26	0	2	8	2	6
May	13	11	21	18	16	3	4	30	3	4
June	4	7	12	22	—	5	3	17	13	—
July	8	5	9	36	—	9	8	6	3	—
August	5	24	13	11	—	21	0	9	4	—
September	8	18	22	24	—	38	24	3	7	—
October	11	15	29	33	—	24	5	12	4	—
November	8	8	48	17	—	16	16	8	3	—
December	9	9	33	22	—	10	10	1	2	—
Totals	93	131	253	347	105	131	114	111	59	33

Regular exams as % of total exams						Preemployment exams as % of total exams				
	41.5	37.6	39.7	62.0	53.0	58.5	32.8	17.4	10.5	18.6

	Insurance Exams					Disability Exams	
	1974	1975	1976	1977	1978	1977	1978
January	—	—	20	19	11	—	1
February	—	—	32	18	9	—	0
March	—	—	25	20	14	—	1
April	—	7	24	16	10	—	2
May	—	14	13	13	12	—	0
June	—	15	27	10	—	—	—
July	—	13	28	14	—	—	—
August	—	22	28	10	—	—	—
September	—	11	16	9	—	—	—
October	—	21	34	6	—	—	—
November	—	0	14	8	—	2	—
December	—	0	13	8	—	1	—
Totals	—	103	274	151	56	3	4

Insurance exams as % of total exams					Disability exams as % of total exams	
	29.6	42.9	27.0	28.3	.005	1.2

NOHMC. With this information it will be possible to build a marketing strategy to promote the use of your services."

After Dr. Randolph completed the explanation of his work to date, Dr. Stephen Drengle voiced the general sentiments of the board, "Well, there is no harm in getting an idea of how others are operating."

"We sure could use some feedback from our own area, also," McDonald added. The rest of the board nodded approval of both men's comments.

"It might be necessary to begin a more active marketing and promotional program at the center," Dr. Randolph continued. "Tom has informed me that you are not affiliated with any hospital or outside organization and are just not receiving the referrals that you feel you should be."

"In the past we have never allocated finances for promotion," Dr. Meyers noted, "because we have felt that it would be considered an unethical practice for a medical facility to promote its services."

"But perhaps we need to do a little changing," McDonald interrupted. "At least we could start to follow up our present patients. Dr. Randolph and I have discovered that not nearly as many patients return for annual examinations as could be expected. Can't we at least start something there?" McDonald passed out a sheet with data on repeat visits (Table 4-3). "That couldn't do too much harm, I guess," Dr. Drengle added.

"Now, let's be careful not to go in too many directions at once," Dr. Randolph said. "We need a plan of action with specific objectives first. Maybe something can be done in this area. But first let's find out where you currently stand and then we will be in a better position to formulate an integrated marketing program that will be efficient and compatible with your medical image."

"If all goes smoothly, by the June meeting, I should have a marketing program for the center pretty well fleshed out," he continued. "From the surveys, we will also be able to determine what types of doctors the center will be able to work with best and whether they need the services you

Table 4-3 Patients Repeating 2nd, 3rd, or 4th Regular Exams

	Total Regular Exams	Number of Repeaters	%
1974	93	0	0
1975	157	40	25.5
1976	253	51	20.2
1977	347	84	24.2
1978 (through May)	89	56	62.9

offer. Once we find out in what direction our potential lies, it will be possible to arrange the means of reaching that potential. Perhaps from the other AMHTSs, we can discover other potential markets we could be reaching and formulate a means of doing so.

"Finally, two things have occurred to me that I feel you as board members might need to think about. First, do you think there might be any conflict of interest by physicians owning the center? How do your patients feel about coming to you for a checkup, then being sent to the center you own, and then making an appointment with your office to review the results? Second, I noticed tonight that the center is far removed from most other health facilities and it is located in a suburban area that is accessible primarily by expressway. This could affect a doctor's decision to refer patients here and more than likely it cuts down on the number of walk-in patients quite drastically.

"That should give you a couple of things to consider during the next month. Rest assured that progress is being made on an integrated marketing plan for the center and that as more data are received, there will be more to go on."

Dr. Randolph was instructed to continue the research, with a report to the board at its June meeting.

By the middle of May results from the surveys were beginning to be tabulated. It was time for Dr. Randolph to start sifting out the facts from the assumptions. A couple of days later, McDonald visited Dr. Randolph to discuss progress. Dr. Randolph started by explaining that 22 of the 57 clinics nationwide had responded to the questionnaire. He had analyzed these by using primarily frequency distributions for the responses to the self-administered survey. Where it was appropriate, he calculated mean scores. He showed McDonald the results of the survey (Exhibit 4-2).

On the second survey, out of 200 physicians contacted in the Toledo area, 75 usable responses were returned. Dr. Randolph had analyzed the data by class tabulations and applied a chi square test to ascertain if the information varied significantly by physician characteristics and by the level of public awareness and acceptance of the concept of AMHTS (Table 4-4).

"Notice," Dr. Randolph said, "that a large proportion of the doctors recommend periodic physicals for their patients, even though nothing is wrong. Yet a large percentage do not have the equipment with which to administer a thorough examination. For starters, that is a pretty good indication that there is a need for your clinic's services in Toledo."

"Now, look at the type of doctors who are most favorably inclined to the AMHTS concept," he continued. "General practitioners are one group

Exhibit 4-2 Highlights of Responses to Questionnaire Sent to Successful AMHTS Clinics

1. The average clinic served about 240 patients weekly.

2. Only 13 percent of the patients were referred by private physicians; insurance examinations accounted for less than 1 percent of the total number served.

3. About 75 percent of the patients were referred by social service agencies, government, or industrial health programs, etc., and 10 percent were walk-ins.

4. General practitioners were the most frequently identified source of referrals.

5. General practitioners and internists considered multiphasic health screening centers as very useful, in contrast to 56 percent of the general surgeons who believed they were not very helpful.

6. In general, the tests given by the surveyed AMHTS were very similar.

7. Thirty-five percent provided standardized tests, 47 percent offered only specific tests.

8. Overwhelmingly, these centers were perceived as being for detection rather than diagnosis.

9. The promotional activities generally were limited, including direct mail to patients, insurance companies, and businesses, and infrequently to the medical profession.

10. Almost 90 percent employed no outside sales force.

11. Fifty-eight percent were financed privately.

12. About three-fourths had some form of affiliation with hospitals, prepaid insurance plans, social service agencies, labor unions, or industry, thereby suggesting a perceived ingredient for success.

Table 4-4 Results from Metropolitan Physician Survey on Attitudes toward NOHMC

	Unfavorable	Somewhat Favorable	Favorable
All physicians	47%	33%	20%
Family practice	33	27	40
Internal medicine	34	34	32
Surgeons	55	31	14
		Unfavorable	Favorable
FPs under age 55		26%	74%
Internists under age 55		71	29
Physicians born in U.S. or Canada		52	48
Physicians born in other countries		38	62
Less than a 3-year residency		39	61
More than 3 years of residency		56	44
Physicians in solo practice		45	55
Physicians in other practice arrangements		62	38
Physicians without hospital admitting privileges		33	67
Physicians with hospital admitting privileges		49	51
FPs referring no patients to other doctors		44	56
FPs referring more than 14 percent of patients to other doctors		24	76
Physicians with office personnel under $500/month		39	61
Physicians recommending a periodic physical every year or two, even if nothing is wrong		29.7	70.3

Machine in Office	% Having Machine
X-ray	21.3
Electrocardiogram	49.3
Equipment costing more than $50	57.3

Affirmative Responses for Each Type of Test Performed	
Anthropometry: height, weight,	78.7%
skin fold thickness	13.3
Vision	42.5
Tonometry	32.0
Pupillary escape	34.7
Audiometry	22.7
Pulse	84.0
Blood pressure	81.3
Electrocardiogram	54.7
Vital capacity	32.0
Forced expiratory	20.0

Table 4-4 continued

Affirmative Responses for Each Type of Test Performed continued

Chest x-ray	64.0
Vibratory sense	57.3
Women—breast palpation	86.7
Women—Pap test	88.0

Blood Tests

Glucose	68.0%		
Cholesterol	57.3	Alkaline phosphatase	42.7
Albumin	46.7	SGOT	41.3
Total protein	37.3	Hemoglobin	72.0
Urea	45.3	Hematocrit	65.3
Uric acid	50.7	White cell count	64.0
Acid phosphatase	14.7	Creatinine	23.3

Urine Tests

Specific gravity	68.0%	Red blood cells	68.0
pH	70.7	White blood cells	68.0
Glucose	81.3	Occult blood	52.0
Ketones	70.7	Casts	54.7
Protein	74.7		

Awareness of Clinic by Years in Practice

	Aware of Clinic		Unaware of Clinic		Total	
Years	#	%	#	%	#	%
0– 4	3	50.0	3	50.0	6	100
5– 9	2	28.6	5	71.4	7	100
10–14	8	88.9	1	11.1	9	100
15–19	10	66.7	5	33.3	15	100
Over 20	16	53.3	14	46.7	30	100
Totals	39	(Avg.) 57.5	28	(Avg.) 42.5	67	100

Tests Found Most Useful in Doctors' Follow-up Exams

Lab tests	59%
Cardiovascular measurements	37
Chest x-rays	19

No other test was mentioned by more than 9 percent of physicians.

Tests Mentioned as Being of No Use

Medical history questionnaire	33%
Audiometry tests	10

No other tests were mentioned frequently.

(continued on page 84)

Table 4-4 continued

Doctors Finding False Results	
False positives	40%
False negatives	32
One or both	53
Most frequently found false positive tests:	
Glucose tolerance	64%
Other blood chemistries	37

Medical History Questionnaire Usefulness	
	Feel It Is Not Very Useful or Worthless
FPs	52%
Internists	62
Surgeons	66

This appears to be the most disliked of the patient summaries.

Further Survey Results

1. As medical income increases, favorability to AMHTS decreases.
2. The more county medical society meetings physicians attend, the more they favor AMHTS.
3. The fewer professional societies specialists belong to, the more they favor AMHTS. Among GPs there is no difference.
4. Physicians who earn the least or who treat the most patients are most favorable. Physicians who earn the most money and treat the fewest patients are least favorably inclined to use this service.
5. The fewer referrals specialists receive from other physicians, the more they favor AMHTS.
6. Physicians who think computers are a good thing in the practice of medicine are consistently more favorable to AMHTS than those who do not. GPs are most impressed by the use of computers to aid in early detection of symptoms.
7. Cross-tabulation of endorsement of computers by year of graduation from medical school shows that older graduates who are most favorable to computers also are most favorable to screening (80 percent). Least favorable to screening are the most recent graduates (26 percent).
8. Physicians who recommend a checkup to their own patients every year or two are more favorable to screenings than those who do not so recommend.
9. FPs feel that computers are valuable in symptom detection.
10. Physicians with one to nine years of medical practice are in favor of AMHTS.
11. Physicians who spend little or no time reading medical literature are more inclined to favor AMHTS.
12. Physicians with no postgraduate training indicate a pro-AMHTS attitude.

highly in favor of the concept of preventive medicine and they really like the idea of having a computer to aid in early detection of symptoms."

"Oh, but we don't have a computer yet," McDonald remarked. "We have talked about it several times. I think I even mentioned to you once that we had talked of purchasing one. But they are expensive, more than I'm afraid we can afford to spare right now."

"Yes, now that you mention it I do remember that conversation," Dr. Randolph replied. "However, let's go on. I want you to notice that doctors with less than ten years in residency are in favor of your type of service also."

With this, the two continued their analyzing of groups that were most inclined to support the AMHTS concept.

"It's also important to note that other AMHTSs receive only 13 percent of their referrals from physicians," Dr. Randolph said. "Most successful clinics are affiliated with hospitals or other organizations. That helps assure them of business. It also enables a hospital to offer a new service that is recognized as being important."

"Do you think we could start having someone go around selling our service to interested parties?" McDonald asked. "Well, that is one possibility for increasing the awareness level. But remember, Tom, that care must be exercised in any promotional activities the center plans. Even your board members are not enthusiastic about the idea."

The two men spent several hours sorting data. As he left, McDonald remarked, "If only we had taken time to plan our strategy out in the first place, perhaps we would not be in the position we are now."

"Isn't it nice to have 20-20 hindsight," Dr. Randolph joked. "Right now, though, we just need to try to improve our foresight so the situation can be rectified. It's going to be a hard task, but not an impossible one."

NOTE

1. U.S. Department of Health, Education, and Welfare, *Provisional Guidelines for Automated Multiphasic Health Testing Services*, Vols. 1 and 2 (Washington, D.C.: DHEW, 1970), p. 2.

OVERVIEW OF CASE 5

Issues to Consider

1. What marketing issues are involved in this case other than a need for promotion?

2. Is market segmentation applicable for this health maintenance organization? If so, how? Has it overlooked any major segments?
3. Is there an issue of ethics, since this center is owned by physicians, and will they be violating this code? How can ethical issues be resolved if they decide advertising and personal selling are essential?

Discussion

1. Marketing Factors

In the realm of services offered, the NOHMC must project an image of a sophisticated medical clinic with high-quality services. Unfortunately, a substantial number of physicians said they had received inaccurate reports, especially involving glucose tolerance and other blood chemistries. Many were not impressed with the Medical History Questionnaire used. The NOHMC must be certain it is offering reliable information in a format that can help physicians improve both their diagnosis and their efficiency.

Personal contact is probably the most effective technique for reaching the physician and agencies. This enables the sales representatives to present full details of the operation and benefits of the AMHTS program and answer questions. This should be done in a professional manner without pressure for purchase. It should be basically informative, since awareness levels concerning NOHMC are low.

It probably is not an appropriate time for a full-scale advertising campaign aimed at the mass consumer market. But it is time for an educational campaign with booklets and brochures available for distribution through the offices of cooperating physicians. The concept of preventive examinations was new, since most patients went to a doctor only when they were ill. NOHMCs should prepare the public to perceive preventive medicine as an essential personal health care activity as opposed to relying solely on physicians for assistance when ill.

Convenience is an important factor. A location near other physicians' offices or a hospital can encourage patronage. Easy access and visibility are important for walk-in patients as they are discouraged easily if the location is inconvenient. Physicians whose offices are close to the NOHMC would seem to be the most likely users of the center. It does little good to convince individuals to utilize the NOHMC's services if they have trouble getting to the clinic. Its location near the expressway system is highly advantageous as it provides rapid and easy access even for those who reside more than ten miles away. The time it takes to reach the center is relatively more important than the distance.

No detailed information is presented concerning the appropriateness of the clinic's pricing structure for the physicians and the institution. These costs generally are not covered by third party coverage so they should be reasonable to the patient. Since they are in addition to the physician's fees, the "well" patient will forgo the clinic on economic grounds if the total is too high.

2. Segmentation of the Market

The Toledo survey provides strong evidence that a potential market for AMHTS does exist. The majority of doctors responding indicated they favored such a clinic and most of its related concepts. But the physicians who were most in favor of AMHTS were those least aware that an example existed in their area. This is attested by the finding that the younger doctors who had lived in the area less than ten years and were receptive to the concept also were the least aware of such a service center there. This suggests that the NOHMC has not informed the medical profession effectively that it exists. It especially must elevate the awareness level of physicians who favor the concept of preventive diagnosis. This group also includes the FPs who are especially receptive to the use of computers in early detection of symptoms. However, the NOHMC does not offer this important service, thereby limiting its appeal.

One of the most useful ways to segment the physician market is to differentiate between those who have the equipment necessary for giving thorough examinations and those who do not. A very obvious market is physicians who favor regular examinations yet cannot provide them because they lack the equipment. The NOHMC needs to convince these doctors that the clinic's function is to enable them to provide better service for their patients.

The Toledo area survey demonstrated that the two broad categories of physicians most in favor of the AMHTS concept are FPs and internists. Other factors such as the type of practice arrangement, length of residence, hospital admitting privileges, age, and attitudes concerning computer use in medicine all can be used to segment the physician market for cultivation for this service.

One technique for educating these physicians is to offer them a tour of the facility. This could be combined with a free screening that could demonstrate the thoroughness of the examinations.

But if Toledo is in any way similar to other AMHTS cities, there are other markets that have a much larger potential for building the clinic's business. Other centers (Exhibit 4-2, supra) report 85 percent of their patients come from sources other than physician referrals—governmental agencies, industrial health programs, social service agencies, or walk-ins. Three-fourths of the successful AMHTS centers were affiliated with hospitals, prepaid insurance plans, social service agencies, labor unions, or industry. These could be educated by tours, salespersons, literature, and mail campaigns.

Another market is the present users of the center. As the clinic builds its clientele, it should be able to assure a given volume simply by encouraging repeat examinations. This could be accomplished easily by sending out reminders that a person's annual checkup is approaching or even scheduling it when the initial examination is completed. Repeat volume should be above 25 percent a year. If it is not, the users may be dissatisfied. The reasons could be discovered through patient follow-up questionnaires.

3. Ethical Issues

In 1847, when the American Medical Association (AMA) was established, it included a ban on physician advertising as part of its original code of ethics. In the years since then, great disapprobation was shown toward physicians who in any way attempted to attract business away from colleagues.

Some physicians—particularly young ones—became concerned when their attempts to advertise met with rebuke. So also did community health plans, which need to advertise to inform the public about their new concept in care. The AMA attempted to block their advertising but the Federal Trade Commission (FTC) intervened, asserting that the association ban affected community health organizations' activities by hindering or preventing these efforts to deliver new health care services.

Ultimately, the U.S. Supreme Court struck down the AMA ban against prescription drug advertising, which by extension has had a major effect on the medical profession as a whole. The basis for the contention is that advertising denies the public information that the free market makes available to consumers in other areas of business. The Justice Department has contended consistently that ethical codes banning advertising violate the First Amendment.

As a result of the court decision, AMA control over medical advertising was reduced sharply. The FTC continued to be the regulator of physician advertising where it deemed there are cases involving misleading or fraudulent claims.

In 1977, the American Hospital Association (AHA) reevaluated its stand on advertising and issued its tenets to insist on truth and accuracy, fairness, and no comparisons, claims of prominence, or promotion of individual professions. At the same time the AHA recognized five ethical purposes for advertising: public education concerning available services, public education about health care, accounting to the community, efforts to obtain financial and/or political support, and employee recruitment.

It appears that new attitudes are emerging over the ethics of medical advertising as a result of court and governmental actions. This is especially important as health maintenance centers attempt to educate the public about their services. But care must be exercised to make sure that advertising is not misleading or fraudulent. If prices are quoted, the promotional copy must state exactly what is included and excluded for that amount, and the advertising physician must in no manner make medical claims that cannot be substantiated. While any business must take great care when it advertises, a higher degree of factuality and truthfulness is demanded from the medical profession in any form of marketing efforts. Yet for the first time the option is available and it should be permitted unless it is misused.

CASE 6. SOUTHLAND HMO: THE NEED FOR
QUALIFICATION—AN OPPORTUNITY FOR A MARKETING
APPROACH

Lance Galsworthy, president of the Southland Health Maintenance Organization (HMO), prepared to telephone Axel Drummond, chairman of the HMO Advisory Committee, who would expect a forthright and thorough review of the major problems facing the HMO and their prospective outcome. The Advisory Committee, composed of representatives of the local political, economic, religious, and social establishment, had been organized recently through Galsworthy's personal solicitation of its members. The committee served as a promotional organ by lending respectability to the infant HMO. As the vanguard of efforts to market the HMO, the committee expected Galsworthy to keep it informed, although he was given a free hand in daily planning and administration.

Certainly, the most pressing issue was qualification. The then U.S. Department of Health, Education, and Welfare (HEW) required a series of formal reports and evaluations before an HMO could be qualified, which meant that it was certified by the federal government as having met all the regulatory requirements for operation. Without formal qualification, an HMO could not invoke the federal mandate that required employers of 25 or more personnel to offer the HMO alternative to their employees. And without the support of the legal requirement, Galsworthy felt that Southland HMO would be a nonstarter.

In any case, the organization had successfully completed the first two review steps: acceptance of its feasibility study and approval of its planning document. Both these steps and a forthcoming proposal (request for an initial development grant) were funded entirely by HEW. Initial development would consist of the first efforts to recruit enrollment staff, provide facilities, and interest customers in the HMO product. To obtain the development grant, the Southland HMO marketing approach would have to be approved by HEW. Then would come the effort to obtain qualified status. The HMO then would have to draw against an HEW loan account specifically created to finance capital investment and cover operating losses for new entities. The loan would be available through the fourth year of operation, after which the HMO would be expected to break even and begin payments. However, before HEW would invest in the development effort, Southland HMO would have to establish its credibility—in other words, its potential viability.

Origins of Southland HMO

During the late 1960s and the 1970s, the metropolitan location of South-land HMO had become conspicuous for controversy and confrontation among aspiring blacks, progressives, and other protagonists of the New South, and the city's traditional and conservative social and financial oligarchy. Leaders and community interest groups who had joined in the battle for civil rights continued to take liberal and reformist positions on other social issues. Religious figures were particularly active.

Among the problems isolated by the reform leaders was that of rising health care delivery costs. Worried by the impact of these astronomically soaring expenses on family incomes, they sought alternatives. One organization, the Southern Religious Association (SRA), began an evaluation that eventually called the health maintenance organization (HMO) concept to their attention. In 1976, the SRA filed a feasibility study with HEW. Since the major reason for HMO failures usually had been unsuccessful marketing, HEW insisted upon a preliminary analysis of marketing potential. The SRA study concluded that a prepaid health provision alternative, to be entitled the Regency Health Plan, would be marketable. That is, the plan would be able to enlist the participation of sufficient providers (physicians) and would be purchased by enough customers to make it a break-even or better proposition. HEW accepted the SRA submission in 1977.

The Regency Health Plan called for the recruitment of providers into an individual practice association (IPA). An IPA consisted of local physicians loosely organized to provide health care services. In 1977, the SRA also began looking for an experienced health administrator to be the president of the plan. After an extensive search, the SRA selected Galsworthy. From 1970 to 1976 he had been director of health services, research, and development in a major southern city. He also had completed an intensive one-semester program to train HMO managers at the Wharton School of Business of the University of Pennsylvania. Galsworthy, 33 years old, was intelligent, articulate, hard-working, and a veteran of health administration in a large southern community.

Upon assuming his new position, Galsworthy began to recruit a staff and develop a budget (Table 4-5). The field of eligible candidates was not large, since HMOs still were relatively small in number and size of coverage. Nevertheless, the recruitment effort bore fruit. By late 1977, Galsworthy had hired Timothy Hanley as director of marketing, Winslow Harris as finance officer, and Mrs. Evelyn Sneed as research assistant.

Galsworthy quickly made two changes. After interviewing several local physicians who had expressed interest in the Regency Health Plan IPA,

Table 4-5 Planning Budget for 1978

SOUTHLAND HMO

Budget Category	Total Amount Requested
Personnel Services	
Project director	
Coordinator	
Legal director	
Marketing director	
Finance director	
Research assistant	
Secretary	
FICA	
Fringe benefits	
Total Personnel Services	$126,885
Equipment	4,485
Other	
Consultant costs	
Marketing	3,100
Financial	5,000
Legal	9,900
Medical	5,000
Office supplies	2,180
Travel	6,850
Rental:	
Office	10,300
Communications	
Postage	1,400
Telephone	3,500
Printing	3,200
Other	
Audit	600
Bookkeeping	1,240
Duplicating	1,800
Insurance	2,500
Meeting costs	700
Membership fees	800
Publications	1,550
Recruitment	2,400
Registration fees	860
Relocation expenses	5,600
Total Other	72,965
Total	199,850

he concluded that, while sympathetic to the plan's goals, they would invest only a small part of their total labor in the project. He therefore insisted that the plan discard the IPA model in favor of a closed panel staff model. That is, contracting physicians would be full-time employees of the plan. Galsworthy hoped to be able to recruit young, idealistic physicians attracted by a regular salary. Faced with the capital investment expenses necessary to establish their own practices, they might be willing to forgo hopes of rapid income growth if offered an opportunity to practice medicine in an already capitalized facility. Time would tell whether these expectations would be justified.

The other change Galsworthy instituted was to change the plan's name to Southland HMO. He gambled that the name change would give his organization a distinctive brand in the health care delivery market and that the HMO label would encounter at least a neutral if not mildly positive reaction from the general public.

Qualifications Revisited: A HEW and Cry

Galsworthy recalled a telephone conversation with Ben Masierelli, the HEW liaison officer for Southland HMO. Masierelli would be in-house protagonist for the HMO during evaluation of its marketability and professionalism before approval of the initial development grant. Masierelli had made it known that his support would depend upon two factors:

1. The HMO would be expected to prove its marketability by soliciting and collecting data on a sufficiently large sample of the local employee population. Although HEW did not specify any set percentage or amount, Masierelli indicated he doubted the grant application would be approved unless information on at least 120,000 area employees was obtained.
2. The nature of the data collected would have to convince HEW that the HMO would be able to determine: (a) the population and composition of local employers; (b) its potential impact on the need for revision of specific terminology in union/employee contracts to comply with federal law; (c) the breakdown of local industry by types, varieties of health coverage, and likely penetration by the new entity; (d) the availability and pricing of traditional health cost programs in the area; and (e) the internal breakdown of currently available health cost coverage according to product mix and ratio of employee/employer contributions. In essence, Masierelli was demanding that the HMO develop a marketing research program.

The Problem of Researching the Market

The marketing research problem posed several dilemmas for the staff of the Southland HMO. While faced with the necessity of satisfying Masierelli and HEW, Galsworthy was far from clear about the best way to obtain the marketing information.

The SRA recently had conducted a local health costs survey for the HMO. The SRA was forced to acknowledge a problem common to most health care delivery providers, including HMOs—they must compete in a two-level market: employers and employees. Health care is provided through the employer, who jointly contributes with employees to their health care insurance. Providers must obtain the support or acquiescence of management to obtain any leverage with the employee pool. Blue Cross, Blue Shield, and the 30-odd other coinsurance agencies and health care providers in the local area had years of experience with and exposure to the employer market. Their names and services were familiar.

How should the HMO overcome this promotional obstacle? Although by law employers of a certain size must offer the HMO option (180 days after formal qualification of and notification by an HMO), such an entity cannot afford to assume employers' good intentions. Employers, like anyone else, tend to accept the inertia of established procedures and familiar brands. To interest them to the point of changing or offering change to their employees, instead of just going through the motions, would require an energetic and persuasive approach. A general public attitude of positiveness and acceptability toward HMOs might be cultivated in the media, but the actual sales effort must be undertaken with the cooperation of employers. Any competitor who fails to observe this dictum probably would have difficulty obtaining working time, space, and cooperation to address its appeal to employees.

Given these considerations, the HMO was compelled to conduct an initial survey of employers, not employees. Approximately 400 local employers were contacted by the letter shown in Exhibit 4-3, and asked to complete a questionnaire (Exhibit 4-4). The mailings were addressed individually to the president or senior executive of each organization. The responses were used to collect surrogate data on covered employees. The mailout was followed by repeated phone calls from HMO staff members. Nevertheless, only 35 responded. Galsworthy had been disappointed with that and with what he perceived as the research staff's failure to usefully collate what information had been received. Believing that the HMO's credibility was at stake with the SRA and the Advisory Committee, Galsworthy instructed Timothy Hanley, director of marketing for the Southland

Exhibit 4-3 Letter for the First HMO Survey

Dear Sir:

One of the problems concerning both business and the consumer is the spiraling cost of health care.

In the interest of identifying the severity of the health cost problem in our community and in the interest of identifying means by which these cost increases can be contained, the Southern Religious Association, a nonprofit organization which has served the needs of our city for a decade, requests that you or one of your staff complete the attached questionnaire.

This information, combined with information previously provided by the local business community, will enable us to prepare a cost-containment plan. You will receive a summary of this plan in January.

This brief questionnaire can be completed from information in your files. A stamped, addressed envelope is enclosed for your convenience. Your help in completing this survey and returning it to us as soon as possible is deeply appreciated.

Sincerely,

Axel Drummond
Chairman
HMO Advisory Committee
Southern Religious Association

Exhibit 4-4 Health Costs Survey Form

BASIC INFORMATION

Company Name: _____

Name and Title of Person Responsible for Health Care Benefits: ____

_____ Phone Number: _____

Is This Site a Division or Subsidiary of Another Company? _____

Total Number of Local Employees: _____

Are Any Employees Members of Bargaining Units? _____ If Yes,

　　Please List Organization(s) That Represent Them: _____

_____

Current Health Insurance Carrier(s): _____

Anniversary Date(s): _____

　　Policy(ies) Include(s):　　　　Hospitalization _____

　　　　　　　　　　　　　　　　Major Medical _____

Other—Please Specify: _____

MONTHLY PREMIUMS

(Excluding Life Insurance)

Type of Coverage	Number of Covered Employees	Company Contri- bution	Employee Contri- bution	Total Premium
Individual	_____	$_____	$_____	$_____
Family* (Including Individual)	_____	$_____	$_____	$_____

　　*Or Other Designation. Please Specify: _____

If You Have Any Employees Not Covered by This Plan, Please Indicate
Reason:

　　Elected Not to Be　　　　　　　Covered by Separate Union
　　　　Covered _____　　　　　　　Plan　　_____
　　Not Eligible_____　　　　　　Covered by Separate Manage-
　　　　　　　　　　　　　　　　　　ment Plan _____

Please Provide a Distribution of Employee's Residence By Zip Code
or, If Not Available, Estimate by Community:

Exhibit 4-4 continued

> Please Enclose a Brochure, Certificate, Booklet and/or Sample Policy of Your Company's Health Care Benefits.
>
> If You Have Any Questions About This Survey, Please Contact Evelyn Sneed or Timothy Hanley at 555-1212.
>
> Your Response Will Be Considered Confidential. Thank You for Your Cooperation.
>
> Please Return To: Mr. Timothy Hanley
> Director of Marketing
> Southland HMO

HMO, to prepare and promote a larger survey and to develop appropriate forms for organizing the information obtained.

Five months after the first survey, the second survey effort began. The chief executives of more than 1,200 local employers received the letter shown in Exhibit 4-5. Enclosed with the letter were the health costs survey form and an article from *The Wall Street Journal* headlined "HMOs Can Hold Down Health-Care Costs Elsewhere in Field, FTC Study Indicates," which maintained that HMOs had broad cost-reducing effects when competing with traditional health care carriers. The HMO staff again followed up the mailout with intensive phone contacts and onsite visits. Coincidentally, two weeks before the mailout, the largest local newspaper carried a highly favorable front page lead article headlined "HMOs Attempt to Check the High-Cost Epidemic." All in all, Galsworthy expected the survey to attract enough response to meet Masierelli's goal of 120,000 employees.

Hanley designed several new forms to organize the response data so as to meet Masierelli's specifications. A summary sheet (Figure 4-1) was prepared to collate insurance data obtained from each employer contacted. The sheet would serve both as a display in the initial development review planned for the fall of 1978 and as a planning document in analyzing the pricing structure of competitors.

A breakdown sheet (Figure 4-2) was developed for displaying employee pool size vs. type of industry. This matrix was expected to demonstrate to HEW that the HMO staff had contacted and obtained responses from a cross-section of local employers.

Yet another form (Exhibit 4-6) was intended for use in preparing a general comparison of types and extent of coverage offered by health insurance carriers to local employees. Again, the data were to be arranged on an employer-by-employer basis.

Finally, Galsworthy asked Mrs. Sneed to obtain a list of local unions and their officials from the AFL-CIO labor council. By contacting these representatives, HMO could learn how specific employment contracts were worded. HEW requires a qualified HMO to give an employer 180 days' notice before the company can be required to offer the HMO alternative to its employees. Then the specific terms of any new coverage options must be inserted in existing union/employer labor contracts. Galsworthy intended to include a contract impact statement in the initial development application.

Three months after the survey mailing, responses had stopped coming into the Southland HMO, where Hanley and Mrs. Sneed recorded the information on the new data forms. The HMO staff pursued the data collection process, making up to seven phone calls to the same employer

---

Exhibit 4-5 Letter for the Second HMO Survey

SOUTHLAND HMO

In October of 1977, the Southern Religious Association (SRA) conducted a health costs survey in this area. The survey reveals: 1) escalating health care premium increases for local employers, and 2) a lack of employer/insurer programs to control these premium increases. SRA has determined that a health maintenance organization should be developed whose inherent efficiencies will—in its operation and as an example to others—do much to contain the rise in health care costs in this area. The SOUTHLAND HMO has been formed as a private, non-profit corporation.

A health maintenance organization (HMO) is a prepaid medical group practice. There are 180 HMOs in the U.S. with over 6 million people enrolled. The SOUTHLAND HMO, currently in its planning stage, will provide comprehensive, quality health care to its members (you and your company's employees and dependents) while containing the rapidly rising cost of health care. The SOUTHLAND HMO offers employers a welcome alternative to the usual method of providing employee health benefits.

We appreciate your response to our October survey. The information that you and other employers provided allows us to tailor our health care delivery system to the needs of this community. For those of you who did not respond, we have enclosed a copy of that Health Cost Survey. We ask you to complete and return it to us in the enclosed postage-paid envelope. Thank you for your assistance.

Exhibit 4-5 continued

We will keep you informed of the SOUTHLAND HMO's progress and of other developments in health care cost containment through a bi-monthly newsletter and reprints of relevant articles appearing in national publications. Also, in the near future, a member of our staff will contact you to provide you with an opportunity to ask questions about the ways in which health maintenance organizations benefit you as well as your employees. In the meantime, if you have any questions, please call Lance Galsworthy at 555-1212.

Thank you for your cooperation in the past. We look forward to working with you in the future.

Sincerely,

Axel Drummond
Chairman
HMO Advisory Committee

in the effort to obtain the desired response. Yet, despite the more thorough preparation for the second survey and despite the solicitation efforts of the staff, only 144 responses out of 1,200 queried were obtained—just 12 percent. The data represented information on 85,000 employees, far short of the target of 120,000. Galsworthy estimated that 50 to 60 more employer responses would be required to obtain the necessary data.

Interpreting the Response to Marketing Research

Galsworthy was concerned as to the reasons he could give Drummond and the HMO Advisory Committee on the results of the second survey. Could the employer unresponsiveness be attributed simply to inertia? Was there an underlying public distaste for, or opposition to, the HMO concept? What about the handful of complaints to Mrs. Sneed that the HMO was "fronting" for labor unions by seeking information on insurance coverage? Were these comments indicative of a broader employer sentiment? What was the source of such suspicions? Galsworthy also wondered whether there might not be better ways to collect the information. For that matter, was the HMO collecting current information? Any survey approach involved use of surrogate or proxy variables. Would Masierelli and HEW accept the format developed by the HMO?

Figure 4-1 Summary of Employers Contacted

No.	Name of Employer Contacted	Number of Employees in HMO Service Area	1978 Rates	Premium Structure			Insurance Carrier and Anniversary Date
			Total Contri-bution	Contract Type/Emp.	Employer Contri-bution	Employee Contri-bution	

Figure 4-2 Category and Industry Breakdown

No.	Employer	More Than 5,000 Employees	4,999-2,500	2,499-1,000	999-750	749-500	499-400	399-0	Public Utilities	Manufacturing	Government	Retail	Wholesale Trade	Transportation	Service	Finance
1																
2																
3																
4																
5																
6																
7																
8																
9																
10																

Exhibit 4-6 General Comparison Form for Types of Carrier Coverage

Employer _____	Premium: Single ____ ____
Carrier _____	Employer Contribution: ____ ____

Inpatient Coverage:	_____
	_____
	_____
	_____
Outpatient Coverage:	_____
	_____
Emergency Coverage:	_____
	_____
Maternity Coverage:	_____
Mental Health Coverage:	_____
Home Health Services:	_____
Preventive Care Coverage:	_____
Dental Coverage:	_____
Drugs and Appliances:	_____
Exclusions and/or Limitations:	_____
Deductible and Premium Coverage:	_____

The Marketability Issue

Galsworthy then turned to the broader issue of whether or not the HMO's product would be marketable. He saw Southland HMO as the purveyor of at least two sequenced products: (1) in the preliminary stage of development, the primary product was the HMO concept itself; (2) in the future, the product would be the organization's services. To market these products effectively, Galsworthy believed that Southland would have to identify and eventually satisfy the needs of several publics. Many of these publics were obvious; others, less so. Had he identified all of them— the general public, employers, employees, HEW, the regulatory agencies, SRA? And how could the HMO determine whether the competition already was meeting those publics' needs? The rising concern about health care costs suggested that the general public was dissatisfied with current services, but how could Southland pinpoint gaps between client needs and available health care delivery?

Hanley had prepared an Analysis of Competition questionnaire (Exhibit 4-7). He felt that by having Mrs. Sneed research the survey responses with the questionnaire as a guide, the HMO could obtain the answers to the significant questions about competitors and then be able to identify a new or vulnerable market segment. Hanley, on his own, further analyzed the issue of carrier/industry trends by breaking down survey data on an industry-by-carrier (Figure 4-3) and carrier-by-industry (Figure 4-4) basis.

Other Concerns

There also was the problem of satisfying the various commissions and agencies with power to approve or prohibit new competitors in the market for health care services. Foremost of these was HEW with its formal review process. But two state regulatory agencies also posed potential obstacles. The state insurance commissioner might decide that the HMO qualified as an "insurance" company, in which case the infant organization would have to post $750,000 in security reserves. To legally challenge the commissioner's decision after the fact would be costly and damaging to the HMO's image. How could the commissioner be persuaded to a favorable position? In addition, a certificate of need would be required from the state health facilities commissioner before the HMO's physical facility could be built.

Galsworthy saw qualifications by HEW as crucial in the effort to ensure the good will of the two state commissioners. Neither could be expected to risk political capital in support of a shaky proposition. Qualification would be prima facie evidence of federal government confidence in the

Exhibit 4-7 Analysis of Competition

Objectives

1. Produce outline of each employer's health benefits. (To assist HMO in preparing employer-specific marketing materials.)
2. Identify the major inadequacy(ies) in each employer's health benefits package. (To assist HMO in identifying market targets.)
3. Identify existing benefits for each employer that exceed HMO basic benefit package. (To assist HMO in determining whether to add supplemental benefits or to create high option coverage.)

Subject: Conclusions on Corporation Benefit Analysis

1. What percent of the corporations have Major Medical?
   What percent of the corporations do not have Major Medical?
2. What percent of the corporations have deductibles?
   What percent of the corporations do not have deductibles?
   What is the high, low, and medium range of deductibles?
3. What percent (number as well) of corporations use usual, reasonable, and customary charges to determine reimbursement?
   What percent of corporations do not?
4. What percent (number) of corporations have first dollar coverage?
   What percent of corporations do not?
5. What percent (number) of corporations cover prescription drugs, and to what extent?
   What percent (number) of corporations do not?
6. What percent (number) of corporations have maternity coverage?
   What percent (number) of corporations do not?
   What is the dollar allowance for maternity coverage and range—high, medium, and low?
7. What percent of the corporations use a fee schedule?
   What percent of the corporations do not?
8. What percent of the corporations have preexisting conditions and limitations on coverage?
   Where are these conditions and limitations most often found?
   Are there any trends in this area? Be specific.
9. What are the maximum limits on (dollar amounts)?
   What percent of maximum falls in high, medium, and low categories?

Exhibit 4-7 continued

10. Is there a correlation between industry and carrier?
11. What percent (number) of corporations have mental health coverage?
    What percent (number) of corporations do not?
12. Are there any trends in benefits, deductibles, major medicals, etc., in the corporation comparisons analyzed?
13. Are physician office visits covered or not covered—what percent of corporations?
14. Are outpatient lab and x-rays covered or not—what percent (number) of corporations?

Figure 4-3 Survey Data Breakdown Form: Industry by Carrier

Industry _____

Carrier	Employer	Anniv. Date	Elig. Emp.	Premiums			Ratio
				1	2	Fam.	

Figure 4-4 Survey Data Breakdown Form: Carrier by Industry

Name of Carrier _____

Employer	Anniv. Date	Type of Industry	Premiums			Ratio between Single Premium vs. Two-Person & Family
			1	2	Fam.	

marketability of the HMO. The state commissioners would not have to go out on a limb by themselves.

Site Selection Controversy

Another basic issue would have to be discussed with Drummond—the HMO's site. Originally, the HMO had planned to extensively renovate and equip a site somewhere in the northeast to southeast portion of the city (Figure 4-5, hatched area) in 1979. A medical group practice, which would use this primary care facility beginning in early 1980, was to be developed simultaneously. Eventually (in about 1983), another primary care center would be built in the growth area of the eastern suburbs (dark area at bottom)—at least ten miles from the initial center.

Galsworthy's rationale for selecting these potential sites was complex. The transportation system, in his view, was more effective in the suburban east than elsewhere. At least it would be more effective for the thousands of public and private employees living and working in the eastern part of the city and its suburbs. Demographic analysis showed a definite shift in population density and affluence toward the east over the preceding two decades. Many flourishing middle-sized corporations had arisen in or relocated to the eastern suburbs. The HMO's appeal would be accentuated by its location on the doorstep of the businesses and agencies whose employees would become members. Therefore, it made good sense to locate where paying subscribers could obtain services readily and save on the real and intangible (aggravation, time lost) costs of transportation to the treatment center.

The HMO also had a responsibility to the city's low-income citizens, most of whom lived closer to the river. The HMO would allocate some fraction of its resources to health care for the indigent, as evidenced by plans to enroll Medicare and Medicaid subscribers. The presence of the huge Memorial Hospital, the State University Medical Center, and several other hospitals and health care facilities in the city proper ensured a high quality of medical care for the central urban population. Galsworthy therefore was confident of his good judgment in selecting a site for the east.

However, the Rev. Avery Bannister of the local chapter of the NAACP, a board member of the SRA, disagreed strongly on the location and had so informed Drummond. The Rev. Mr. Bannister saw Galsworthy's site selection as an evasion of the HMO's social charter—to provide the public with a cost-efficient health care alternative. Were not the poor and minorities those most victimized by rising health costs? Hadn't their plight motivated the SRA's involvement with the HMO in the first place? And was not Galsworthy aware that many of the medical personnel in the city's

Figure 4-5 Southland HMO Service Area

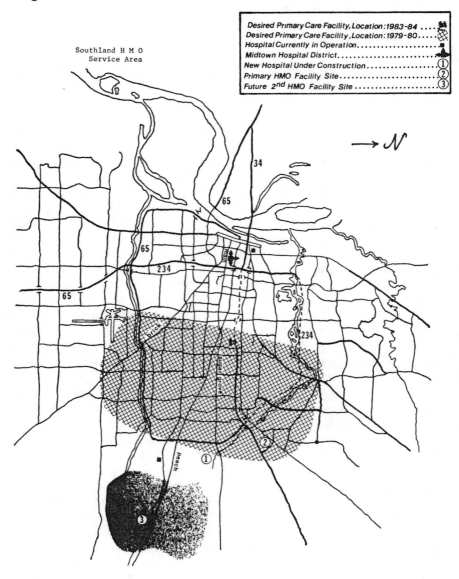

hospitals were academics, researchers, or specialists, with little impact on the health of the general public? The Rev. Mr. Bannister was willing to bet that any fair analysis of how and where the university and hospital physicians spent their working hours would show that many, if not most, at best were involved only marginally in primary care delivery. To maintain its precious credibility with the public and fulfill its initial inspiration, he agreed that the HMO must locate its first facility in the downtown or midtown areas.

Galsworthy recalled a recent discussion with Wilbur Fine, the president of Blodgett Realty Corporation. Blodgett held title to several hundred acres of prime commercial property in Black Oaks Corporate Park (No. 2 in Figure 4-5) on the northeast fringe of the city. The park was just beginning to attract builders and corporate entrepreneurs. Should the city continue to experience economic growth, the park was well-situated to attract or capitalize on part of such expansion. But Fine was eager to sustain the momentum of the park's initial success. A health facility that catered to an employee clientele right on its doorstep seemed a promotional opportunity too good to be true. So Fine had jumped at the HMO's initial feelers with the offer of a highly favorable leasing rate. Galsworthy was inclined to accept the offer. Such an attractive site at such reasonable cost would be unlikely to reappear in the future. The cost certainly would be far less than for building or renovating in the downtown or midtown areas. But how to respond to the strongly opposed views of the Rev. Mr. Bannister?

OVERVIEW OF CASE 6

Issues to Consider

1. What is the real impact of the effort by the Southland HMO to become qualified and how important is qualification to the organization's strategic goals?
2. How should Southland formally evaluate future facility sites?
3. What major marketing issues have been overlooked as the president prepares a status report to the HMO Advisory Committee?

Discussion

1. Survey Good, Follow-Up Weak

The key to success or failure at the Southland HMO may very well be the attempt to obtain qualification. Without it, the infant organization would have to mount a prohibitively expensive advertising campaign to open up the employer market. Once an HMO is qualified and has made formal notification, employers by law must permit access. Then the HMO can go after the employee market.

To become qualified, Southland has been challenged by HEW to come up with certain information on 120,000 employees, their employers, and their current health care providers. Simply put, HEW expects a demonstration of credibility and preliminary market penetrability.

The problem with Southland's approach to marketing research is not the questions asked or even the use of the survey technique. The HMO stumbled by not combining the survey with a more aggressive follow-up. Instead of bemoaning the failure of the second survey to bring in enough responses, Galsworthy should realize that the survey approach actually has succeeded. It has saved time and money by bringing in data on the most responsive part of the employer market without requiring substantial personal sales effort. If the employer market is envisioned as a multilayered entity, then the uppermost responsive layers have been peeled off by the surveys. Now, a different approach is required to penetrate the less responsive underlayers. These employers would be expected to own or manage smaller, more conservative private businesses. This type of business executive sees red when asked to fill out forms (thanks to the Occupational Safety and Health Administration, Equal Employment Opportunity Commission, Environmental Protection Agency, and other regulatory form-consuming agencies). These individuals also would be suspicious of novelty per se, would resent/resist disruption of their pattern of management, and, perhaps most importantly, would be untouched by the impersonal survey approach.

In fact, the HMO staff should devote more attention to the entire issue of cultivating employer receptivity to the HMO concept. Ideally, employers will be amenable to providing company time for a company-backed introduction to the HMO and its product. To the extent that this ideal goes unfulfilled, the marketing staff's task will become more difficult. Just because the federal government requires employers to offer the HMO option does not guarantee success. The employers can weaken and even completely frustrate the marketing effort through their indifference or active hindering efforts. The HMO could be reduced to the unpromising extreme of simply posting bulletin board notices if the employers get their danders up. So, Southland HMO must devise specific techniques for gauging and then nourishing the responsiveness of the immediate target market—the employer.

The question of marketability is dependent upon obtaining qualification. Galsworthy, in addition to listing the HMO's publics, should develop (or direct Hanley to develop) a marketing network chart that illustrates the precise sequence, timing, and coordination of the HMO's interaction with the various publics. In other words, the amorphous entanglements of the marketing environment should be reduced to a manageable marketing model.

2. Future Site Evaluation

If Southland is successful and becomes a growing enterprise, more facility sites will have to be selected. How should the HMO go about selecting these sites? The formal evaluation process must consider at least the following factors:

- actual and perceived accessibility
- perceived quality of the site neighborhood
- proximity in terms of travel time to potential member residences
- proximity to consulting hospitals and specialist providers
- topographical features—intervening rivers, mountains, or other physical features that pose real or perceived obstacles for potential members
- area zoning requirements
- terms of purchase or lease
- the qualities and appearance of the building, if purchasing or leasing an existing structure

Of these factors, the lease/purchase terms and building characteristics should be the last to be considered, not the first. Only after the more important, if less tangible, preceding elements have been examined closely, should the Southland management focus on lease/purchase terms. It would be a Pyrrhic victory to obtain advantageous terms on a beautiful building in an inaccessible or unattractive part of the city.

Finally, before any of these site selection factors are analyzed, Southland management should ask and answer an even more fundamental question: How will the selection of the next site fit in with the organization's master plan or marketing strategy? The marketing director will be able to identify neighborhoods or industrial areas that a growing HMO should attempt to penetrate. The strategy for enrollment growth, therefore, will involve a sequence of targeted marketing opportunities. As these opportunities arise and enrollment exceeds the current capacity for membership, several additional facilities may be required. Their mutual locations must be planned as much as possible in advance and be part of an integrated site selection strategy.

3. Overlooked Issues

Among the marketing topics Galsworthy has not confronted directly are staff training, product development, and pricing.

A staff training program, prepared by the marketing director, should be in place already when the first sales personnel are hired. This program will have both classroom and field sales components. The former might cover such general subjects as:

- the HMO concept
- the HMO Act of 1973—P.L. 93–222, as amended
- the local insurance industry
- the traditional health benefits package
- the Southland HMO benefits package
- the underwriting and legal requirements
- the HMO financial system/claims processing

Product development involves the creation of new or expanded benefits to meet competition and sustain member satisfaction. Federal law stipulates the basic benefits that qualified HMOs must offer but does not require a wide range of supplemental benefits. For example, HMOs are not required to provide a pharmacy benefit. The marketing director should prepare a product development strategy for evaluating these potential supplemental offerings as Southland's revenues increase and a richer benefit package becomes feasible.

There are strict federal regulations governing the price-setting procedures of qualified HMOs. For example, they must set most of their prices at a "community rate" instead of using the traditional experience rating of the insurance industry. The major difference is that qualified HMOs cannot discriminate among customer groups on the basis of experience factors such as age, sex, and previous illness.

Chapter 5

Market Segmentation

CASE 7. THE GEORGIA MEDICAL PLAN: MARKET SEGMENTATION FOR AN HMO

The Georgia Medical Plan (GMP), a health maintenance organization (HMO) in the Atlanta market, is in the feasibility stage of formation, awaiting approval for federal qualification. Larry Pett, executive director, and Debbie Nelson, administrative assistant, are reexamining GMP's marketing plan. While a fairly sophisticated strategy has been devised, they are particularly interested in refining their method of market segmentation—that is, of identifying accounts that are perceived to offer the most cost-effective results for their marketing efforts.

Industry Concept and Background

The health maintenance organization is a medical care delivery system that provides organization, financing, and delivery of services for a specific population. It provides an alternative to traditional fee-for-service health insurance programs, of which Blue Cross and Blue Shield are the largest.

The distinguishing features of HMOs are prepayment as the financing mechanism and group practice as the mode of delivery. The managerial-administrative organization assures a constant source of supply of health services through contracts with providers (physicians), and most plans offer a complete range of benefits. The typical product, such as GMP, includes these services:

- hospital room and board
- hospital ancillary services
- extended care

113

- emergency room
- hospital outpatient
- ambulance
- physician visits
- physician office services
- physician consultation
- surgery
- anesthesia
- obstetrics
- outpatient psychiatry
- radiology
- pathology
- vision care
- home health

The advantages of HMOs are reduced cost as a result of less need for hospitalization by emphasizing preventive treatment and early diagnosis, assurance of access to care, and more control over the quality and appropriateness of care received by enrollees in the program.

The first group practice prepayment program in this country was in a small clinic in Elk City, Okla., in 1932, while the Kaiser Foundation Health Plan on the West Coast was the first sizable implementation of the concept. As of this writing, there are more than six million HMO enrollees in the U.S., and the data indicate that HMOs can supply a comprehensive benefit package of health care for substantially less cost than the predominant fee-for-service system.

Georgia Medical Plan: Market Segmentation Strategy

If it receives all approvals, GMP plans to conduct its marketing campaign through an in-house marketing staff and by direct sales. During the early years, it proposes to direct its marketing efforts primarily toward large, stable, healthy employer groups to maximize enrollment and minimize financial risk. Because two other HMOs will begin operations in the Atlanta metropolitan market area (Clayton, Cobb, Gwinnett, DeKalb, and Fulton

Counties), employers' willingness to offer more than one HMO plan becomes a critical factor in estimating GMP's potential for success.

GMP used survey techniques to identify its primary market. Market segmentation was perceived to include the following:

- governmental groups
- large employers (100 or more employees)
- small employers (25 to 99 employees)
- individual subscribers (although not considered a cost-effective target during the first two years)
- Medicare
- Medicaid (year 4)
- unions

For years 1 and 2, groups considered most likely to produce cost-effective enrollment are governmental organizations and large employers. Smaller employer groups and possibly unions are looked upon to provide backup if enrollment of the primary target groups does not produce the desired results.

Preliminary selection of target accounts is based on these criteria, which can have an impact on enrollment:

1. group size, since larger units offer the potential for greater return on marketing effort expended
2. employer attitude toward GMP
3. accessibility to employees, a key factor in maximizing enrollment
4. level of health benefits, since HMOs usually provide a higher level of benefits than group insurance coverage and there is a direct relationship between this difference and enrollment
5. premium differential
6. degree of unionization
7. location of decision making, since local corporate headquarters or local management with decision-making authority can eliminate red tape
8. account prestige, which is a possible spillover effect from important accounts
9. adverse industry characteristics, since high employee turnover, seasonality, and many locations with few employees each create undesirable administrative problems

10. other HMO experience in the industry, since certain groups have established themselves historically as good potential sources of enrollees
11. dissatisfaction with current insurors' service, since groups unhappy with their present service are better prospects
12. financial condition of the organization
13. employer's experience with HMOs, important because the GMP must deal with a general unfamiliarity with the HMO concept
14. employer contribution

All groups in the primary target market are evaluated according to these criteria. Next, groups not eliminated are analyzed individually to determine their value as prospects. At this stage of analysis, several factors are considered:

Rate Differential

A point value (based on savings or additional out-of-pocket charges to the employee) is assigned to the employer and combined with other assigned values on the segmentation variables form (Exhibit 5-1), including:

Employer Attitude

Employer attitude is rated from 0–6 based on willingness to promote HMO to employees.

Enrollment Supervision and Control

A scale of 0–4 is used to rate the ability of local management to make decisions as to how HMOs are presented to employees.

Benefits Comparison

A scale of 0–2 is used to summarize the differences between the benefits under the HMO plan and benefits of the group insurance plan.

Competition Factor

The dilution of enrollment if other HMOs are offered to the same group of employees must be considered by the GMP.

Values derived through this analysis are then compared to a penetration rate percent scale:

Exhibit 5-1 Segmentation Variables

I. *Family Rate Differential*

PENETRATION MATRIX

Monthly premium difference

Less costly HMO premium	$15	15-11	10-6	5-1	HMO	0-5	6-10	11-15	$15	More costly HMO premium
			Points							Employee Contribution Value
	28	24	20	16		12	8	4	0	

	POINT VALUE
II. *Employer Attitude*	
1. Favorable toward HMO concept. Company will allow on-site, on-time presentations.	6
2. Favorable attitude toward concept. Employer will not permit onsite, on-time presentations but will cooperate on mailings, onsite space for questions, etc.	4
3. Neutral attitude. Company will not bend over backward to facilitate accessibility but will not cast unfavorable light on HMOs either.	2
4. Unfavorable attitude. Employer will do no more than required under HMO law.	0

III. *Enrollment Supervision and Control*

1. Enrollment procedure is designed and supervised by local management.	4
2. Enrollment procedure is designed by home office out of state but local management has some flexibility.	2
3. Enrollment procedure is totally out of local hands.	0

IV. *Benefits Comparison*

1. HMO benefits are superior to group insurance plan in several major areas.	2
2. HMO benefits will be perceived to be about the same as insurance plan.	0

V. *Competition Factor* (to be multiplied by total point value)

1. GMP is only HMO offered.	1
2. GMP is offered with HealthCare (closed panel) and company is located within 15 minutes of facility.	.6
3. GMP is offered with Metro (IPA).	.5
4. GMP is offered with Metro (IPA) and HealthCare (group) and group is located within 15 minutes of facility.	.4

Segmentation Variables Scale

40–38	18
37–33	16
32–28	14
27–23	12
22–19	10
18–14	8
13–10	6
9–6	4
5–1	2
0	0

The appropriate rate for a company or employee group is then multiplied by the competition factor (1–4).

This process was applied to each selected account and formed the basis for enrollment projections for marketing and financial planning. As a result, 48 primary target accounts were identified, representing for GMP 100 percent of the projected group enrollment for the first two years of operation.

While this market segmentation technique is quite thorough, GMP's management is anxious to heighten its present awareness of changing factors affecting identified groups, allowing for adjustments and substitutions to produce more favorable enrollment results.

The market segmentation technique used by GMP had helped management focus its sales efforts on those employees likely to enroll. The process was highly subjective, yet seemed effective. Pett decided to review the technique to determine if it could be improved without major revision.

OVERVIEW OF CASE 7

Issues to Consider

1. Evaluate the objectivity and utility of the Georgia Medical Plan segmentation scale.
2. Has Georgia Medical Plan determined the market demand for health maintenance organization services in the delivery area?
3. Are the identified market segments satisfactory for GMP's penetration objectives?

Discussion

1. Refining Target Market Definition

The Georgia Medical Plan (GMP) of Atlanta is facing the common problem of refining its target market definition with the objective of increased enrollment. Initially, GMP's in-house marketing staff surveyed its service area to identify desirable markets. The staff concluded that the first two years would be devoted to recruiting government organizations and large employer groups (of at least 100 employees). If penetration efforts were unsuccessful, the marketing staff would then focus their resources on the smaller employer groups and the union organizations.

To further define their target markets large employers were rated on the basis of 14 factors: size, HMO accessibility, attitude toward GMP, level of health benefits, premium differential, degree of unionization, location of decision maker, account prestige, adverse industry characteristics, other HMO experience, dissatisfaction with current insurers' service, financial stability of organization, employers' experience with HMO, and employer contribution. By weighting these factors, the marketing staff rated the overall attractiveness of employers and targeted selected companies.

Critics have challenged the rating scales and factors as being overly subjective. There appears to be little basis for selection and weighting of the employer characteristics. Still, as long as the approach serves to screen out unattractive employers, the system should be useful.

2. Demand Evaluation

HMOs are the preventive health alternative to the traditional delivery system. However, national research demonstrates that the overwhelming majority of the public is not familiar with this type of care. Because of this ignorance, HMO marketers need to identify target market demand for the service before initiating the adoption process. If the demand is nonexistent, then the market needs to be stimulated before the product will be adopted. Demand must be preceded by awareness, product interest and knowledge.

The marketing staff has made no attempt to define the total market. An attempt has been made, however, to categorize large employers among the actual market, the potential market, and the non-market. The actual market represents those individuals who are attracted to the product or service due to a match of the product attributes and individual needs. The potential market represents individuals who may become interested in a product or service under certain circumstances. The non-market is comprised of those individuals who under no circumstances will be interested in a product.

Market definition and segmentation provide the marketer with criteria for the allocation of limited resources and direction for market penetration. GMP will benefit from redefinition of the total market to determine the actual, potential and non-markets. Those industries and individuals comprising the actual market can then be delineated and marketing strategies developed.

3. Satisfactory Market Segment Definition

The HMO concept is appealing to various segments of the population and is unacceptable for other segments. The key factor is the level of satisfaction with the current system and the perceived benefits of the HMO alternative. Targeting all large employers may be unwieldy. An alternative to segmenting based on employment size would be to select variables that directly affect the decision process, such as benefits, income, education, family size, length of time in community, and accessibility to care.

This tool was developed to provide the marketer with a viable prospect list. To determine if the tool was beneficial one would evaluate the ratio of adopters to non-adopters. This examination will help to evaluate the criteria used to select one employer over another.

CASE 8. SOUTHERN JAMAICA PLAIN HEALTH CENTER

The Southern Jamaica Plain Health Center (SJPHC), after five and a half years of operation as a noncomprehensive neighborhood health center offering pediatric and gynecological/family planning services, was planning two major changes in October 1975: (1) to move to new, larger quarters, and (2) to add internal medicine and dental services. The addition of these services would fulfill its long-awaited goal of becoming a fully comprehensive primary care health center.

Marketing Needs of the SJPHC

The SJPHC had achieved a total registrant population by May 1975 of 3,000 but of these only 2,000 were active registrants. The remaining 1,000 were adult males to whom the center had few direct services to offer but who were registered as family members of active registrants. The 2,000 active registrants had utilized approximately 6,000 visits in the previous year. John Cupples, SJPHC administrator, felt that to fully utilize the revamped and expanded center, he would need to increase his registrant population to 10,000 (6,000 to 7,000 active) within the next 18 months, and these registrants would have to make 18,000 to 20,000 visits annually once the center offered fully comprehensive services.

Cupples, who had directed the SJPHC for a year, believed that insufficient attention had been paid in the past to the marketing aspects of the center's operation. Moreover, he felt that, for the registration and visit goals to be realized, a marketing strategy had to be considered. The lack of a formal strategy was thought to be a problem for other neighborhood health centers as well. In response to this perceived need, the Massachusetts League of Neighborhood Health Centers in September 1974 had released a statement, "Neighborhood Health Center Marketing Needs," calling for the establishment of a Leaguewide marketing/publicity program that should address, among other things:

- "the need to maximize utilization of neighborhood health centers as a means toward fiscal self-support;

- "(the need to) identify service needs which neighborhood health centers should and could plan to meet;

- "(the need to) identify underserved groups, and the means to attract them to neighborhood health centers."

History of Neighborhood Health Centers

Neighborhood health centers originated in the mid 1960s when the Johnson administration inspired expansion of and concern for the provision of social services. The first centers essentially were experiments in the War on Poverty, which sought to address a wide range of social service needs of the poor that included nutrition, mental health, family planning, and drug counseling; the need for community self-participation and determination; and the provision of direct primary health care such as pediatrics; internal medicine; and obstetrical, gynecological, and dental services.

Initially the centers provided only free care, being prohibited by governmental grant terms from charging for any services. This fact, coupled with the location of many in center city and rural ghettos and enclaves, led to a distinct "charity" or "welfare" image for any facility that bore the neighborhood health center label. However, the utility of the concept of a comprehensive neighborhood-oriented, community-governed, family-centered, preventive health care ambulatory facility led to centers' being established in other than strictly ghetto or truly severe poverty areas. The great amounts of money poured into them made it easy to forget the necessity of organizing for or thinking about the future as self-sufficient health care facilities.

In the early 1970s, however, federal funds for the centers began to dry up and the future had to be faced. In 1972, neighborhood health centers receiving federal grants were allowed to charge fees and bill third party insurers. Some centers established sliding scale fee schedules, others set minimal charges for noninsured users. Many of the grant-supported services, however, still had specific restrictions against fees. As the mid-1970s arrived, therefore, most centers were faced with the problem of becoming more self-sufficient by reducing the dependence on grants, but they remained plagued by the image and organizational problems that were the legacy of the early development of their concept.

SJPHC—1969 through 1974

The SJPHC opened on November 9, 1969, providing pediatric and gynecological services on a half-time basis. The center was located on the third floor of the Curtis Hall municipal building built in 1912, a site previously occupied by the Jamaica Plain Health Unit of the Boston Department of Health and Hospitals. The unit had existed there for 25 years before the center's opening and had operated a well-baby clinic one afternoon a week in addition to providing public health nursing services such as home visits and health education.

The impetus for the center had begun in late 1968 when the Southern Jamaica Plain Health Committee (SJPHComm) was formed to look into ways of getting better health care services in the area. At that time, the existing neighborhood health centers—Martha Eliot Health Center, which was located in a housing project in the extreme northern end of Jamaica Plain, and what was to be renamed the Brookside Park Family Life Center in eastern Jamaica Plain—both excluded southern Jamaica Plain area residents because of federal funding constraints on their geographical service areas.

The committee worked for a year and a half on various plans to get a center operating, and eventually settled on the concept of forming a satellite clinic to the Martha Eliot Health Center that would be located at Curtis Hall and would expand the well-baby services previously offered there. The Boston Department of Health and Hospitals agreed to transfer the well-baby clinic funds to this effort; Action for Boston Community Development offered to establish a family planning gynecological clinic at the center; and the Health and Hospitals Department, Children's Hospital Medical Center, Peter Bent Brigham Hospital (PBBH), Faulkner Hospital, and the Boston Hospital for Women all agreed to help get the center running through the donation of services and money.

Until early in 1973, the center had no onsite administration; administrative tasks were taken care of primarily by the Martha Eliot staff, although for a time the Peter Bent Brigham Hospital Office of Community Medicine did maintain a staff member at the center to deal with administrative work. This was at the request of the SJPHComm. In 1973, an onsite administrator was hired, and in May 1974, Cupples became the full-time director. In July 1974, the satellite relationship with the Martha Eliot center was severed.

Community Demographics[1] and Health Status

Jamaica Plain as a whole was a diverse neighborhood consisting of four quite distinct populations: in northern Jamaica Plain, there was a small but concentrated (3 percent in 1970) poor black segment; in eastern and central Jamaica Plain, there was a growing group of Spanish-speaking residents (7 percent of the population in 1970 but estimated to be growing rapidly). In the southwestern part was a relatively affluent group, and finally, by far the largest segment, were the working-class Irish Catholics who were spread throughout the community. Children under 15 constituted 23 percent of the population. The elderly (65 and over) formed 17 percent of the total, a percentage that exceeded the city average.

Residents had a median income of $9,618 per year. Of these, 36 percent had incomes in excess of $12,000, 10 percent fell below the poverty level (approximately $4,000) and 26 percent were in the "medically indigent" category with incomes below $8,000. The average resident was a high school graduate (12.1 years of schooling). Further demographic information is contained in Figure 5-1, Table 5-1, Figure 5-2, and Exhibit 5-2.

General mortality in Jamaica Plain exceeded national levels, but infant mortality was much lower. The 1974 ABT study showed that Jamaica Plain used in the range of −6 percent to +8 percent of the expected medical visits based on similar populations, and −9 percent to −31 percent (considerably fewer) dental visits than would have been expected. A primary health need of the community was indicated to be dental care for adults.

Rationalization of current services was seen as a major problem. There was a widespread feeling that the elderly had distinctly complex needs (health care, transportation, health education) that had long been neglected. Working adults also were seen as a neglected group as were teenagers in the areas of sex counseling and alcoholism. The rapid growth of the Spanish-speaking population presented another area of need because of language and cultural barriers.

Community Organization and Control

Jamaica Plain was somewhat unusual among Boston neighborhoods because of its large number of organized community groups. Over the past few years there had been, in addition to the Jamaica Plain Wide Health Coordinating Committee and the SJPHComm, which were concerned with health care issues, a variety of other community groups involved with zoning, banking, highway construction, and schools. James Warram, chairman of the SJPHComm, was not sure of the origins of all these groups since he felt that "the neighborhood had an ambient distrust of such 'do-good' agencies." On the other hand, he felt that their existence demonstrated a "rampant attempt (on the part of the community residents) to control events within the community."

The community group with the greatest influence on the SJPHC was the Southern Jamaica Plain Health Committee. While the SJPHComm was an incorporated body, SJPHC was not and no legal relationship between the two existed. Warram characterized the relationship between the SJPHComm and the center director as a "gentlemen's agreement." This agreement was implemented through the committee's exercise of interviewing and hiring authority for center staff members whose funding authority agreed to this procedure, i.e., some of the grants that paid staff salary allowed the center hiring discretion and the center director in turn deferred to the SJPHComm. Cupples, the administrator, made certain that the committee was aware

Figure 5-1 Southern Jamaica Plain Health Center Map

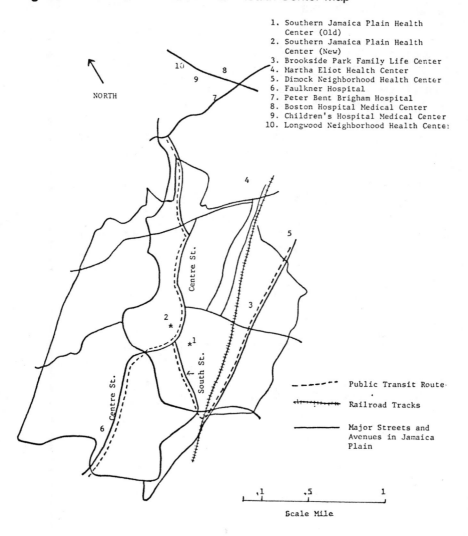

1. Southern Jamaica Plain Health Center (Old)
2. Southern Jamaica Plain Health Center (New)
3. Brookside Park Family Life Center
4. Martha Eliot Health Center
5. Dimock Neighborhood Health Center
6. Faulkner Hospital
7. Peter Bent Brigham Hospital
8. Boston Hospital Medical Center
9. Children's Hospital Medical Center
10. Longwood Neighborhood Health Center

NORTH

Public Transit Route

Railroad Tracks

Major Streets and Avenues in Jamaica Plain

Scale Mile

Table 5-1 Age and Sex Census Tract Data for Jamaica Plain Area and Two Centers

Census Tract		Age 0–14		Age 15–64		Age 65 +		Census Tract Totals	SJPHC Totals	BPFLC Totals
		Total	SJPHC	Total	SJPHC	Total	SJPHC			
1101	M:	1,070	40	2,309	27	464	0	3,843	67	114
	F:	927	31	2,537	45	771	0	4,235	76	150
								8,078	143	264
1106	M:	1,149	6	2,602	5	714	0	4,405	11	10
	F:	1,143	7	3,135	5	1,244	0	5,522	12	13
								9,927	23	23
1201	M:	904	63	1,942	47	446	0	3,292	110	129
	F:	814	61	2,679	80	833	0	4,326	141	169
								7,618	251	298
1202	M:	564	70	1,289	51	233	0	2,086	121	324
	F:	573	67	1,441	86	323	0	2,337	153	383
								4,423	274	707
1203	M:	710	10	1,479	13	308	0	2,497	23	1,077
	F:	740	11	1,691	12	639	0	3,070	23	1,276
								5,567	46	2,353
1204	M:	696	82	1,981	70	665	0	3,342	152	303
	F:	645	61	2,300	94	1,010	0	3,955	155	346
								7,297	307	649
1205	M:	369	5	651	8	102	0	1,122	13	82
	F:	354	10	792	11	130	0	1,276	21	113
								2,398	34	195
1206	M:	435	9	1,015	14	169	0	1,619	23	124
	F:	428	12	1,107	19	289	0	1,824	31	121
								3,443	54	245
1207	M:	189	1	750	2	136	0	1,075	3	31
	F:	169	3	830	5	234	0	1,233	8	41
								2,308	11	72
Totals		14,018	237	3,237	0			23,341	523	2,194
		16,512	357	5,473	0			27,778	620	2,612
								51,119	1,143	4,806

6,086 286 ----Males Registered at SJPHC
5,793 263 ----Females Registered at SJPHC
Females in Census Tract
Males in Census Tract

Table 5-1 continued

SOUTHERN JAMAICA PLAIN HEALTH CENTER

Age	0-4	5-9	10-14	15-19	20-24	25-34	35-44	45-54	55-64	65+	Totals
Males	302	214	126	174	125	212	71	28	6	0	1,258
Females	253	216	135	111	215	333	96	34	2	1	1,396
Totals	555	430	261	285	340	545	167	62	8	1	2,654

BROOKSIDE PARK FAMILY LIFE CENTER

Males	715	966	828	660	618	913	528	351	213	412	6,204
Females	735	887	820	742	889	1,373	592	418	238	528	7,222
Totals	1,450	1,853	1,648	1,402	1,507	2,286	1,120	769	451	940	13,426

Note: The data presented for SJPHC and BPFLC are based on the *known* tract registrants of these facilities. Since the computerization of the registration forms does not always yield a census tract assignment, the totals in the first part of this table do not equal the total registrants of the centers. The second part presents a more fine-grained breakdown of the age distribution of both centers' registrant population, and the totals represent *all* early 1975 registrants. Neither part of this exhibit identifies registrants as active or inactive.

Source: 1970 U.S. Census data.

of the center's budget and that the panel was involved in program definition and budgeting. The committee in the past had sought to legalize the relationship and continued to attempt to do so.

The committee consisted of 15 active community residents, of whom only five had been born and raised in Jamaica Plain. Ten members were women, and Warram thought the ages ranged from 25 to 40. He freely admitted that the committee was not entirely representative of the community but he thought that it included a wide diversity of opinion, and that it "would be impossible to represent the whole community and get anything done." However, he felt that the committee was conscious of its composition and often discussed how it might recruit new members such as elders and professionals.

Goals and Objectives of the SJPHC

Both Warram and Cupples were keenly aware of the diverse nature of the community and both indicated a desire to serve the multiple populations. Neither felt they had yet figured out the optimal strategy for doing this; however, Cupples said the overall goal of the center was to provide accessible, comprehensive, high-quality care.

Figure 5-2 Census Tracts and Locations of Providers

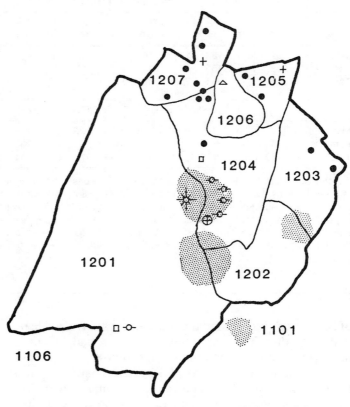

Source: 1970 U.S. Census data.

Exhibit 5-2 Description of High Density Census Tracts

Census Tract	
1101:	Females, who outnumber males, are found in three modal ages (10–14, 25–34, and 65 +, comprising 49 percent). Males are found in three modal ages (10–14, 25–34, and 65 +, comprising 34 percent). Modal family income is $9,000–$12,000 (24 percent); lesser modes are at $3,000–$4,000 and $6,000–$7,000 (6 percent and 8 percent) and one larger mode is at $15,000–$25,000 (13 percent). Jobs tend to be clerical and service in manufacturing, retail, and health. Those 25 and older have modal educational achievement of four high school years (37 percent). The most common ethnic groups are Irish and Canadian.
1201:	Females, who outnumber males, are found in two modal ages (20–24 and 65 +, comprising 29 percent). Males are found in three modal ages (10–14, 25–34, and 65 +, comprising 34 percent). Modal family incomes are $9,000–$12,000 (19 percent) and $15,000–$25,000 + (38 percent); lesser modes are at $0–$1,000, $2,000–$3,000, and $4,000–$5,000 (1 percent, 3 percent, and 4 percent). Jobs tend to be professional and clerical in manufacturing, retail, finance/real estate, health, and education. Those 25 and older have modal educational attainments of four high school years (34 percent) and four-plus college years (21 percent). Ethnic groups most common are Irish and other or not reported.
1202:	Females and the slightly less numerous males are found in three modal ages (0–4, 25–34, and 65 +, comprising 36 percent of all females and 38 percent of all males). Modal family incomes are $6,000–$9,000 (26 percent) and $15,000–$25,000 (16 percent); lesser modes are at $7,000–$8,000 and $10,000–$12,000 (10 percent and 14 percent). Jobs tend to be clerical and service, in manufacturing, retail, health, and public administration. Those 25 and older have modal educational achievement of four high school years (33 percent). Ethnic groups most commonly found are Irish, Italian, and Canadian.
1204:	Females, who outnumber males, are found in two modal ages (25–34, and 65 +, comprising 36 percent). Males are found in

(continues)

Exhibit 5-2 continued

> four modal ages (0–4, 10–14, 25–34, and 65 +, comprising 47 percent). Modal family incomes are $6,000–$9,000 (20 percent) and $15,000–$25,000+ (24 percent); lesser modes are at $3,000–$4,000, $5,000–$6,000, and $7,000–$8,000 (6 percent, 6 percent, and 7 percent). Jobs tend to be professional and clerical, in manufacturing, retail, finance/real estate, and health. Those 25 and older have modal educational achievements of four high school years (30 percent) and four or more college years (11 percent). The most common ethnic groups are Irish and other or not recorded.

Warram, while agreeing that comprehensiveness of care was a primary goal of the center's existence, perhaps reflected the different role he filled as a representative of the SJPHComm when he suggested a second equally important goal: keeping control of the center in the hands of the community. He also saw the SJPHC as an attempt to alter the welfare care image that neighborhood facilities such as the Martha Eliot Health Center had developed. This was further evidenced by a statement that appeared on a center brochure that the SJPHComm "was organized by a group of community residents who wanted *reasonably priced*, quality health care available in their community."

The planned expansion of SJPHC services was in consonance with center's goals and was targeted specifically to begin to deal with the health problems and to meet the need for dental services of southern Jamaica Plain's population.

Current Organization

The legal status of the SJPHC was undergoing changes at the time of the case writer's visits because its request for a Determination of Need from the Massachusetts Public Health Council (required of any facility that expanded or added programs) was being processed. In May 1974, the SJPHC had asked the Peter Bent Brigham Hospital (PBBH) to include the center under its licenses to provide medical care. Since plans for relocating also were being considered, a certificate of need was required. Once the certificate was issued, the center would be a professional and fiscal responsibility of the PBBH, according to Dr. Harold May of the PBBH Office of Community Medicine.

As with most neighborhood health centers, the SJPHC gathered resources from wherever it could. This led to a somewhat amorphous management situation, wherein center staff members were paid from a variety of sources, and functions such as purchasing and financial data reports were handled by different institutions. The license to operate under PBBH authority was expected to be granted in June 1975, however, and once that was received the majority of administrative support functions would come from PBBH. Cupples's liaison with the PBBH was through the hospital's Office of Community Medicine, which had been established in 1969 to assist in the coordination and planning of primary health care in Jamaica Plain. An idea of the complexity of the origin of resources for the center may be gathered from Table 5-2.

There were referral agreements for any necessary inpatient services with Massachusetts Mental Health Center, Children's Hospital Medical Center, Boston Hospital for Women, PBBH, and the Washingtonian Center for Addictions. In addition, these institutions provided monetary, staff, and/ or service support to the center. Cupples commented that, by and large, the backup hospitals were quite happy to provide administrative support for the center and serve as professional referral sites (Children's Hospital Medical Center had determined that 15 percent of its outpatient visits were from neighborhood health centers), but that when it came to dollars, they were considerably less beneficent.

The center had no formal organization chart in May 1975, but Cupples planned to establish a more formal setup, including a director of professional services and program coordinators once he moved into the new site in October.

Services Offered by SJPHC

The services offered by SJPHC are illustrated in Exhibit 5-3.

Pediatrics

The center employed a three-quarter full-time equivalent pediatrician who held seven four-hour patient encounter sessions per week, including one on Tuesday evenings. Working with him was a full-time pediatric nurse practitioner paid by one of the supporting hospitals. She carried her own patient load and was always available to deal with walk-ins when the pediatrician was not present. Four community health nurses represented additional resources. They were employed by the Department of Health and Hospitals and were available for home visiting, health education, and well-baby care. Altogether these pediatric practitioners were capable of 20 patient encounters per day and had been having 15. New patients could be seen within two weeks and routine follow-up visits usually could be

Table 5-2 Southern Jamaica Plain Health Center: Grant Summary

Source and Title	Amount of Grant	Terms
Private Hospital Matching Grant	$10,000	Free care is provided for Southern Jamaica Plain residents who are inpatients there at the hospital or for laboratory services there.
Private Hospital Matching Grant	$10,000	The services of the SJPHC's pediatrician are underwritten in part.
Private Hospital Matching Grant	$13,333.33	The hospital agrees to place an R.N. on its payroll from the SJPHC.
Family Planning Project/ ABCD	up to $10,200	An HEW grant pays for a Gyn physician @ $60 per session to work at the SJPHC.
Health and Hospitals City of Boston Matching Grant	up to $50,000	Personnel and equipment are provided under a contract to match grants from the private sector.
Private Hospital Matching Grant	$11,935	An in-kind grant covers salaries of personnel working at the SJPHC.
Private Hospital Matching Grant	$17,111.80	Physician, other staff, and overhead are paid.
Private Hospital	$4,856	Physician, other, and supplies are paid.
Public Health Nursing Department of Health and Hospitals	--------	In-kind service is provided by public health nurses.
Well-Child Clinic Department of Health and Hospitals	$25 per session @ one session per week	Boston's Health and Hospitals Department pays for time spent by a pediatrician in well-child checks.
Private Hospital	$42,000	Three staff, phone, supplies, and equipment are provided.
Family Alcoholism Program National Institute on Alcohol Abuse and Alcoholism	$67,744	This program is licensed through the Washingtonian Center for family therapy, outreach, building of community awareness, and agency consultation.

Exhibit 5-3 Program/Services Outline

Program and Provider	Mon am	Mon pm	Mon eve	Tue am	Tue pm	Tue eve*	Wed am	Wed pm	Wed eve	Thu am	Thu pm	Thu eve	Fri am	Fri pm	Fri eve
PEDIATRICS															
Pediatrician		x		x	x			x			x		x	x	
Nurse Practitioner	n	n		x	x		o	x		o	x		n	n	
Public Health Nurse	n	n											n	n	
GYNECOLOGY															
Gynecologist				x						x					
Nurse Practitioner				x	o		n			x	o				
Family Planner	o	o		x	o		x			x	o				
MENTAL HEALTH															
Mental Health Social Worker				x	x	x	x	x		x	x		x		
Mental Health Social Worker				x	x	x	x	*		*	*		x	x	
Psychiatrist				x	x								x	x	
NUTRITION															
Nutritionist													x		
ALCOHOLISM															
Therapist	x	x		x	x		o	x		x	x		x	x	
Social Service	x	x		x	x		o	x		x	x		x	x	
SUPPORT SERVICES															
Receptionist/ Supervisor		x		x			x			x			x		
Receptionist	x	x			x		x	x		x	x		x	x	
Lab Tech		x		x	*			x		x	*			x	
Unit Secretary		x		x			x			x			x		
Clinic Aid				x											

Services to be added in October, 1975

Program and Provider	Mon am	Mon pm	Mon eve	Tue am	Tue pm	Tue eve*	Wed am	Wed pm	Wed eve	Thu am	Thu pm	Thu eve	Fri am	Fri pm	Fri eve
ADULT MEDICINE															
Internist		*			*			*			*			*	
Nurse Practitioner	*	*		*	*	*	*	*		*	*		*	*	

(continues)

Exhibit 5-3 continued

Program and Provider	Monday			Tuesday			Wednesday			Thursday			Friday		
	am	pm	eve	am	pm	eve	am	pm	eve	am	pm	eve	am	pm	eve
DENTAL															
Dentist		*		*	*			*			*		*		
Hygenist	*	*		*	*		*			*			*	*	
Asst/Reception	*	*		*	*		*	*		*	*		*	*	
SUPPORT SERVICES															
Social Worker	*	*		*	*		*	*		*	*		*	*	
Family Health Worker	*	*		*	*		*	*		*	*		*	*	
Intake Specialist	*				*			*		*				*	
Receptionist	*			*				*		*				*	

Key: x = now operative
    n = patient sees nurse only (now operative)
    o = nonpatient encounter session (now operative)
    * = sessions to be added by October 1, 1975
Note: Evening sessions run until 7 P.M.

scheduled the same day. The pediatrician maintained a private practice in Newton, an upper-middle class suburb of Boston, but was quite accessible for emergency calls.

Barbara Hohman, the pediatric nurse practitioner, noted that most families brought their toddlers and infants to the center but not their adolescents as often as they should. She said this was a common reality of pediatric medicine since adolescents tended not to want to see the "baby" doctor. Ms. Hohman felt that they saw a variety of classes of families but that the predominant group was working-class white. Dr. Leber, the pediatrician, was well liked by the families and local school authorities, a fact which led to his being called on to do a number of camp physicals and the state-mandated medical examinations of learning disabled children each year.

Gynecology

Gynecological services were provided by a team consisting of a female gynecologist, a nurse practitioner, and a family planning counselor, all of whom were subsidized by an HEW Family Planning Project grant administered by Action for Boston Community Development (ABCD). They held two sessions a week during which they provided 15 to 18 patient visits; utilization had been about 85 percent. Both the nurse practitioner and the family planning counselor were available at times other than the scheduled session, and Cupples said ABCD could rotate an additional nurse into the center if need be. A new patient desiring an initial visit had to wait no more than two weeks.

Marion Isner, the family planning counselor, felt that 80 percent of the patients the team saw were working class women in their 20s and the remaining 20 percent were older women coming in for annual gynecological checkups. Ms. Isner thought that 90 percent of their patients came for family planning assistance because SJPHC was the only well-identified source of such information in the community. The Family Planning Project provided free birth control supplies (devices, pills, etc.) to all patients. A six-month supply of pills usually was given to patients. Ms. Isner believed that about half of the young mothers the team saw also brought their children to the center for pediatric services.

Mental Health

Mental health services were provided by two mental health social workers and one psychiatrist, all of them employed by the Massachusetts Mental Health Center and assigned to work in Jamaica Plain. At least one of them was available every day of the week except Monday, and an evening session was held on Tuesday. They had a capacity to treat 25 patients per week and actually were seeing 10 to 15. Utilization of this service usually was on a relatively long-term basis, and once a client was seen initially (one- to two-week wait for an appointment), the person usually appeared weekly for 50-minute therapeutic sessions.

Nutrition

A nutritionist held one session per week at the center, on Friday mornings. This individual was on the PBBH payroll and provided service to Brookside Park Family Life Center as well as the SJPHC and PBBH. The nutritionist could see six patients per session and had been seeing an average of three, who were referred by other staff members.

Family Alcoholism Program

The Family Alcoholism Program began operation in January 1975 with a therapist, community liaison staff member, and unit manager, all of whom were supported by the Washingtonian Center for Addictions (a specialized hospital in Jamaica Plain) through a National Institute on Alcohol Abuse and Alcoholism (NIAAA) grant. The grant called for the following: direct family therapy services, increased awareness of alcoholism as a disease in the Jamaica Plain community, outreach to families affected by alcoholism, and consultation with agencies dealing with alcoholics and their families.

Stanley Rusnak, the therapist, said they were seeing 34 persons on a consistent basis. The program also dealt with a number of crisis stage walk-ins who did not establish a continuing relationship with the program. He characterized this as rather typical of the problem of providing alcoholism services; he considered the program underutilized. About 50 percent of the individuals who visited the program returned; spouses of alcoholics were more likely to avail themselves of the services than the alcoholics themselves.

The program was geared to deal with alcoholism as a problem that disrupted the entire family system, requiring family therapy and other supportive services to the group as a whole. To this end, the program provided space for Al-Anon meetings (for the spouses of alcoholics) as well as offered links to other necessary social services. The community liaison worker, Nancy MacDougall, spent 10 percent of her time addressing the social service needs of the clients and their families, such as enrolling them for welfare or veteran's benefits.

Rusnak felt that the program was seeing primarily working or lower class Irish-Americans and commented that they were in large part first- or second-generation immigrants.

Laboratory and Radiology

The center maintained a small laboratory facility capable of carrying out routine blood tests, urine analysis, and cultures. The longest of these tests had a 24-hour turnaround but many could be done while the patients waited. The center had to send any radiology work or other more complex diagnostic procedure to its referral hospitals. Cupples was quite satisfied with the 24-hour turnaround these hospitals provided.

General

Cupples characterized medicine at the center as "modified team practice" in which staff members, while not working in formally established teams, did conduct weekly case conferences on patients. Any staff member could participate.

The center discouraged walk-in patients, as did most neighborhood health centers (a procedure the Massachusetts League of Neighborhood Health Centers wanted to study further to determine whether it was appropriate), and tried to keep a tight appointment schedule. About 8 percent of scheduled appointments cancelled, but center staff attempted to reschedule the appointment immediately. Some three to five percent of scheduled appointments failed to show up; these individuals were the target of a vigorous telephone follow-up program. Cupples felt that the average waiting time once a patient arrived rarely exceeded 20 minutes. For the hours that the center was not open, a 24-hour answering service was maintained.

Planned Services

As shown in Exhibit 5-4, the SJPHC planned on occupying its new quarters in October 1975. At that time adult internal medicine services, dental services, and a full-time social worker and a full-time family health worker were to be added. Adult services were to be provided by a half-time internist and a full-time adult nurse practitioner. Cupples estimated that this staffing would provide capacity to see 90 patients per week.

Dental services were to be provided by a six-tenths full-time dentist and an eight-tenths full-time hygienist whose hours would be arranged so that at least one staff member would be available during all the hours the center was open. Primary funding was to come from the City Department of Health and Hospitals, which once had run a dental clinic at the present site of the center but which the SJPHComm had succeeded in closing down because of its poor quality a number of years ago. Mental health services would be expanded by adding three more sessions of mental health social worker availability. The laboratory technician would add two sessions per week.

Users

According to Cupples, the SJPHC had little active registrant dropout; this was attributed to the highly personalized care delivered at the center. He cited the fact that a significant number of users (25 percent) came from outside Jamaica Plain and that previous southern Jamaica Plain patients who had moved out of the area continued to travel long distances to use the center.

Once a year, the record of every registrant was reviewed; a telephone call was placed to all inactive registrants to determine whether they wished to remain in the center's files. Those who could not be reached by telephone were sent two letters. Any inactive registrant who could not be reached through this process or who wished to be dropped from the files then was terminated as a client.

Cupples estimated that the 75 percent of the users who came from Jamaica Plain were primarily of lower middle class working whites with a significant minority of higher level professionals and a few Spanish-speaking people and blacks. Table 5-2 (supra) presents age, sex, and census tract data on area residents and SJPHC registrants.

Serving the Elderly

The SJPHComm was much interested in meeting the health needs of the elderly. Both Cupples and Caral Mpontsikaris, southern Jamaica Plain

Exhibit 5-4 Space Utilization Plan

Room No.	Room Function	Percent Utilization (44-hour week)
Ground Level 687 Centre St.		
1.	Waiting room	100
2.	Reception, self-pay collections	100
3.	Laboratory	63
4.	Consultation, intake, social work	100
5.	Medical exam	100
6.	Consultation, medical consultant, social work	100
7.	Medical exam	81
8.	Medical exam	90
9.	Medical exam	81
10.	Medical exam	81
Basement Level 687 Centre St.		
11.	Conference, staff lounge (nonprogrammed space)	0
12.	Storage	100
13.	Consultation, mental health	72
14.	Consultation, alcoholism, family therapy	90
15.	Consultation, mental health	36
16.	Consultation, mental health, family therapy	81
17.	Consultation, alcoholism, social service	90
18.	Office space, chart review	40
19.	Consultation, training, observation, play therapy	0
20.	Office space	100
21.	Janitor's closet	100
22.	Mechanical equipment	100

Exhibit 5-4 continued

Room No.	Room Function	Percent Utilization (44-hour week)
Second Level 687 Centre St.		
23.	Office, community liaison	100
24.	Office, billing	90
25.	Office, administration	100
Curtis Hall		
26.	Dental suite	72
27.	Dental suite	72
28.	Dental suite	72
29.	Office	0
30.	Office	0
31.	Office	0
32.	Dental reception	75

community organizer at PBBH, noted, however, that medical care was only one part of the service package the elderly required. They also needed education in primary preventive care, in proper nutrition, and on their diseases (such as arthritis). And they needed assistance on transportation and access to other social services such as getting food stamps and signing up for Medicare.

A number of area organizations had formed what was called the Jamaica Plain Geriatric Provider Group to begin to provide the necessary services for the elderly. A consumer organization was founded through the efforts of Ms. Mpontsikaris, the Faulkner Hospital Department of Community Services, and the Jamaica Plain Mental Health Outreach program's geriatric social worker. This group was called the Jamaica Plain Senior Council and, according to Ms. Mpontsikaris, had a core of 8 to 20 participants who met at the new site of the SJPHC. She felt that if the seniors' needs were to be met, it would be crucial for the Geriatric Provider Group and SJPHC to see outreach as a goal separate from the simple establishment of services. She believed that only in this way could service providers really make contact with the seniors and understand their unique problems. Even with outreach, Ms. Mpontsikaris noted that the seniors who responded and were active in groups such as the Senior Council were the articulate and relatively mobile ones, and that a goodly number would be much less responsive to outreach. It was a constant battle to keep the Senior Council interested in dealing with the problems of this other group of the elderly, she said.

Cupples said that a student fieldworker from Boston College had visited a number of community senior groups and discussed the role the SJPHC could play in meeting their needs.

Pricing

The center classified pediatric and gynecological visits in three categories—initial, comprehensive, and routine—that carried charges of $30, $30, and $18 respectively. The same prices were expected to be charged for internal medicine services. These also were the prices charged to third party payers such as Medicaid and Blue Cross. In establishing the center, the SJPHComm had decided that for those who had no insurance and would have to pay the bills themselves, the charges would be discounted by 80 percent to produce self-pay prices of $6, $6, and $3.60, respectively. There was no sliding scale based on income but the possibility of using one when the center relocated was being considered. The Family Planning Project grant constrained the center from billing Medicaid or self-paying patients for gynecological services but it could bill Blue Cross. Pediatric well-child visits for children up to the age of 5 were free since they were paid for by the Department of Health and Hospitals.

A visit to the nutritionist was priced at $18 for third party charges and $3.60 for self-pay patients. Patients who saw only a nurse were charged $3.12 if they were self-payers and $15.60 if they had third party coverage. Mental health visits were not categorized as above, but carried a third party fee of $30 and a self-pay charge of $6.00. Laboratory fees ranged from $3 for a hematocrit determination to $21.60 for a glucose tolerance test, and were discounted by 80 percent to self-paying patients.

The Family Alcoholism Program grant specified that all services had to be free during the first year of the funding. Rusnak, the therapist, felt this was a negative factor in attracting patients since he believed that community residents tended to view free services as suspect and charity oriented. However, the terms of the grant permitted charging the same fees as the Washingtonian Center in the second year of the program. Ms. MacDougall, the program social services and community liaison worker, felt that price was not a major consideration when someone came in seeking aid in a crisis state of an alcoholic problem.

Fiscal Information

Financial information on SJPHC operations was not readily available since PBBH still was debugging the computerized reports it was providing the center. Cupples's May 1975 administrative report, however, indicated that the center's total operating budget for fiscal year 1975 (October 1, 1974, to September 30, 1975) was projected at $197,016.58. The FY '76 budget was projected to be:

Personnel (salary and fringe benefits)	$157,812.58
In-kind salary and services grants	115,168.82
Nonpersonnel costs	37,000.00
Total	309,981.40

This represented a 157 percent increase over FY '75. Cupples anticipated that the center would be approximately 70 percent grant subsidized in FY '75 with the rest of its income coming from third party and self-paying billing. He gave the following breakdown for his billable population:

Medicaid	34%
Blue Cross	34%
Self-Pay	25%
Commercial	7%

The center did not bill commercial insurers, however, and Cupples felt that it received only 50 cents on the dollar net of charges on combined billing to all parties, and only 40 cents on the dollar on billing to self-payers. The center could not bill Medicare yet but was attempting to obtain certification to do so and expected to receive it upon the opening of the new location. For self-paying users, the center followed a dunning cycle that consisted of sending out four bills and then dropping the matter—no collection agency was used. However, if the patient came in again, the billing began anew, including the old charges.

Through the expansion of services and projected increases in utilization, Cupples hoped to reduce the grant support to 50 percent within 18 months.

Facilities and Location

The center was located on the third floor of a 1912 vintage municipal building (Curtis Hall) a quarter of a mile from downtown Jamaica Plain. It housed a pool and gym along with some city government offices. The facilities were cramped, noisy, and accessible only by stairs. When the center was in the planning stages, the SJPHComm had not wanted to locate there, but no other site could be found. Cupples and all of his staff felt that the facilities were a major problem in marketing the center. However, a new site, 687 Centre Street, in the heart of downtown Jamaica Plain, had been leased, and the alcoholism program had in fact been operating out of that location since its inception. This was to be remodeled in the late summer and early fall of 1975 with a planned opening date of October 1, 1975. Exhibit 5-4 is the planned space allocation for the new building. Curtis Hall was to be retained for use by the dental providers, and repainted and renovated to a certain extent before they moved in.

Figure 5-1 (supra) shows the location of the old and new facilities in relation to the community, transportation routes, and other health care resources. Both were felt to be excellent locations and the Centre Street site was in an area that would facilitate multipurpose trips, thus enhancing the ease of using it. Parking was available at both sites.

The elderly did not find it particularly difficult to get around in the community unless their mobility was restricted. There was a possibility that this could be resolved by the acquisition of a special van solely for transporting them.

One of the staff noted that the Centre Street site had been functioning as a place where people would drop in and ask about the center, but she felt that this would not continue to be true when the center moved its complete operation into the Centre St. building.

Promotion of SJPHC

All persons who utilized the center were asked to indicate how they had heard of it. More than 95 percent cited word of mouth. Cupples suggested that this explained the pockets of SJPHC registrants that had developed in certain parts of the community (see Figure 5-2, supra).

There was no exterior identification of the SJPHC at Curtis Hall, and on the day of the case writer's first visit the building attendant was not sure where the center actually was situated. Cupples said that, until recently, there had been a sign in the lobby identifying the location but that it had been removed so that people would begin to think of Centre Street as the center's primary location. In the window, a large sign identified the center and its services. Coffee was provided to anyone who visited the center, even if they only wanted to pick up information on its services. The coffee cost the center $5 per week.

Cupples felt that the health committee (SJPHComm) was quite active in promoting the center to the various sources of funding and was aware of the importance of this activity. The committee was not involved, however, in formally promoting the center to potential users.

The SJPHC had three major pieces of promotional literature. The first was a single-page brochure (folded in thirds) for distribution by the center. It had been printed and paid for by the Peter Bent Brigham Hospital at no cost to the SJPHC. The brochures, containing information concerning the center's services, were given to all SJPHC users and were distributed by staff members when they called on community groups and by SJPHC public health nurses on home visits. There had been no direct mailing of these brochures or any other SJPHC promotional material to residents of southern Jamaica Plain. There also had been no broadcast advertising. Ten community organizations had been addressed by Cupples, Ms. Mpontsikaris, or a mental health social worker in the past year. They would have liked to have visited more groups but felt that demands upon their time did not permit them to do so.

The second promotional piece was a flyer describing the mothers' groups held at the SJPHC, focused on child-rearing problems. Participation in these groups was sought mainly from among center registrants. However, announcements also were placed in the local newspaper, the *Jamaica Plain Citizen,* flyers were distributed throughout the community, and SJPHC staff members visited local schools to speak to mothers' groups and sign their members.

The third promotional piece dealt with the family alcoholism program. Five hundred copies of a short blurb explaining the nature of the program were printed by the Washingtonian Center for $40.50, a cost covered by the program grant. The blurb was handed out to the program's clients and was sent to referral agencies. In addition, Stanley Rusnak, the program's therapist, wrote a biweekly column on alcoholism and alcohol education for the *Jamaica Plain Citizen*; in most other weeks, there was an article from the SJPHC that mentioned the center.

The staff of the family alcoholism program was acutely aware of the difficulty of marketing that service. Nancy MacDougall, community organizer for the program, said the community's residents were fearful of discussing emotional, mental health, alcoholism, or family planning problems—these were topics about which one did not talk. The result was that Ms. MacDougall felt that her job was primarily to "make the program acceptable and/or known to other organizations and agencies" in the community and thus to generate referrals from these agencies.

To this end, the program had conducted a direct mailing to 400 community agencies and organizations, and Ms. MacDougall spent 90 percent of her time establishing contacts with them. She estimated that 98 percent of all Jamaica Plain residents came in contact with one or more of these organizations at some time or another. She identified the police as a particularly interesting target for her efforts. In 1973, Massachusetts had repealed the crime of public drunkenness. This left the police in a difficult position. For years they had been locking up drunks; now they had to establish relationships with programs such as this to deal with them, and the change in police behavior was slow in coming.

Rusnak agreed that the center's main effort had to be in cultivating referrals. He recognized, nevertheless, that this required outreach to agencies and organizations was expensive from a cost/benefit standpoint. For example, Ms. MacDougall estimated that an average of ten agency contacts (five by telephone, one by letter, and four by personal visitation) were necessary to produce one referral.

Internal Communication

Cupples identified the role of intake worker as a crucial factor in any internal marketing program, particularly in relation to the elderly. There was general agreement among the staff as to the importance of the first contact with the patient or client but there was some disagreement over exactly what was required of a general intake worker.

The issue was a live one and was considered in staff meetings in planning for the move to the new facility. Representatives of the alcoholism and mental health services reflected their concern for identifying possible referrals and pinpointing problems in their areas by their desire for a well-developed intake evaluation. Other staff members, however, felt that it would be more successful in the end to gain patients' confidence slowly and have all staff members sensitive enough to the individuals' problems to be able to refer them to the appropriate service once a relationship had been established. Most of the providers seemed to feel that when they all started functioning in the same location on a comprehensive basis, a good internal referral pattern would evolve.

Other Health Care Resources Serving the Community

The sources of health care for Jamaica Plain residents were as follows:

Private physicians	38%
Hospital outpatient departments	29%
Neighborhood health centers	22%
Hospital emergency rooms (nonacute)	10%
Other	1%
	100%

The primary hospital sources were Children's Hospital Medical Center, the Peter Bent Brigham Hospital, and Boston City Hospital. The Faulkner had no outpatient department or emergency room and thus was not used. The neighborhood health centers most used were:

Martha Eliot Health Center	41%
Brookside Park Family Life Center	37%
Dimock Community Health Center	9%
Longwood Clinic	9%
Southern Jamaica Plain Health Center	4%
	100%

Dental care was delivered as follows:

Private dentists	74%
Hospital outpatient departments	14%
Neighborhood health centers	12%
	100%

There were 23 private physicians and 14 private dentists in Jamaica Plain, but in neither case did the majority of their patient visits go to residents. Figure 5-2 (supra) shows the locations of the private physician offices in Jamaica Plain. Cupples believed that an increasing number of physicians were leaving the Jamaica Plain area. He felt that the more affluent residents (seniors and others) continued to use the private physicians but that the other populations received a greater proportion of their care from hospital emergency rooms and outpatient departments and from neighborhood health centers.

Cupples and other members of his staff felt that the three neighborhood health centers were used by distinctly different market segments. Brookside Park Family Life Center had a large Spanish-speaking population and drew most of its people from the other side of the Penn Central railroad tracks. (Table 5-2 shows general registration data for Brookside.) Brookside had a number of specialties available but did not participate in the family planning project. Martha Eliot Health Center was not used by southern Jamaica Plain residents because of its low-income housing project location and image.

In general Cupples felt that he had good working relations with the primary health care resources in the area.

Summary

Cupples was faced with the task of marketing his new location and services. He wanted to increase billable utilization so as to reduce his dependence on grant support but at the same time to seek some more substantial grants, both federal and private. He felt he could increase registrants by some 3,000 in the first six months at the new location and by 4,000 in the ensuing 12 months, winding up with 18,000 to 20,000 patient visits per year for an average encounter rate of three visits per active registrant. He was particularly interested in meeting the needs of the elderly population of southern Jamaica Plain.

NOTE

1. Information on health status and needs in the fourth and following sections is drawn from *Ambulatory Health Care in the City of Boston*, ABT Associates, Inc., Cambridge, Mass., April 1974.

OVERVIEW OF CASE 8

Issues to Consider

1. How does the SJPHC define itself? What business is it really in, and whom does it serve?
2. What has attracted registrants to the center in the past and what have been the real limitations to utilization?
3. Are the SJPHC's service expansion plans appropriate in light of current registrant rolls?
4. Is financial viability a realistic goal?
5. Does the promotion of the SJPHC deal with the major issues?

Discussion

1. Definition, Organization, and Clientele

Like many organizations that just kept on growing after responding to an initial need, the SJPHC has lost its grip on what it is and who it serves. Although a community health center is unlikely to want to think of itself in terms of a business, its long-term need for financial viability forces a hard look at its capacity to meet its markets' needs.

A community's needs develop over time along with its changing demographics. Although the case identifies general demographic patterns for the area, the SJPHC does not have a mechanism for collecting accurate and updated data on its present registrants and potential users.

The case sets the SJPHC in a transition period, evolving from a noncomprehensive neighborhood health center into what its directors hope will become a comprehensive primary care health center. Its present amorphous organization and management make real leadership difficult and impede a unified image. Operation from two sites probably further confuses the public. And the center's lack of status as a legal entity cripples the administrator's authority in decision making. In fact, decision by committee (the SJPHComm) is a disadvantageous approach to the center's management.

The market segmentation presented in the case does not provide adequate information to design a marketing approach. For example, the age and sex data by census tract do not tell anything about income level, health status, ethnic group, or other critical factors. Yet the service providers attempt to categorize their patients as "working class males" and "working age females." The principals in the case seem to have made plans for the future based on assumptions of community needs and on present registrants who come from an admittedly small segment of the service area.

Combining resources from several different facilities and funding sources adds to the SJPHC's identity and management problems. And rather than determine an effective organizational structure, the administration prefers to let it evolve as the expanded staff functions in the new facility.

2. Attraction and Utilization

The center has always been identified with ob-gyn and pediatrics, so the high percentage utilization of these services is to be expected. Service levels provided were responding to historical patterns. The low utilization rate for mental health, nutrition, and alcoholism services may stem from a lack of promotion or convenient service hours, as indicated in the case. However, the level of service may be in excess of the population's needs. Although this may be unlikely, the point is that needs assessment must precede the decisions on levels of service.

The census tract map indicates that proximity to the center is a factor for many users. But what is it that attracts former residents to return for health care? Is it the quality? The personal service? The low price? The lack of competitive services in the vicinity? The answers could provide much insight in evaluating the center's services.

Many assumptions can be made about the reasons for low usage. For example, the elderly face a physical barrier in the three flights of stairs at the present facility. Working men may find the hours inconvenient. Teens may reject the "baby care" stereotype. Spanish-speaking and black community segments may be served adequately by other centers. But these are only assumptions. Until the SJPHC gathers concrete data on user and nonuser preferences, it cannot assess its services adequately.

Other sources of information are inactive registrants. Those who do not wish to continue with the center are dropped from the files. This is an efficient weeding-out procedure, yet those who drop are not asked why.

Table 5-3 Utilization of Services

Service	Capacity	Use	Percent Utilization
Pediatrics	20/day	15/day	75
Gynecology	30–36/week	25–30/week	85
Mental health	25/week	10–15/week	40–60
Nutrition	6/week	3/week	50
Alcoholism	n.a.	34 clients	Under-utilized

Along with the center's long-standing identity with limited services has been its link to the Martha Eliot Health Center and a welfare care image. The SJPHC's difficulty in developing an independent identity and a broader range of clients will continue to be a problem as long as its definition of itself is unclear.

3. Expansion and Underutilization

The SJPHC appears uncertain of its direction. Its existing services are underutilized (Table 5-3) yet it is expanding both types of services and number of hours offered to meet what seem to be community needs. Cupples's objective, to increase the registrant population to 10,000 within 18 months, would more than triple registrants without clearly identifying which population segments they will be and how demand will be stimulated.

The SJPHC's present active registrants average three visits per year. New registrants would be expected to visit the center with the same frequency. However, Cupples has not investigated whether an appropriate objective in meeting the full utilization goal might be to increase visits per registrant, not just total number of patients. In fact, users of new services, such as dental, may well be drawn from the center's existing registrants.

The case repeatedly states SJPHComm interest in meeting the needs of the elderly. Census tract data show a substantial number of persons over 65 in the center's service area. However, it has virtually no elderly on its present rolls. Offering of special services is not the total solution; locating, attracting, and then making services accessible to the elderly must be addressed.

4. Financial Viability

Many issues are tied to the SJPHC's ability to sustain grants and improve collections for a financially sound operation. The center's definition of itself and its image in the community may affect user attitudes about the necessity of paying bills. Collection policies play an important role, too, in its receipt of only 50 cents on the dollar on all billings and only 40 cents on the dollar on billing to self-payers. Pricing policies may affect users' impressions of the worth of the services.

Another factor is whether services are reimbursable by third party payers. Maximum use of the facility does not translate into fiscal self-support if bills for services go unpaid and therefore yield insufficient revenue. Increases in personnel without adequate assurance of greater revenues could easily produce a budget deficit.

Cupples hopes to reduce grant support from 70 percent to 50 percent in the next 18 months through service expansion and increased utilization. Given a FY '76 budget that is 157 percent of the FY '75 budget, it is unclear how expenses will be met on reduced grant support and uncertain collections. A policy of improving collections would be in order. Most important, however, is the development of a sound basis for projecting revenue increases.

A related issue is the role of the neighborhood health center in providing care to the medically indigent (26 percent of Jamaica Plain's population). Whether the center's goal of financial viability and a nonwelfare image can accommodate this population segment must be determined.

5. Segmentation and Marketing

The center suffers from the dilemma facing many organizations that must attract two separate markets: resource providers and service users. The SJPHC is straddling the issue as it attempts to move toward fiscal self-support. However, until it is entirely free of grant support, it must deal with these two major markets.

The SJPHComm has been active in promoting the center to funding sources but plays no role in reaching potential users. With greater reliance on revenue from service in the future, the SJPHComm must reexamine its role. Brochures and fliers have been developed to reach users of specific services. However, their distribution has been limited, and direct public contacts slim.

Given the center's lack of clear segmentation, it is easy to understand why a promotional plan has not been developed. The difficulties in finding users for the family alcoholism program may reflect the center's lack of a basic understanding of who it is trying to serve.

Part III

Elements of a Marketing Plan: The Health Care Marketing CAPS

The cases in this section focus attention on four controllable elements in health care marketing management. In consumer goods marketing these elements are referred to as the four Ps: product, promotion, place, and price. The environment in which the health care system operates differs substantially from consumer goods. Health care marketing CAPS recognizes key differences between the two environments. The acronym stands for:

C—Considerations or costs exchanged for health care
A—Access and/or availability
P—Promotion
S—Service development

Considerations or costs exchanged for health care (Chapter 6) go beyond the dollar price or cost to the consumer. They include things of value that often are nondollar costs: time waiting, opportunity costs, handing control of one's body over to another, having to admit to being sick, discomfort, inconsideration, loss of personal interaction, perceived lowered social status or self-esteem. If understood, some of these costs can be controlled or minimized, thus increasing satisfaction. This element is similar to "price" in goods marketing except that price in health care often is controlled by external forces such as reimbursement mechanisms and regulations.

Access and/or availability (Chapter 7) in the health delivery system are similar to the "place" or physical distribution element in goods marketing. Ironically, the common health care terms of "access" and "availability" contain a greater notion of consumer orientation (a component of the marketing concept) than the traditional consumer goods marketing term of "place" or physical distribution.

151

Promotion (Chapter 8) is another controllable element in the health care marketing mix that has caused serious problems. While promotion is an important element, it too often is assumed to be synonymous with marketing—thus ignoring all the other elements that make up marketing. In consumer goods marketing, the promotional element is composed primarily of personal selling and advertising. In the health care industry, the focus is on public relations and atmospherics. Advertising has become more important. The cases in the promotion section address two issues and types of organizations. Case 13, "The ABCs of CPR," considers how a public relations idea might be positioned in terms of the objectives of the total organization. Case 14 reviews some typical problems of fund raising in a health care setting.

Service development (Chapter 9) parallels product development in goods marketing. Many health care services are derived from technological advances rather than from the needs of certain market segments. Service development is a critical part of strategic marketing. Case 15, Colonial Manor Hospital, presents an opportunity to match various market segments and their potential to certain hospital outpatient services. Case 16, Good Samaritan (B), explores the use of marketing research to determine the possibilities for a new technological service. Case 17, Mount Carmel, deals with a decision to eliminate obstetrical services. Service elimination in the health area industry often is a reaction to the development of a problem rather than the result of a continuing evaluation.

Chapter 6

Cost

CASE 9: ADAMSVILLE HEALTH CENTER: THE COST OF HEALTH CARE IN A FREE WELL-CHILD CLINIC

In May 1980, free well-child clinics in Fulton County, Ga., were to convert to fee for service. The County Board of Commissioners and Health Department officials approved the transition to bring the county into compliance with guidelines of the Medicaid program (see organizational chart, Figure 6-1). Under Medicaid, the federal government reimbursed the county $25 per complete physical examination for eligible children. The agreement provided that if the federal government subsidized physicals for Medicaid children, it would not provide money for them.

On March 26, 1980, the receptionist at the Adamsville Health Center, one of 24 physical health centers in Fulton County (Figure 6-2), sorted the day's incoming mail. Opening a long, cardboard container, she unrolled a poster that read: "Remember. . . Starting May 1st we must charge for family planning and children's exams. Your charge will depend on your income and family size. See the receptionist for details." Walking into her supervisor's office she exclaimed, "I knew we were going to fee for service from that meeting last November, but this says, 'See receptionist for details.' What am I supposed to tell people?"

For the supervisor at Adamsville, the receptionist's query was the first of many posed by the 14-member staff at the clinic. At a meeting the preceding week, she had been informed of the impending change and could allay staff anxiety on some aspects of it. In addition, a class had been scheduled for April 24 to instruct the staff in handling various aspects of fee for service such as billing, etc.

Among the staff concerns was a question for which there was no ready response. As the primary care providers, public health nurses wondered whether imposing a charge for physical assessment would cause a major

Figure 6-1 Fulton County Health Department Organizational Chart

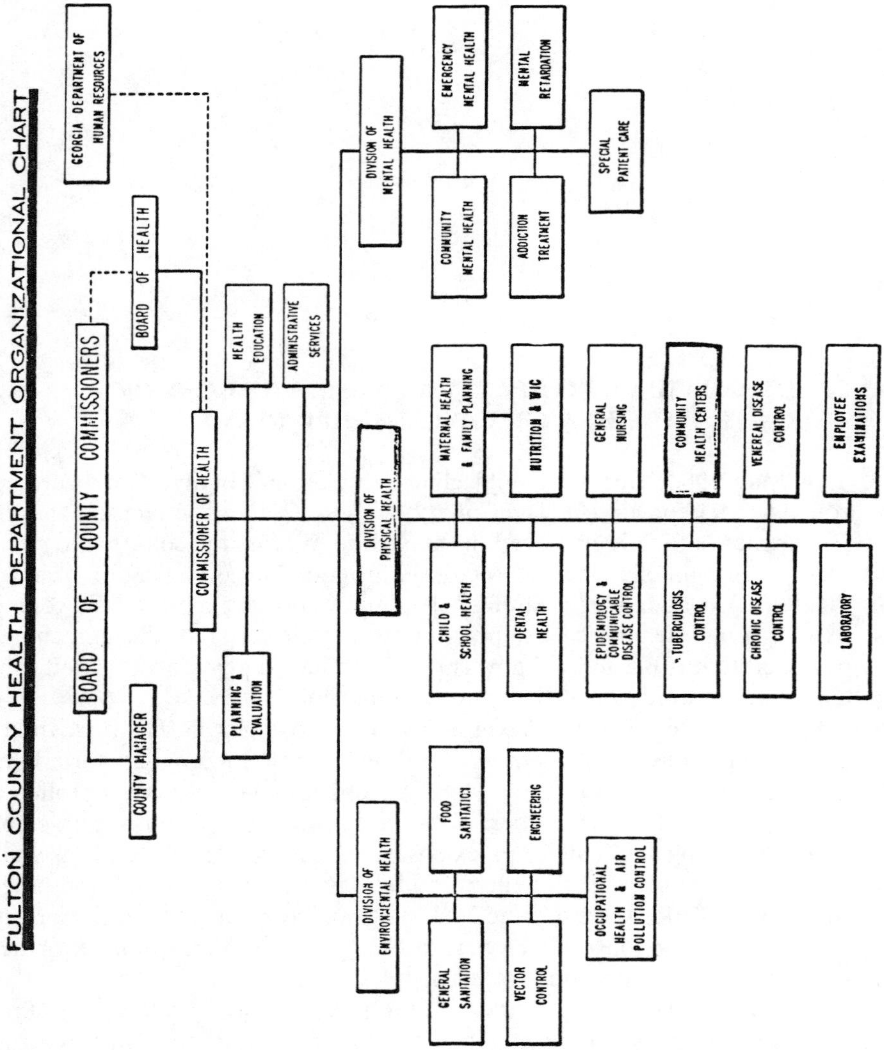

Source: Fulton County Health Department Annual Report 1978, Atlanta.

Figure 6-2 Fulton County Public Health Centers

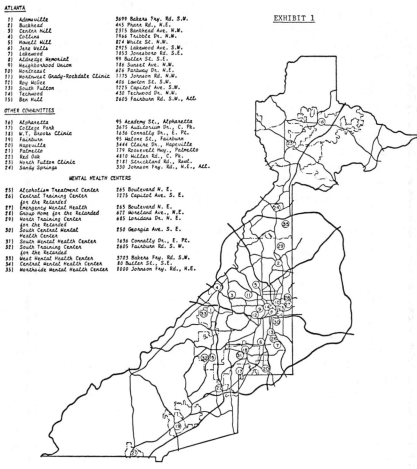

PHYSICAL HEALTH CENTERS

ATLANTA

1)	Adamsville	3699 Bakers Fry. Rd. S.W.
2)	Buckhead	445 Pharr Rd., N.E.
3)	Center Hill	2515 Bankhead Ave. N.W.
4)	Collins	1966 Tribble Dr. N.W.
5)	Howell Mill	824 White St. N.W.
6)	Jere Wells	2925 Lakewood Ave. S.W.
7)	Lakewood	1853 Jonesboro Rd. S.E.
8)	Aldredge Memorial	99 Butler St. S.E.
9)	Neighborhood Union	186 Sunset Ave. N.W.
10)	Northeast	626 Parkway Dr. N.E.
11)	Northwest Grady-Rockdale Clinic	1175 Johnson Rd. N.W.
12)	Roy McGee	406 Lawton St. S.W.
13)	South Fulton	1225 Capitol Ave. S.W.
14)	Techwood	430 Techwood Dr. N.W.
15)	Ben Hill	2605 Fairburn Rd. S.W., Atl

OTHER COMMUNITIES

16)	Alpharetta	95 Academy St., Alpharetta
17)	College Park	3675 Auditorium Dr., C. Pk.
18)	W.T. Brooks Clinic	1636 Connally Dr., E. Pt.
19)	Fairburn	95 Malone St., Fairburn
20)	Hapeville	3444 Claire Dr., Hapeville
21)	Palmetto	179 Roosevelt Hwy., Palmetto
22)	Red Oak	4810 Miller Rd., C. Pk.
23)	North Fulton Clinic	2181 Strickland Rd., Rswl.
24)	Sandy Springs	330 Johnson Fry. Rd., N.E., Atl.

MENTAL HEALTH CENTERS

25)	Alcoholism Treatment Center	265 Boulevard N. E.
26)	Central Training Center for the Retarded	1275 Capitol Ave. S. E.
27)	Emergency Mental Health	265 Boulevard N. E.
28)	Group Home for the Retarded	672 Moreland Ave., N.E.
29)	North Training Center for the Retarded	685 Loridans Dr. N. E.
30)	South Central Mental Health Center	250 Georgia Ave. S. E.
31)	South Mental Health Center	1636 Connally Dr., E. Pt.
32)	South Training Center for the Retarded	2605 Fairburn Rd. S. W.
33)	West Mental Health Center	3703 Bakers Fry. Rd. S.W.
34)	Central Mental Health Center	80 Butler St., S.E.
35)	Northside Mental Health Center	1000 Johnson Fry. Rd., N.E.

EXHIBIT 1

Fulton County Public Health Centers

Source: Fulton County Health Department Annual Report 1978, Atlanta.

target market to drop out of care. They reasoned that persons with incomes just above the level that would exempt them from paying for care might perceive even a small fee as prohibitive.

The client census could not be relied upon to assess the type of individual attending child health conferences. Persons made medically indigent by inflation were entering the clinic population. Therefore, if the client census remained constant, it could mask persons leaving service. The nurses feared that clients most dependent on the clinic for health care also would be most sensitive to monetary cost and that many would stop attending.

For the nurses at Adamsville, the health marketing issue was to determine the most effective means for gaining acceptance of fee for service. In light of known barriers to care, how could the present clientele be maintained and expanded? How might the organization enhance client perception of care? What would be the least costly and most effective means of reaching the target population?

History of Well-Child Clinics in Fulton County

The well-child clinics in Fulton County began in the late 1940s as an outgrowth of the Works Progress Administration (WPA). The WPA was a federal employment program to find jobs for (among millions of others) out-of-work nurses. It put nurses to work in home health care and at Grady Memorial Hospital. When the WPA went out of existence in 1940, the Fulton County Health Department began to use those nurses to set up well-baby, obstetrical, and venereal disease clinics around the county. By 1980, there were 24 physical health centers and 11 mental health centers in the department.

The health clinics were held in office buildings, schools, and churches, with local physicians conducting the physicals at a nominal fee. The clinics worked in coordination with Grady Memorial Hospital to serve the medically indigent. Their primary function was to provide immunization and health screening, referring persons with medical problems to Grady.

Over the years the child health clinic concept evolved into a child health program, adding services for illness prevention, health maintenance, and the treatment of minor health problems. In 1952 the City of Atlanta and the Fulton County Health Departments combined, increasing the number and quality of services. In the late 1940s and early 1950s, permanent health centers were built, staffed by public health nurses.

Expanded Role of the Nurse

Nursing responsibility and accountability grew with the expansion of the child health program. This trend also produced more clients to be seen and more difficulty in obtaining physicians to staff the clinics. In response to this need, a formal program to teach nurses the physical assessment of well children was begun in 1969. Since that time, specially prepared nurses had assumed an expanded role in the clinics by doing physical assessments. Physicians at the clinics saw only children who had been identified as having problems.

Advent of the Medicaid Program

The proposed change to fee for services in the well-child clinics had its origins in the Medicaid act of 1972. Among numerous other things, Medicaid offered financial incentives to provide well-child screening for the medically indigent. The significant difference of this aid from other programs was its specificity: $25 per well-child physical assessment.

In 1974–75, when Fulton County adopted the Medicaid program, it also instituted an elaborate system of recordkeeping in accordance with federal guidelines. In addition, certain tests, such as audiometric screening and urinalysis, were added. And, the upper age limit for children seen in clinics was raised from 6 to eighteen. In 1980, the county was expected to come into compliance with the provision requiring a fee for the well-child physical. Table 6-1 shows the method used to determine fees charged to each family for services.

History of Adamsville Health Center

When the clinic at Adamsville was founded in 1948, it was a rural health center with only one nurse. The public nurse spent most of her time in the community visiting families with newborns, infants, and chronic and communicable diseases, and conducting immunization programs. As the community grew, so did the staff and services at the center. More clients utilized the clinic for services such as child and maternal health and family planning.

As the community increased in population, it became part of urban Atlanta. A predominantly white area became predominantly black. A strictly residential area became combined residential, apartments, and commercial buildings. Concomitantly, the caseload and types of services at the public clinic increased.

In recent years, Adamsville was the second busiest physical health center in Fulton County. The center served a community of 40,000 residents. More than 200 children were seen in health conferences each month, slightly less than half of them Medicaid recipients. According to the Fulton County Office of Planning and Evaluation, 2,527 children were examined at Adamsville in 1978 at a cost of approximately $53 per physical assessment.

Table 6-1 Eligibility Determination

TOTAL ANNUAL GROSS INCOME
(Pay Category)

Family Size		0% (Under)	20%	40%	60%	80%	100% (Over)
1	Annual	5,340.15	5,340.16 – 6,140	6,141 – 7,010	7,011 – 7,890	7,891 – 8,770	8,771
	Monthly	445.01	445.02 – 512	513 – 584	585 – 657	658 – 730	731
	Weekly	102.70	102.71 – 118	119 – 135	136 – 151	152 – 168	169
2	Annual	6,983.27	6,983.28 – 8,010	8,011 – 9,160	9,161 – 10,300	10,301 – 11,450	11,451
	Monthly	581.94	581.95 – 667	668 – 763	764 – 858	859 – 954	955
	Weekly	134.29	134.30 – 154	155 – 176	177 – 198	199 – 220	221
3	Annual	8,626.39	8,626.40 – 9,900	9,901 – 11,310	11,311 – 12,730	12,731 – 14,140	14,141
	Monthly	718.87	718.88 – 825	826 – 942	943 – 1,060	1,061 – 1,178	1,179
	Weekly	165.89	165.90 – 190	191 – 217	218 – 244	245 – 271	272
4	Annual	10,269.51	10,269.52 – 11,780	11,781 – 13,470	13,471 – 15,150	15,151 – 16,830	16,831
	Monthly	855.79	855.80 – 981	982 – 1,122	1,123 – 1,262	1,263 – 1,402	1,403
	Weekly	197.49	197.50 – 226	227 – 259	260 – 291	292 – 323	324
5	Annual	11,912.63	11,912.64 – 13,480	13,481 – 15,410	15,411 – 17,330	17,331 – 19,260	19,261
	Monthly	992.72	992.73 – 1,123	1,124 – 1,284	1,285 – 1,444	1,445 – 1,605	1,606
	Weekly	229.09	229.10 – 259	260 – 296	297 – 333	334 – 370	371
6	Annual	13,555.75	13,555.76 – 15,550	15,551 – 17,780	17,781 – 20,000	20,001 – 22,220	22,221
	Monthly	1,129.65	1,129.66 – 1,295	1,296 – 1,481	1,482 – 1,666	1,667 – 1,851	1,852
	Weekly	260.69	260.70 – 299	300 – 341	342 – 384	385 – 427	428
7	Annual	13,863.84	13,863.85 – 15,910	15,911 – 18,180	18,181 – 20,450	20,451 – 22,730	22,731
	Monthly	1,155.32	1,155.33 – 1,325	1,326 – 1,515	1,516 – 1,704	1,705 – 1,894	1,895
	Weekly	266.61	266.62 – 305	306 – 349	350 – 393	394 – 437	438
8	Annual	14,171.92	14,171.93 – 16,439	16,440 – 18,705	18,706 – 20,974	20,975 – 23,240	23,241
	Monthly	1,180.99	1,181.00 – 1,370	1,371 – 1,559	1,560 – 1,748	1,749 – 1,936	1,937
	Weekly	272.54	272.55 – 316	317 – 360	361 – 403	404 – 446	447
9	Annual	14,480.01	14,480.02 – 16,797	16,798 – 19,114	19,115 – 21,430	21,431 – 23,740	23,741
	Monthly	1,206.67	1,206.68 – 1,400	1,401 – 1,593	1,594 – 1,786	1,787 – 1,978	1,937
	Weekly	278.46	278.47 – 323	324 – 368	369 – 412	413 – 456	457
10	Annual	14,783.09	14,788.10 – 17,154	17,155 – 19,520	19,521 – 21,886	21,887 – 24,250	24,251
	Monthly	1,232.34	1,232.35 – 1,430	1,431 – 1,627	1,628 – 1,824	1,825 – 2,020	2,021
	Weekly	284.39	284.40 – 330	331 – 375	376 – 421	422 – 465	466

Effective 2/8/80

Source: Georgia Department of Human Resources.

The federal government paid $25 per examination for Medicaid recipients, the rest of the cost being borne by the county.

The staff was composed of a nursing supervisor, nine public health nurses, a clinic nurse, a nursing assistant, and two clerks. Three of the public health nurses had advanced training in the physical assessment of children. There also was a dental clinic on the premises and a mental health center next door.

The Child Health Conference

Persons up to the age of 21 were seen in child health conferences. As part of the check-up, parents were offered information about nutrition, child growth and development, childhood diseases, and the treatment of minor health problems. Sick children were referred to a physician for treatment and other problems were referred to the appropriate resource for follow-up. The child health conference was in the business of prevention via health education, health screening, and intervention and referral for problems.

When a child visited the clinic, an overall health status evaluation was obtained. Height and weight were measured and iron levels in the blood (hematocrit) were tested in the laboratory. The public health nurse then obtained a medical history to identify risk factors. This was followed by a dietary review and a developmental test to determine whether or not the child could perform tasks appropriate to the age group. Specific problems identified during the interview or expressed by the parent were addressed by the nurse, and were evaluated further on the physical assessment. The assessment also included vision and hearing tests and (in older children) blood pressure readings. Finally, immunizations were given as required for diphtheria, tetanus (lockjaw), pertussis (whooping cough), rubella, rubeola, mumps, and polio. Families identified as needing further public health nurse supervision were rescheduled for clinic appointments or home visits by the nurses.

The Cost of Health Care in a "Free" Well-Child Clinic

At 10:45 a.m., a mother sits with her two young children in the waiting area at Adamsville Health Center. She is one of many mothers lining the rows of plastic chairs who have taken their children for check-ups. Waiting an hour or so, she mentally runs through the tests and interviews yet to come, the long bus ride to the nursery, and clocking in at work late.

Despite the hassles inherent to the visit, this mother was motivated to take her children to the clinic. She may recognize the benefit of health screening for the prevention and early diagnosis of problems. Perhaps one of her children has been complaining of an ailment or has shown a change in behavior. She may be interested in qualifying for Women-Infants-Children, a government supplemental food program. Or she may be present to fulfill a requirement to receive specific other Medicaid medical benefits or for a recommended physical for her child to enter first grade.

Whatever motivated the mother, her perceived benefit of a child health conference outweighed the barriers such as transportation, waiting time, and being away from her job. Other important influences on clinic attendance are the client's perception of staff attitude and treatment at the center.

In addition to these "invisible" costs of health care, a visible cost to be added in 1980 was that of fee for service. Up to then, health care at public clinics was provided at no cost to the recipient. However, beginning in that year, a system of billing the client was to be instituted. No one would be turned away if they could not pay; however, clients would be expected to pay for services according to their incomes and family size (Table 6-1, supra).

Fee for Service

It was generally recognized that preventive health services, such as the child health conference at Adamsville, could offset a high monetary and personal cost of illness. At the same time, the direct benefit associated with the cost of medical care for an illness was not as obvious in preventive care. Indeed, paying for health services without the motivating factor of an illness might keep some persons from attending the clinic.

Families with low incomes that are not eligible for Medicaid and are most dependent on the public clinic for primary health care are most vulnerable to fee for service. Payment for service may give these persons a sense of proprietorship and increased involvement with the community clinic. Conversely, it might be perceived as an obstacle to care for children, "when they're not even sick." Therefore, a marketing plan to increase acceptance of fee for service should be targeted to reach this group.

Methods available to the health department for reaching the public or influencing its perceptions differ somewhat from those in private business. There is no advertising department and only a limited budget for advertising. Programs to reach clients are coordinated through the health education department and may involve the offices of nursing, planning and evaluation, and administration. The responsibility for promotion should not be divided because that could dilute the impact of such efforts. There are many opportunities to contact the public such as television and radio

Exhibit 6-1 Example of News Release on Program Fees

Fulton County Health Department
Press Release
March 27, 1980

COUNTY TO START CHARGING FOR FAMILY PLANNING, CHILD
HEALTH SERVICE

Effective May 1, 1980, the Fulton County Health Department will begin charging for family planning and well-child services, including screening of children for health problems.

The federal government now requires all health departments to charge for certain services. Fees will range from 0 to 100 percent of the cost of services and supplies provided the client. The amount charged will be based on family size and income unless the client is eligible for Medicaid or Title XX.

Family planning services include a complete medical examination with breast and pelvic examination, lab work, counseling, and contraceptives. Well-child services include physical examination, dental screening, laboratory work, and immunizations (if required).

"The Fulton County Health Department hopes that our clients will understand the necessity for making these charges," says Dr. William R. Elsea, County Commissioner of Health. "We urge you not to allow these small fees to keep you from receiving these important health services. No one will be denied service because of inability to pay."

For further information call the Fulton County Health Department, 572-2927.

---

public service announcements and newspaper articles, community organizations such as clubs and churches, and direct patient encounters (Figure 6-3, Exhibits 6-1 and 6-2).

In summary, the Adamsville Health Center is a community-based, prevention-oriented, public health clinic. Prevention and early intervention for problems is the objective of the child health conferences. The service is open to everyone and was to be converted to a sliding scale charge in 1980. The future utilization and success of the clinic will be determined in part by client acceptance of fee for service.

Figure 6-3 Example of Program Fee Announcement

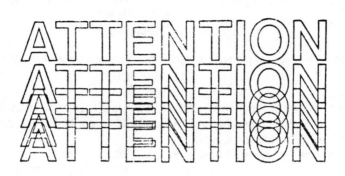

Starting May 1st we must charge for the following services.

FAMILY PLANNING: CHILD EXAM:

Initial/annual visit   Complete
Medical revisit   Partial
Supply visit (including supplies)
Pregnancy test

The amount charged will be based on family size and income unless the client is eligible for Medicaid or Title XX. You will not be denied service if you cannot pay.

For information call........ 572-2927

FULTON
COUNTY
HEALTH
DEPT.

Source: Fulton County Health Department.

Exhibit 6-2 Examples of Broadcast Announcements

ANNOUNCEMENT NO. 1:
COUNTY TO CHARGE FOR SOME HEALTH SERVICES

Beginning May 1st, the Fulton County Health Department will start charging for family planning and well-child services. Family planning services include the initial and annual visit, the medical revisit, the supply visit, and the pregnancy test. Child exam services include the complete physical exam. You will not be denied service if you cannot pay. For further information call the Fulton County Health Department at 572-2927.

ANNOUNCEMENT NO. 2:
COUNTY SETS CHARGES FOR SOME HEALTH SERVICES

The Fulton County Health Department will start charging for family planning and well-child services, beginning May 1st. Family planning services include a complete medical examination, lab work, counseling and contraceptives. Well-child services include physical examination, dental screening, laboratory work and immunizations. No one will be denied service because of inability to pay. For further information call the Fulton County Health Department at 572-2927.

This is Judy Stevens for the Fulton County Health Department at WPLO, together on your kind'a radio..

OVERVIEW OF CASE 9

Issues to Consider

1. Has the target market for the Adamsville Health Center been segmented to identify the population affected by the sliding fee scale?
2. Will the promotion techniques presented in the case bring about the desired outcome?
3. What strategy can be outlined for the marketing of the sliding fee scale and demarketing free care? How are the various internal and external personnel who may assist implementation of the strategy identified?
4. Is the sliding fee scale acceptable?

Discussion

1. Segmentation and Notification

Management and staff are concerned about the effect of implementing the sliding fee scale. It is mentioned in the case that there is concern "whether imposing a charge for physical assessment would cause a major target market to drop out of care." It is evident throughout the case that the public has been notified of the billing change. The problem has arisen in the area of understanding who this billing change will affect and what the impact will be.

It is possible to segment the target market by family size and income. By analyzing those currently utilizing the services, the population affected will become obvious. Only the market that will be affected by the change needs to be notified through promotional and advertising techniques. Management should take the time and effort to conduct this analysis since this program will affect the image of the center, the staff's confidence in handling the situation, and the consumer mix that will continue to utilize it.

2. Promotion Techniques

The message of the promotion campaign is that business is as usual except that those that are financially able to pay will do so based on the size of their family and its income. The desired outcome is that utilization levels not be impacted adversely.

Two items should be considered in the promotion campaign:

1. There may be an opportunity to increase the target market and include various groups who previously had rejected the services because the clinic had a welfare image.
2. Communication efforts need to be different for the various market segments that obtain their information in various ways. That is, different promotions should be addressed to clients affected by the sliding fee scale and to those not affected.

3. Marketing and Demarketing

The Adamsville Health Center case represents the marketing of one service and the demarketing of another. The service population may not be pleased with the sliding fee scale. Implementation of this change should include monitoring the competition and analyzing the services offered that will keep the consumer. The center does not want to lose its customers;

therefore, the program implementation must be sensitive to how the fee for services plan is accepted by its patients.

There always will be barriers to care. To compensate for this, the provider must understand the barriers and provide the consumer with appropriate compensation. For example: an increase in monetary cost requires a similar reduction in other barriers to care (waiting time, cleanliness, quality, personal attention). A major barrier is a misunderstanding of how the change will affect decision makers and their families.

Internal and external personnel are necessary to implement the strategy. The internal personnel are obvious: the medical and nursing staffs, laboratory assistants, and administrative individuals. The external personnel are community workers, county workers, neighborhood support groups, and community groups that have been advocates for the program.

To develop the marketing and demarketing strategies, management must communicate with the target population to understand the problems that will arise as well as how this change will impact on utilization and on consumer attitudes, perceptions, and preferences for the clinic.

4. Acceptability of Sliding Fees

Any review of the sliding fee scale should focus on the question of acceptability. Acceptability can be measured from the viewpoint of both the provider and the consumer. Providers will want to verify that this scale is comparable with others in regard to income and family size. Public acceptance of the sliding fee scale can be answered only by the consumer and therefore is an empirical question.

CASE 10. SUNRISE HOSPITAL: AN INNOVATIVE MARKETING STRATEGY

David R. Brandsness, administrator at Sunrise Hospital in Las Vegas, Nev., had just looked at figures that indicated that the hospital was underutilized on weekends. The figures revealed that the 486 beds at Sunrise had only 60 percent occupancy on weekends, compared with turnaway business on weekdays. This was a recurrent problem. Brandsness, in frustration, said to himself, "Our weekend census is below 300 and I know that by Tuesday night we will be turning patients away." He wondered, "How can we have increased utilization of our outstanding equipment and skilled personnel on weekends so as to eventually reduce patient costs and allow us to offer health services at the lowest rates of any private acute care hospital in Las Vegas?"

Background

Sunrise Hospital is a fully accredited private acute care hospital with a licensed capacity of 486 beds. Since it opened in 1958 with 62 beds, it had shown a consistent growth in both capacity and census, as shown in Table 6-2.

These expansions were accompanied by the development of an extensive range of ancillary services designed to meet both inpatient and outpatient demands. As a result of these programs, the hospital's share of the Las Vegas market had grown to approximately 46 percent of the total patient days recorded for the first half of 1976. This growth was expected to continue.

Market Demographics

Over the previous 15 years, the population of Clark County (Las Vegas), Sunrise Hospital's primary service area, had increased 162 percent for a

Table 6-2 Sunrise Hospital Bed Capacity and Average Daily Census

Year	Bed Additions	Licensed Capacity	Average Daily Census
1958	—	62	—
1961	66	128	82
1963	14	142	117
1965	174	316	124
1972	170	486	263
1976	—	486	363

Table 6-3 Population Growth of Clark County (Las Vegas)

Year		Population
1960		127,016
1970		273,288
1975		332,497
1980	(estimated)	435,000
1985	(estimated)	520,000

Source: Clark County (Nevada) Regional Planning Center.

compound annual growth rate of 7.12 percent. Clark County was the largest and fastest growing in Nevada and projections indicated its population would continue to expand at a 5 percent rate through 1985. Table 6-3 indicates that approximately 188,000 new residents were expected by 1985.

A survey conducted in 1975 of 5,584 admissions to Sunrise Hospital revealed the geographic dispersion shown in Table 6-4.

Market Share

Perhaps the most important measure of success Sunrise Hospital used was that its average daily census had increased at an 8 percent compound average rate between 1972 and 1975 (264 average daily census to 333) while total patient days recorded for all Las Vegas hospitals had risen at a compound rate of 4.74 percent. Sunrise had come to dominate the Las Vegas market, as indicated in Table 6-5.

Sunrise had achieved its market position by marketing its services aggressively to the medical and general communities. Recent innovations such as a satellite outpatient testing center, 24-hour pharmacy, and a laboratory pickup and delivery service for physicians' offices were indicative of the marketing efforts.

As Sunrise Hospital's market share approached the 50 percent level it gave a significant degree of stability to operations. The broad base of

Table 6-4 Patient Origin of Inpatients—Sunrise Hospital, 1975

Residence	No. of Admissions	Percent
Clark County (Las Vegas)	5,127	92.0
Other Nevada	88	1.5
Other states & foreign	369	6.5
Total	5,584	100.0

Table 6-5 Licensed Hospital Beds in Las Vegas Metropolitan Area

Hospitals	Licensed Beds	Percent of Total	1973	1974	1975	1976
Hospital A	211	16	9%	10%	11%	11%
Hospital B	278	21	27	26	23	22
Sunrise	486	37	43	45	45	46
Hospital C	269	21	15	13	16	16
Hospital D	62	5	6	6	5	5
Total	1,306	100	100	100	100	100

support required to sustain this dominance indicated that Sunrise was not overly dependent on any single group of physicians and could continue to exercise leadership in providing medical services over a broad range of specialties.

Sunrise had always been a financially stable operation. Some factors that contributed to this success were:

- The maintenance of a prestigious position as "the" hospital in Las Vegas.

- The relatively low (35 percent) number of governmental reimbursement type patients.

Medical Staff

The history of the Sunrise Hospital medical staff could be classified into three phases. At its inception, the primary support came from general practitioners, a limited number of internists, and fewer than six general surgeons. During the 1960s, a concentrated effort was made to attract specialists. This thrust, in the initial stages, was directed primarily toward internists and subsequently moved to other areas, including the subsurgical specialties.

In 1976, the medical staff consisted of 403 members. Of these, more than 50 percent had offices within a one-mile radius of Sunrise Hospital. Another major concentration of physicians was located between Sunrise and Southern Nevada Memorial Hospital, a distance of less than four miles. These physicians, like most of those in Las Vegas, had multiple hospital staff memberships. Seventy physicians limited their practice to Sunrise exclusively.

The Rebate Campaign

Brandsness recalled that other industries such as hotels and airlines offered special rates during certain times of the week to achieve overall efficiency, so why shouldn't an investor-owned hospital do the same?

After a careful economic analysis by his staff, Brandsness announced a revolutionary new health care policy: a 5.25-percent cash rebate on the total hospital bill of every patient admitted to Sunrise Hospital on Fridays and Saturdays. The program was advertised in area newspapers (Figures 6-4 and 6-5).

Brandsness stressed that the rebate program "will be paid directly to the patient by Sunrise Hospital and will have no effect on insurance claims." A patient admitted on a Friday or Saturday who is confined for a week, a month, or longer would receive a cash rebate covering the entire length of stay. Brandsness further stressed that the rebates "will amount, in all cases, to 5.25 percent of the entire hospital bill—not just for Fridays and Saturdays."

Within eight months the program had boosted weekend occupancy by 15 to 30 percent. More than 2,200 patient had received $190,000 in rebates, averaging more than $85 per patient. One of the largest amounts paid was to a juvenile involved in an auto accident whose bill totaled more than $22,000. The insurance company provided 100 percent coverage, thus paying the entire bill, and Sunrise rebated $1,164 to the youth.

Almost everyone was most happy with the plan. Doctors who in the past had been only on call on weekends now found themselves on the job. Doctors and nurses knew from the start that they would have to work a seven-day week. The biggest critic of the program, however, had been the insurance industry, distressed that rebates were to patients instead of insurers. Other hospitals in the area seemed skeptical of the whole idea.

The rebate program was abruptly stopped after 11 months. Brandsness said the "revolutionary" cash rebate plan was suspended because large insurance companies were keeping the 5.25 percent rebate for themselves. However, he said the hospital was pursuing legal action and intended to reinstate the program when possible.

"The rebate worked far better than we expected," he reported, adding that Sunrise had no price increases in the program's 11 months. "I don't know of another hospital in the western United States that can say that." He said the rebates amounted to $350,000.

He said the insurance companies believed that since they were insuring the patients, they should be the benefactors of the rebate. But Brandsness said that wasn't true because it was hospital profits that were redistributed

Figure 6-4 Example of Advertisement for Rebate Program

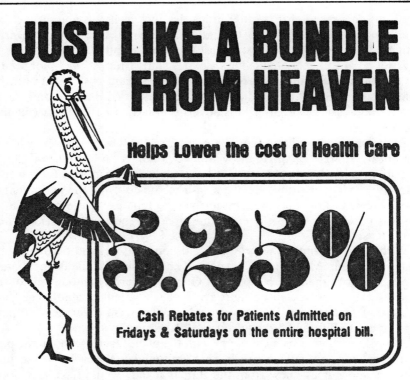

Source: Courtesy of Sunrise Hospital Medical Center.

Figure 6-5 Another Example of a Rebate Advertisement

TOGETHER
SUNRISE HOSPITAL and YOU

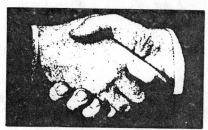

Lower the cost of Health Care

FRIDAY **5.25%** SATURDAY

Cash Rebates for Patients Admitted on
Fridays & Saturdays on the entire hospital bill.

Rebate to Patient NOT to Insurance Company

The purpose of this revolutionary health care innovation is to rebate to the patient the cash savings achieved by Sunrise Hospital if you as a patient choose to be admitted on Friday or Saturday when the demand for hospital services is low.

Our savings are passed on to you. It's as simple as that.

Sunrise Hospital Medical Center
3186 MARYLAND PARKWAY • LAS VEGAS, NEVADA 89109 • TELEPHONE 732-9011

Source: Courtesy of Sunrise Hospital Medical Center.

to the patients, not insurance money. What eventually killed the program, he said, was the insurance companies' deducting the rebate themselves before they paid expenses to the hospital. Some companies, he charged, even conspired to get patients to boycott the hospital.

Brandsness declared that hospitals must be allowed to initiate any cost-cutting innovations they could devise and not be hampered by outmoded concepts in hospital administration. "The health industry just tends to move at a slower rate. Other companies have offered rebates and felt no repercussions," he said.

Brandsness now had to face the same problem over again, i.e., how to get potential patients to check in on Friday or Saturday. In January 1977, he announced in newspaper advertisements (Figures 6-6 and 6-7) that a weekly drawing would be offered to patients who checked in on the previous Friday or Saturday. The Winner of the drawing, to be held on Monday, would win an all-expenses-paid vacation for two worth $4,000 to the vacation spot selected by the successful patient. There would be a drawing every Monday—52 weeks a year. Brandsness hoped this new idea would be as successful as the cash rebate without the repercussions from the insurance companies.

OVERVIEW OF CASE 10

Issue to Consider

1. What alternatives are available to the administration of Sunrise Hospital to increase weekend utilization?

Discussion

1. The Alternatives

The main problem examined in the case is how to increase weekend utilization and thereby improve the hospital's profitability. There are at least four alternatives available to Brandsness:

1. Reinstitute the rebate program and fight the insurance companies in court if necessary.
2. Continue with the drawings as begun in January 1977.
3. Eliminate promotions and use personal selling efforts and advertising to encourage patients to request weekend scheduling.
4. Create a new promotional program to emphasize weekend admittance.

Figure 6-6 Example of Advertisement for Vacation Prize

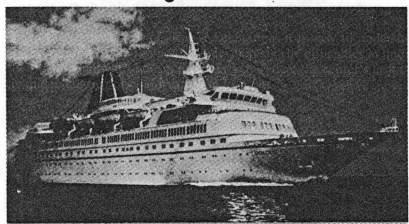

Introducing the Sunrise Cruise.

Win a once-in-a-lifetime cruise simply by entering Sunrise Hospital on any Friday or Saturday

RECUPERATIVE MEDITERRANEAN CRUISE FOR TWO

That's all there is to it! Just schedule your admittance into Sunrise Hospital for any Friday or Saturday. You'll be eligible to win a free recuperative vacation cruise for two. There's nothing to do. No obligation.

Why this offer?

On weekends Sunrise Hospital has an abundance of unoccupied beds. Yet our facilities and staff must operate around the clock on a 7-day schedule. This costs money!

To reduce operating costs we must even out this workload — make greater use of our facilities on weekends. By shifting weekday admissions to Friday and Saturday we can actually reduce per patient expenses. This will help hold down our rates.

Who is eligible to win?

Every patient who checks into Sunrise Hospital on a Friday or Saturday is eligible to win this free luxury cruise for two. There will be a new drawing every Monday.

You can't always select the day to enter the hospital obviously. But in many cases you can. So suggest to your doctor to arrange your admittance on a Friday or a Saturday. You may check out with an expense-paid "recuperative cruise" for two!

What do you have to do?

Just enter Sunrise Hospital any Friday or Saturday. One of the patients who checks in on either of these two days will win the cruise in the Monday drawing.

This is an expense-paid luxury cruise for two. And you'll have your choice of several cruises to be taken within the year. All first class passage!

Most important — there will be a drawing every week, 52 weeks a year! Come aboard.

Sunrise Hospital Medical Center

3186 MARYLAND PARKWAY • LAS VEGAS, NEVADA 89109 • TELEPHONE 731-8000

Source: Courtesy of Sunrise Hospital Medical Center.

Figure 6-7 Example of Another Vacation Plan Advertisement

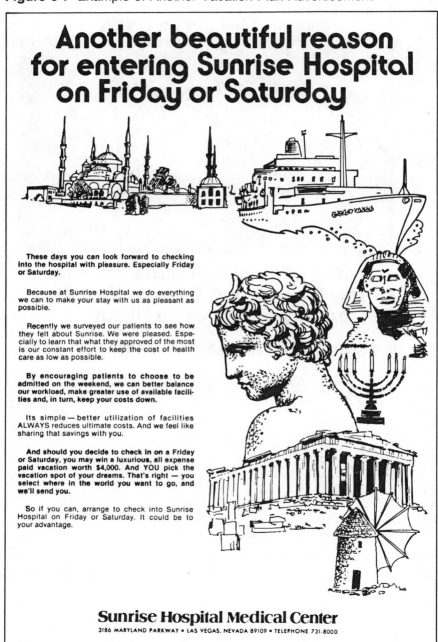

Source: Courtesy of Sunrise Hospital Medical Center.

An evaluation of these alternatives can consider a number of points. For example, although no specific costs were provided, it generally can be assumed that a highly significant part of overall expenses is fixed as opposed to variable. Thus, higher utilization becomes especially important to defray the costs over more patients. Another important factor is that of the sheer novelty of Sunrise's approach to marketing. Not only has the hospital increased profits by raising utilization and reducing per-patient costs, it also has acquired national recognition through its promotional efforts. It may be, in fact, that this will be of greater consequence over the long term. There are other factors:

- Despite the great success of the rebate program, such a confrontation with the insurance companies will entail a costly and time-consuming legal process. In addition, the potentially bad publicity for the hospital may negate any future benefits.

- Although the drawings for vacations have great promotional appeal, the actual attractiveness to patients is uncertain. Expensive, and presumably long, vacations might not be enticing to patients who cannot afford to take time off from work or who know they will be incapable of taking the trip until they fully recover—perhaps months away.

- The distastefulness of high pressuring sick persons could create highly adverse publicity for the hospital. Patients also may react by complaining to their physicians, thus endangering the hospital's present competitive position.

The development of a more broadly based promotional program not only should increase weekend utilization but also should create the favorable image Sunrise desires. Such promotion should feature the convenience and minimal disruptions to personal time schedules that weekend utilization offers to many busy people who require elective, postponable services.

Chapter 7

Access/Availability

CASE 11. WEST OAKLAND OSTEOPATHIC AMCARE CENTER: DEVELOPMENT OF A PROPOSAL FOR A HEALTH CARE FACILITY*

The Detroit Osteopathic Hospital Corporation (DOHC), chartered in 1919, is a Michigan not-for-profit company that owns and operates three hospitals. The original opened in 1919 in Highland Park (400 beds); Riverside Osteopathic Hospital was acquired by the corporation in 1944 (200 beds); and Bi-County Community Hospital in Warren commenced operations in 1966 (250 beds). Thus, by 1979 the corporation had a capacity of 850 beds. A central corporate operation provides centralized services, including materials and purchasing, medical electronics/biomedical engineering, communications, central word processing, and executive functions.

Since 1975, the DOHC had encouraged a merger of several hospitals in Detroit and, since 1977, had taken an active role in involving Detroit Osteopathic Hospital in this program. Detroit Osteopathic, Zieger Osteopathic Hospital, and Arts Center Osteopathic Hospital had approved consolidation and had filed a letter of intent under the Osteopathic Hospital Development Corporation with the intent of forming a hospital separate from the DOHC. A reduction of beds and more efficient use of resources would result. The DOHC would reduce its own beds to 450—a net loss of 400, or 47 percent. Detroit Osteopathic often operated at less than 50 percent of capacity, with resulting high costs per case. The physician staff was aging and there were few younger replacements.

---

* Information for the case taken from application 63-106-1 Michigan Department of Public Health Application for Certificate of Need Act 256, Public Act of 1972.

Proposed Amcare Center

The DOHC proposed development of an ambulatory care (Amcare) center in western Oakland County, outside Detroit, to serve the primary osteopathic health care needs of a six-township region (Figure 7-1). Ultimately, DOHC management saw the possibility of the evolution of the center into a complete hospital facility. Ambulatory and emergency services and a physician office building were to be included in the proposed Amcare Center, which would be on a 53-acre site. The center's main structure would encompass 15,000 square feet and the center itself would occcupy fifteen acres.

The center's thrust would be to coordinate all aspects of an organization designed to meet a perceived need for osteopathic health care delivery. Special concern for prevention and health education programs, in conjunction with diagnostic services and treatment, was emphasized in the planning. Staffing would be headed by a general osteopathic physician, who would maintain a general practice at the center. A pediatrician would be available for consultation. In addition, an obstetrician from the Botsford General Hospital would be available one afternoon each week. Botsford General is 18 minutes from the proposed Amcare site. An emergency treatment center would be located at the center, along with basic laboratory and radiology services.

In all, six physicians would be recruited to staff the center. The cost would be $445,000 for land, $1,575,000 for construction, and $300,000 for equipment, for a total of $2,320,000, with annual operating costs estimated at $1,000,000. It was anticipated that 25 clinic visits would be scheduled per working day and that 30 emergencies could be treated daily.

Amcare Location

The need for emergency services in the Amcare primary service zone, including South Lyon Township, Milford Township, Milford, and Wixom, was clearly evident. No emergency services existed. Moreover, these areas were not included in the primary zone of emergency services to be provided by the proposed Providence Center in Novi or the Ford West Bloomfield Center in West Bloomfield. Driving time to area health facilities is:

30 minutes—Pontiac Hospital, Pontiac
25 minutes—St. Mary's Hospital, Lavonia
30 minutes—Ann Arbor hospitals (St. Joseph's and University)
18 minutes—Botsford General Hospital
25 minutes—McPherson Hospital, Howell

Figure 7-1 Amcare Primary Service Zone (Shaded Area)

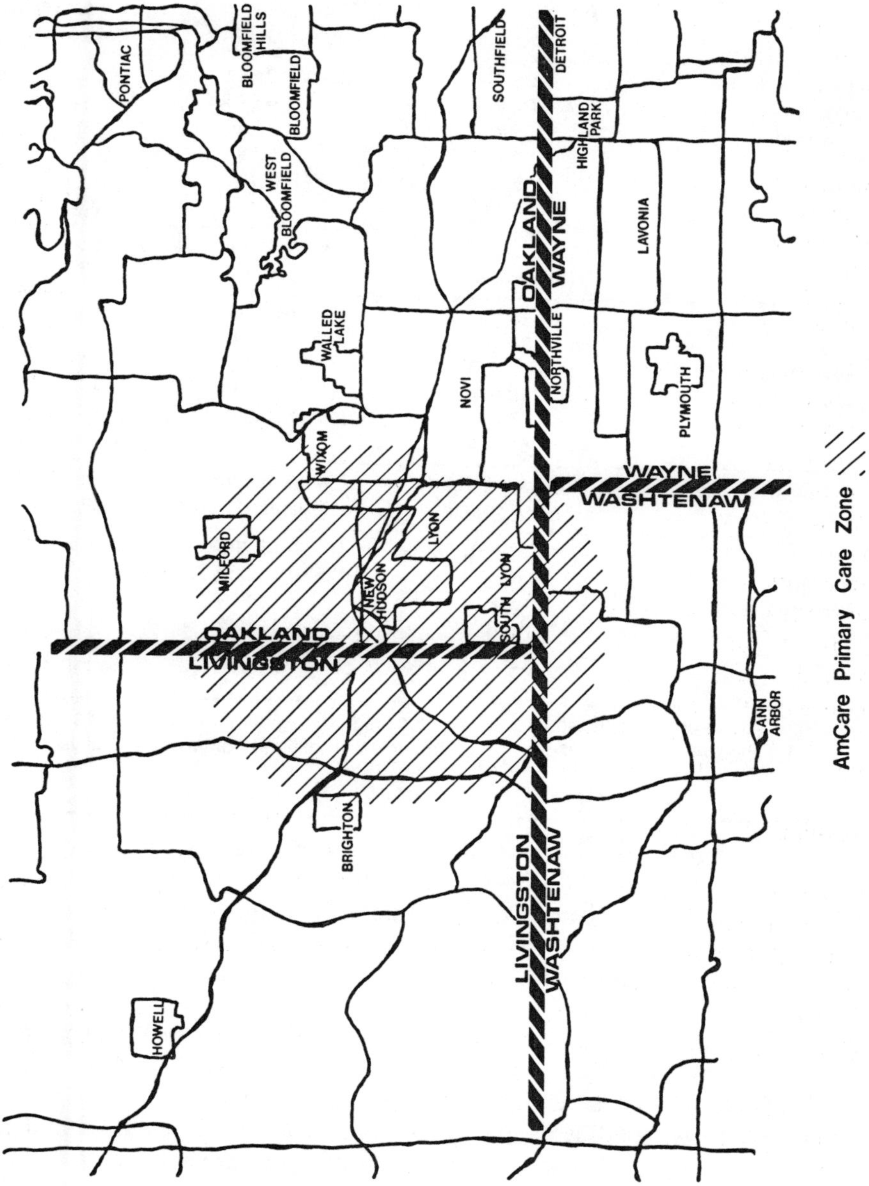

Shadowed section identifies primary service area for proposed Amcare Center.

Table 7-1 Population and Visit Demand for Amcare Primary Service Zone

	Total 1980 Population	Total Adjusted Population*	Visit Demand (3.2)++
Milford	25,774	(50%) 12,887	
Brighton	27,939	(25%) 6,984	
New Hudson	694	694	
South Lyon	10,284	10,284	
Wixom	5,426	(40%) 2,170	
Total	70,117		105,660

	Forecast Total 1985 Population	Total Adjusted Population*	Visit Demand (3.2)++
Milford	28,093	(50%) 14,046	
Brighton	24,142	(25%) 8,535	
New Hudson	763	763	
South Lyon	12,866	12,866	
Wixom	5,888	(40%) 2,355	
Total	81,752		123,408

	Forecast Total 1990 Population	Total Adjusted Population*	Visit Demand (3.2)++
Milford	31,416	(50%) 15,708	
Brighton	40,239	(25%) 10,059	
New Hudson	849	849	
South Lyon	17,042	17,042	
Wixom	9,448	(40%) 3,779	
Total	98,994		151,799

* Populations are adjusted to exclude those outside the Amcare primary service zone.
++ Adjusted population multiplied by 3.2 provides an estimate of yearly ambulatory care visits.

---

19 minutes—Henry Ford Hospital, West Bloomfield Ambulatory Care Center
10 minutes—Providence Center proposed facility, Novi
5 minutes—Providence Hospital proposed Family Health Care Center, South Lyon

The population density of the primary service area was 425.9 persons per square mile in 1975; by 1990 this was expected to reach 704 per square mile. Table 7-1 shows the distribution of population in the primary service zone, along with adjustments for present health care coverage and an estimate of expected visit demand for ambulatory care service.

In view of the perceived need for expanded emergency service facilities, tentative plans had been developed by various hospitals. Residents of South Lyon had encouraged Southfield Hospital to place a center in their area.

Providence Hospital, in Southfield, had long intended to develop a center in Novi and received its certificate of need a few weeks before the DOHC certificate of need was scheduled to be presented to the Comprehensive Health Planning Council of Southeastern Michigan.

The DOHC was quietly planning two additional centers similar to Amcare—one, near the Riverside Osteopathic Hospital in Trenton, was in an area designated as medically underserved, 18 to 20 minutes from Riverside Osteopathic; the other, in northern McComb County, was 30 minutes from the Bi County Community Hospital. The Amcare Center in western Oakland County, as proposed by the DOHC, would be the first to be submitted for certificate-of-need approval.

Planning History of the Amcare Project

From the beginning of the Amcare project, area health providers, physicians, hospital planners, and community representatives at all levels in western Oakland and western Wayne Counties were involved. As early as 1970, the Detroit Osteopathic Hospital Corporation board had authorized ambulatory planning and site reviews were conducted that year. In January 1976, at the urging of community leaders, the DOHC accepted an invitation to discuss mutual interests in providing health services and developing facilities for western Oakland County.

Physician Interviews and Needs Survey

In the fall of 1976, DOHC representatives began to assemble information collected from area physicians. Seventeen primary care physicians from Novi, Wixom, South Lyon, and Brighton were interviewed. The results indicated a consistent professional recognition of the corporation's activity in western Oakland County, with physician reaction ranging from extreme interest to guarded caution.

Following these interviews, the DOHC board of trustees authorized a mail survey of all 4,000 households in the proposed primary and secondary service areas, asking for information on perceived health care needs. Approximately 12 percent of the households responded. Twenty percent of the respondents agreed to serve on a special review board designed to analyze the DOHC plan.

The survey showed that 73 percent of all respondents drove 20 miles or more to see a physician, 47 percent 30 minutes or more, and 17 percent 40 minutes or more. It was concluded that these travel times and distances closely paralleled driving times to major shopping centers. Therefore, it was felt that services provided within shorter distances would not in them-

Table 7-2 Amcare Primary Service Zone by Physician Deficit

Year	Anticipated Visit Demand	Visit Supply 5,688 per year*	Anticipated Visit Deficit	Estimated Physician Deficit
1980	105,660	45,504	60,156	10.5
1985	123,408	45,504	77,904	13.6
1990	151,799	45,504	106,295	18.7

* Includes 70 percent adjustment for Brighton and Milford physicians. Providence Hospital Family Clinic physicians are included. Total of 8 equivalent physicians.

selves necessarily change long-used service patterns. Table 7-2 shows the physician deficit that the DOHC planning staff determined existed in the Amcare primary service zone.

A total public review of the DOHC western Oakland County plan was assisted by the 500 respondents to the survey. After receiving printed copies of the plan, all respondents were invited to attend a series of community meetings in the primary service zone of the proposed center. Dates and attendance were as follows:

Date (1977) and Location	Attendance
July 13: Northville	60
July 26: South Lyon	70
July 28: Novi	70
August 1: Walled Lake	30
August 10: Wixom	70
August 25: Milford	35
Total	335

Two full-time physicians, anticipated to be assigned to South Lyon, the site for the Providence Hospital Family Clinic (nonemergency/family medicine only), are included in the DOHC primary service zone.

Examination of the Providence Hospital data and cross-checking of the DOHC Amcare needs assessment demonstrate clearly that both the Amcare Center and the Providence Hospital Family Clinic are necessary to provide health care needed in western Oakland County. In fact, additional physicians will be required for the region in 1980.

In the series of meetings, the DOHC learned that area residents wanted a major hospital but would accept an ambulatory care center, as proposed. There was consistent support for a regional osteopathic ambulatory care service with an adjacent medical village. The DOHC also proposed development of a senior citizen resident complex, and, while this was received with enthusiasm, it was not adjudged a priority. Consequently, the objective would not be pursued until later. The most enthusiastic support of the

DOHC proposal was received from residents of Wixom and South Lyon. Among the 335 persons attending the meetings, there was a clear pattern of men and women willing to serve on joint advisory committees governing the clinic, with hundreds of others willing to phone, work, and do whatever was necessary to bring these facilities to their area. In all, 20 promotional mailings were distributed to the 500 respondents.

From the beginning, the Amcare project received considerable media attention from the *Milford Times, South Lyon Herald, Novi News,* the *Apinal Column* (Wixom and Walled Lake), the western edition of the *Detroit News,* and the *Medical Center News.*

The Existing Situation

The Providence Hospital in Southfield was hesitant to comment on the DOHC proposal. The Ford Hospital (West Bloomfield Unit) remained distant on the subject, and the McPherson Hospital in Howell, which at the time had a 63 percent occupancy, quietly opposed it. The Pontiac hospitals were openly opposed. While Botsford General Hospital supported the plan, the relationship between it and the DOHC had been clouded by years of conflict and competition, so that mutual trust and the possibility of coalition were lacking. The Greater Detroit Area Hospital Council supported the DOHC and had endorsed the merger of the inner city osteopathic institutions. In addition, the Comprehensive Health Planning Council staff and members were kept informed of the DOHC program.

On May 10, 1977, the certificate of need for the West Oakland Amcare Center was sent to the Comprehensive Health Planning Council for review and approval.

Epilogue

The Amcare project failed to receive approval of either the Comprehensive Health Planning Council of Southeastern Michigan or the State of Michigan. However, DOHC projects similar to Amcare in northern Macomb County and western Wayne County near the Riverside Osteopathic Hospital both were approved within 12 months after the Amcare Center was rejected. The attention attracted to West Oakland, the experience it provided, and the leverage of its failure can be seen as partly responsible for the success of the two additional outpatient centers—Southwest and Northeast. The Amcare project also was hampered by the failure of the inner city hospital merger, resulting from physician dissatisfaction with the proposed terms. Considered a high-risk project from the beginning, the

Detroit Osteopathic Hospital Corporation's West Oakland project placed the company in direct competition with the Henry Ford Hospital and the Providence Hospital, giving DOHC visibility by association with two of the finest health facilities in Detroit.

OVERVIEW OF CASE 11

Issues to Consider

1. Was the DOHC Amcare Center actually needed?
2. Was the research of physicians' attitudes and potential consumers' needs appropriate? Was the research complete? What additional research would have been valuable?
3. Was the promotion appropriate? How might it have been supplemented?

Discussion

1. The Need for a Center

The need for the ambulatory care center in western Oakland County was not established clearly, and both the Henry Ford Hospital and the Providence Novi and South Lyon Centers could easily fulfill the demand for health services in the area. However, primary and secondary service areas' needs were justification enough to warrant serious consideration of the DOHC by all parties, including the competitive hospitals and the news media.

While the Detroit Osteopathic Hospital Corporation was interested in development of the Amcare Center because it hoped that it might eventually become a hospital, it was understood from the beginning that hospital bed additions in the Detroit metropolitan area would be difficult to accomplish. Putting the DOHC in competition with Henry Ford and Providence Hospitals gave it added visibility, not only with the general public but also with the health systems agency and the Greater Detroit Area Hospital Council.

The case should be evaluated in the context of the DOHC and the benefits of a multihospital health system. The merger of the inner city hospitals was extremely relevant to the development of the Amcare Center and the success of that project could have had greater influence on the DOHC proposal. Amcare could have had an important role to play in the overall identity of the DOHC market position. The marketing of Amcare provided visibility in the context of "an honest health care provider trying to do the right things for the people." This context may have helped when the ambulatory centers near the Riverside and Bi-County Community Hospitals were presented to the approving bodies.

2. Adequacy of the Research

The survey of the 4,000 households in the service area suffered several serious deficiencies. First, it appears that it was designed without input from, or understanding of, consumer behavior for ambulatory care. The questions focused on length of time to access medical care when the real issues were what kind of care was desired most and how satisfied the residents were with current options. The 12 percent response rate should be viewed with extreme concern, since nothing is known about the representativeness of this small group. The same criticism can be made of the 17 physician interviews.

Additional research is needed on consumer attitudes and preferences on ambulatory care. Even though the population data suggest a need for a facility, the DOHC must develop an understanding of the factors that motivate consumer behavior in seeking health care.

3. The Promotional Aspects

The promotion of the Amcare Center was relevant only to the overall market position of the DOHC. The news media activity and the attention brought to western Oakland County did not have a significant impact on the success or failure of Amcare there. The statistical analysis of need and the interplay of the powerful health care providers were the determining factors. Community involvement was not sufficient to oppose the more powerful organizations. The "considerable publicity" appears to have been managed poorly. The DOHC did not establish objectives for the promotional efforts and thus did not prepare and disseminate messages that would have had the desired impact on specific target audiences.

CASE 12. GRADY MEMORIAL HOSPITAL: A PLAN TO IMPROVE UTILIZATION OF FOUR SATELLITE CLINICS

Dr. Dan Dragalin, medical coordinator of the Grady Memorial Hospital Satellite System, had been on the job for two months. His position, along with that of Ms. Marguerite Davis, administrative coordinator for the system, had been created to improve the effectiveness of four satellite clinics operated by Grady in Atlanta. The four centers (Figure 7-2) were created in the mid-1970s to provide primary care to patients who previously had used the Grady emergency room for nonemergency visits.

The four satellites had not achieved planned levels of utilization. The newly appointed directors were charged with developing a plan to improve the effectiveness of the centers as measured by utilization, cost per encounter, and possibly a reduction in the level of nonemergency visits at the Grady emergency room.

Development of Hospital Satellite Systems

A unique health care marketing problem concerns the delivery, in a consistent fashion, of ambulatory health care to the medically indigent of large cities. The medically indigent population is defined independently by state and usually includes residents who rely on a variety of city, county, or federal aid sources to support their medical care.

Thirty-one percent of the U.S. population is classified as urban, living in central cities with populations greater than 50,000, while another 21.0 percent live in central city counties and may be considered residents of the inner suburban ring. The population under consideration generally is densely packed, averaging 4,000 to 5,000 persons per square mile. The average central city resident faces a 9 percent greater chance of dying in a given year than one who lives in an adjacent suburban county and a 1.5 percent greater chance than residents of nonmetropolitan counties. Inner-city poor are especially at high risk. They make relatively few routine or health maintenance visits, particularly for their children, since doctors are scarce and costs are high in their areas.

Many cities have addressed the problem of providing health care to their medically indigent populations by establishing large county or county-city hospitals funded by the local government(s). A number of these (more than 500 beds) are affiliated with medical schools, providing mutual benefits: training sites for the medical schools and a relatively inexpensive source of medical personnel for the delivery of health care. In 1979, 53 state or local government hospitals with more than 500 beds were affiliated with medical schools. These totaled 1.3 million admissions and 17 million

Figure 7-2 The Grady Memorial Hospital Satellite System

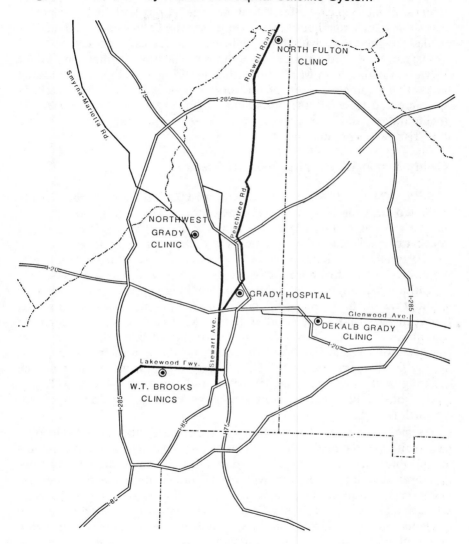

outpatient visits per year. In an effort to increase both the comprehensiveness of medical care offered to their target populations and to decrease access barriers, a number of these hospitals in the 1970s established satellite clinics designed to provide both well-care and sick-care services.

The satellites used a variety of methods to encourage utilization of their services, ranging from word-of-mouth advertising to well-designed formal marketing strategies, more of the former than the latter. The satellites were created to satisfy the outpatient health care needs, both immediate (acute illness) and long term (chronic illness and preventive services) of a high-risk target population (the urban poor).

Grady Memorial Hospital Satellite System

Since 1974, Grady Memorial Hospital, a 1,000-bed county-funded facility affiliated with the Emory University School of Medicine in Atlanta, has used a growing system of satellite clinics to satisfy the needs of its target market of medically indigent patients in the metropolitan area.

The system arose in the mid-70s largely as a result of independent neighborhood demand for more accessible medical services. Neighborhood associations requested an alternative to the "long trip to Grady" for those without means to obtain health care from the private sector. As a result, between 1974 and 1976, Grady satellites were established at preexisting Fulton and Dekalb County Health Department Clinic sites. The clinics were cosponsored by Grady and the county health departments. In addition to the Grady services, each facility houses a health department branch offering well-child, maternal, prenatal, and dental services as well as a variety of specific screenings for tuberculosis, venereal disease, cancer, and so forth (Exhibit 7-1).

As a result of this cooperation between the Fulton-Dekalb Hospital Authority and the health departments of the two counties, Grady patients could obtain a fairly comprehensive set of appointment-based health-related services in a setting removed from Grady's inconvenient downtown location. In addition, the patients have the option of returning to the same physician or nurse practitioner. The health care provider deals directly with patients' broad range of medical needs and also functions as a triage agent attempting to smooth coordination with subspecialty and inhouse needs at Grady. Because a provider repeatedly sees the same patients, preventive education also is enhanced.

By 1980, there had been 40,000 adult and 20,000 pediatric visitors to the satellite clinics. Sixty percent of the patients were classified as "medically indigent," with an additional 35 percent receiving aid through Medicare and Medicaid. Grady's sliding fee scale was applied to determine charges.

Exhibit 7-1 Grady Memorial Hospital Satellite Clinics

NORTHWEST GRADY CLINIC

The Northwest Grady Clinic (NWG) is at 1175 Johnson Road, N.W. It is Grady's first outpatient facility located away from the Butler Street complex. Its purpose is to make health care more accessible to the many eligible patients living in northwest Atlanta. The patient can save waiting and travel time by using this clinic. The clinic operates from 8 A.M. to 5:30 P.M., Monday through Friday. Grady cards are issued at NWG for patients who lack them.

The clinic provides general medical care and laboratory and x-ray services. It also contains a pharmacy. The staff includes internists, general practitioners, pediatricians, pediatric nurse practitioners, adult nurse clinicians, and medical technicians, as well as administrative and ancillary services personnel.

W. T. BROOKS SATELLITE CLINIC

The W. T. Brooks Satellite Clinic, at 1636 Conally Drive, East Point, is open from 8 A.M. to 5 P.M. It is Grady's second outpatient facility away from the Butler Street complex. Its purpose is to make health care more accessible to the many Grady-eligible patients living in southwest Atlanta. The patient can save waiting and travel time by using the clinic.

The clinic provides a pharmacy, laboratory, x-ray, health education, and social services. The medical staff includes pediatricians, internists, general practitioners, nurse practitioners, and public health nurses.

DEKALB/ATLANTA HUMAN SERVICES CENTER

Dekalb/Atlanta Human Services Center is at 30 Warren Street, N.E. The clinic is open from 8 A.M. to 5:30 P.M. Its purpose is to make health care more accessible to the many eligibles living in the Dekalb County portion of Atlanta.

The clinic provides general medical care that is comparable to the two other satellite clinics (NWG & WTB). Services offered are laboratory, x-ray, pharmacy, social services, and health education. The staffing also is equatable to the two other clinics: internists, general practitioners, pediatricians, pediatric nurse practitioners, adult nurse clinicians, and medical technologists.

Exhibit 7-1 continued

NORTH FULTON CLINIC

The North Fulton Clinic (NFC) is at 2181 Strickland Road in Roswell. The clinic hours are from 8:30 A.M. to 5 P.M. Its purpose is to make health care more accessible to the many Grady eligible patients in northern Fulton County.

The clinic offers all other services (limited) comparable to the three other clinics except x-ray. The services include pharmacy, laboratory, health education, and social services. The staffing includes an M.D. and two R.N.s.

The bill to most patients was $2, with small additional charges for medications.

The satellite system operates on an annual budget of about $2 million, provided by the counties and administered through Grady. The medical staff members are drawn from the Emory University faculty under the supervision of the Department of Preventive Medicine. Nursing is coordinated by the Grady Nursing Service.

Utilization of the system was less than anticipated. Many patients continued to use the Grady emergency rooms (250,000 visits per year) instead of going to the more convenient satellite facilities. In addition, several independent federally funded ambulatory clinics were established in the metropolitan Atlanta area, receiving about 40,000 visits per year.

The Development of a Marketing Plan

Dr. Dragalin and Ms. Davis, in their early weeks as satellite coordinators, had become familiar with the distribution, costs, and communications efforts. They believed many improvements were possible and undertook several initiatives in an attempt to increase utilization involving the development of consideration (price), access/availability (place), promotion, and services (product). Dr. Dragalin believed these efforts were essential to the development of a marketing plan that would address the perceived medical needs of the satellite system clients.

Cost (Price)

Price (cost/visit) was addressed through the increased use of nurse practitioners as providers, thereby cutting salary requirements. Heavier reliance on the more inexpensive generic drugs rather than upon brand names was emphasized to providers and pharmacists. Providers were urged to use restraint in ordering laboratory tests and radiographic procedures while still maintaining quality of practice. As one result, a reduction of 16 to 20 percent was achieved in x-ray usage without concomitant increase in morbidity. In addition, a nearly completed cost-benefit analysis of clinic operations was expected to result in the installation of an automated continuing comparison of provider techniques between clinics (laboratory tests, x-ray procedures, drugs ordered, patient volume per provider, etc.). The automated system would allow objective discussion of differing methods of health care delivery. Price also was considered in terms of nonmonetary costs to patients. An automated appointment system under investigation promised to streamline waiting times.

Access/Availability (Place)

Renovation or total reconstruction was planned at each of the four clinics. One clinic already had been totally renovated while another moved from a deteriorating old structure to a new, larger facility a mile from its original site. The larger facility was designed to house many county services (health, welfare, and social) to decrease inconvenience to clients. A free bus operated between the old and new sites, providing transportation from the old catchment area in an attempt to retain patients who might have been inconvenienced by the move.

In addition to structural changes, providers were urged to treat their offices as if they were in private practice rather than in public service. Plants, diplomas, and wall hangings were installed in an effort to replace decor that might remind patients of their welfare status. Future clinic placement was under investigation through a computerized demographic study of community needs based on census.

Random samples of patients were surveyed to determine convenience of clinic hours to the target population. Studies of the utilization of hospital emergency rooms by time of patient arrivals determined the volume of patient run-off from the satellites during nonoperational hours. This information was used as an aid in determining clinic hours.

Promotion

Promotion was handled through a segmented approach aimed at several different publics. The provider public was divided into several different groups. Medical house staff members providing inpatient care at Grady Memorial Hospital were urged to refer patients, once discharged, to satellite facilities for followup. An automated record transferral system was established to shift satellite records to the hospital whenever a satellite patient was admitted. This system contributed to patient care by offering a more complete set of medical data to the house officer. It also continually reminded the hospital physician of the existence of the satellites for future referrals.

In addition, efforts were under way to include satellite physicians in the hospital's teaching rounds. This was expected to decrease the volume of patients seen at the satellites because of physicians' intermittent absences while at the hospital; it was felt that this effort eventually would increase the volume of referrals from Grady. The system automatically referred high-risk newborns from Grady (6,000 deliveries per year) to the satellites for routine care. Promotion also was aimed at emergency room physicians at other hospitals, enabling them to refer medically indigent patients directly to satellites for continuing care. These physicians were provided with brochures that described the services offered by satellite clinics.

Promotion to the patient public used computer analysis of catchment areas for the satellites. Primary areas, which contributed the majority of patients, and secondary areas (urban sections not using satellite services) were identified. Advertising campaigns were directed at the two segments through neighborhood associations and various county agencies seeking to maintain the current market while developing new ones.

In addition, a "case control" survey of patients was under way using patients seen in the satellite clinics as controls. Cases included patients who lived in geographic proximity to the clinics but continued to use Grady Memorial Hospital during satellite operational hours. The study was intended to investigate demographics, health beliefs, accessibility, historical family usage, and perception of services received. Comparative analysis of the survey results was expected to yield information on patient perceptions.

Services (Product)

Finally, and most critically, the service offerings of the satellite system were under review. Formal interclinic peer review systems already in place were to be enhanced by an automated management information system (MIS). Selected clinical and administrative factors were included in the MIS to assist in the peer review process. Joint administrative and medical meetings of all clinic personnel then would be held at regular intervals to facilitate information exchange and problem discussion. These meetings were expected to help providers determine how their diagnoses and prescriptions compared to the rest of the medical staff.

Shared services, both clinical and clerical, were under consideration with the independent federally funded primary care clinics in Atlanta. Dr. Dragalin expected this effort to benefit the target population through improved coordination and communication among clinics.

OVERVIEW OF CASE 12

Issues to Consider

1. Why would a consumer utilize the emergency room over a more convenient satellite center?
2. What is the image of the satellite clinics from the target markets' viewpoint?
3. What single item seems to have the highest potential for success?

Discussion

1. Satellite Utilization

The case lends itself to speculation as to why consumers continue to utilize the Grady emergency room rather than turning to the more convenient satellite clinics. The following factors may be barriers to utilization: waiting time, scheduling, transportation, treatment hours, established patient-physician relationships, financial, facility reputation, and communication barriers.

To understand the actual and perceived barriers to care via the satellite clinic, input from consumers is essential. They are the only individuals who can identify the factors considered when selecting where to purchase the needed care. To understand the processes, and problems of the decision makers, the health care marketer needs to coordinate and conduct focus groups with the various market segments. Further understanding of the concerns of the decision maker can be elicited from personal interviews or mail or telephone surveys.

Surveying patients of both emergency rooms and satellite clinics through personal interviews will identify similar and differing characteristics of the two markets. Grady Memorial Hospital is interested in moving consumers from one source of care to another. An understanding of factors that motivate this behavior change can be answered only by the consumer. The following variables should be addressed in the survey analysis: age, sex, income, employment status, access to transportation, distance from clinic, type of payment used, and severity/immediacy of the medical problem.

2. Public Perception of the Satellites

The target market for the satellite clinics encompasses individuals who utilize the Grady emergency room for their primary care and are "conveniently located" near a satellite clinic. As described in the case, these individuals are characterized as low income, low mobility, and with a long-standing relationship to Grady's emergency rooms for primary care services.

Within this target market are segments to define, based on demographic, geographic, and psychographic characteristics. Distinctions also can be made between the actual market, the potential market, and the nonmarket.

The medical and administrative coordinators lack data on the image of the satellite clinics held by various key publics. An increase in the utilization levels of the satellites will decrease use of the emergency rooms. Therefore, it is essential to consider the image of the facilities as well as marketing and demarketing techniques and applications.

The image of the clinics can be measured by surveying all segments of the target market. Analysis of both satellite and emergency room consumers will permit contrasting the behavior of the two groups. There are many possible reasons why the satellite clinics are not being utilized at acceptable levels:

- The emergency room consumer is not dissatisfied with the service.

- There is no built-in incentive mechanism to change the present behavior.

- Consumers are unaware of services offered at the satellite clinic.

- Many consumers have a negative image of the clinics.

3. The Tool with the Best Potential for Success

The marketing concerns addressed in the case all were directed at the health care provider rather than the consumer. The case presented a marketing strategy addressing the concerns of the organization and the provider. The purpose of the strategy is to modify consumer behavior. However, it is unclear whether the incentives described would bring about the desired behavior change.

The single tool that seems to have the highest potential for success is the case-control survey. Analysis and interpretation of these data will provide an understanding of buyer behavior. Once that behavior is understood, the development of a strategy to provoke a behavior change can be established.

Chapter 8

Promotion

CASE 13. MOUNT ZION HOSPITAL AND MEDICAL CENTER: THE ABCs OF CPR

Mount Zion is a voluntary, nonprofit, teaching hospital and medical center with facilities for patient care, research, teaching, and community service. It is a Jewish-sponsored institution that was started in 1887 but now is utilized by the entire community of San Francisco and by physicians making referrals from all over Northern California.

Mount Zion Hospital and Medical Center has a total operating budget of $60 million, with 2,000 employees. It, therefore, is an important economic resource for the entire community and is one of its largest employers.

Mount Zion is a major heart and cancer center and one of the most complete resources for diagnostic services. It includes the Maimonides Rehabilitation Institute, an innovative Pain Center, and the Claire Zellerbach Saroni Tumor Institute. It has a major psychiatric program with inpatient, outpatient, and walk-in crisis clinic services. Mount Zion provides comprehensive maternal and child health services. Mothers and infants are transported from a very wide area. The Mount Zion Birth Center and the Care with Parent unit were among the first in the area. Mount Zion also is a regional center for renal dialysis. It occupies more than a complete city block, is licensed for 457 beds plus 36 bassinets, and has a large ambulatory service.

The hospital admits 12,000 patients annually and provides care in some 170,000 ambulatory visits as well as in an additional 10,000 home care visits.

The ambulatory services programs include an emergency room, an outpatient department with more than 25 clinics, a home care program, a complete range of ambulatory diagnostic facilities, clinical cardiology and pulmonary function laboratories, and physical and occupational therapy.

The clinical laboratories and diagnostic radiology provide some tests not done anywhere else in the area. Radiology includes new computerized axial tomography (CAT) for brain and whole-body scans.

Geographically, the hospital is in the middle of the city, bounded on one side by the wealthy Pacific Heights neighborhood yet being on the edge of the Western Addition, a predominately poor, minority area. The Western Addition was in transition, though, with new businesses moving into the area and many homes being renovated. The neighborhood was beginning to be seen as up and coming.

Mount Zion administers special programs for the economically disadvantaged, such as the Children and Youth Project sponsored by the U.S. Department of Health, Education, and Welfare. In addition, all of Mount Zion's services are available to the total community—regardless of ability to pay. Its cost for the care of those who cannot afford to pay in full exceeds $3 million annually.

Mount Zion is a major educational facility in the Bay Area, with undergraduate, graduate, and postgraduate training in the health care professions. It supports a house staff program costing $2.5 million a year that includes more than 100 medical students, interns, and residents in all the major medical and surgical specialties.

Under a formal affiliation agreement with the School of Medicine of the University of California, San Francisco, Mount Zion Hospital and Medical Center provide the teaching of certain required core subjects and electives for UCSF medical students as well as for those from schools all over the country. The two institutions also exchange house staff assignments in such fields as dermatology, medicine, surgery, clinical pathology, pediatrics, and orthopedic surgery. Formal departmental affiliations are in medicine, radiation oncology, diagnostic radiology, and psychiatry.

Research is an important aspect of the Mount Zion program with 40 projects supported by research and development grants from HEW and various federal, state, and local foundations and health agencies. Research and administration grants to Mount Zion total more than $2 million annually.

Economic Climate

The competitive environment is sharp in San Francisco. The city has 17 major health care institutions, including two county and two federal facilities. The local Health Systems Agency estimates there are 1,000 extra beds in the city. Occupancy at Mount Zion has been:

1976–77	81%
1977–78	77%
1978–79	73%

At that, Mount Zion's medical-surgical census was the highest of any private hospital in the city. However, generally low occupancy rates, rising costs, and duplication of services have put pressure on all San Francisco hospitals to cooperate more closely and even to merge. Mount Zion was intensely involved in a series of merger discussions with two other San Francisco hospitals between 1975 and 1978 but no agreements were reached.

Approximately 49 percent of Mount Zion's patients are over 65. Seventy-nine percent of its patient population comes from San Francisco. The city's population is roughly 600,000, with more than 20 percent elderly. In response to the needs of this population, Mount Zion has developed an extensive geriatrics program, including a day health care center, a fellowship in geriatric medicine, information, counseling and referral service, home care, health screening, and research into better ways to coordinate services for the elderly in the community.

One of the most serious problems facing the hospital from 1977 to 1979 was the ever-changing regulations involving reimbursement for Medicare and Medi-Cal patients. Some 70 to 75 percent of Mount Zion patients fall into one of these categories, and reduced reimbursements caused serious across-the-board budget cuts for all departments. In addition to reduced funding of government patients, the hospital's psychiatry program faced cuts of hundreds of thousands of dollars from outside funding sources.

Organizational Structure

Mount Zion is governed by a voluntary board of 30 directors. The executive vice president reports to this board; in turn, an administrative staff of 10 reports to that executive. Included in the administrative staff is the community relations director.

The board is guided by a statement of purpose that emphasizes the Jewish identity of the hospital and affirms its commitment to providing health services to the extent possible to persons who cannot afford to pay the full cost of their care. The statement also affirms patient care as the institution's primary purpose, with teaching and research being important functions.

Each year the board of directors approves a set of operational goals for the hospital. Department heads then write departmental goals that support and carry out the hospitalwide goals. Among the goals stated for 1977–78 were: "development of a community health education program."

The CPR Project

In keeping with the hospital's traditional emphasis on education, the community relations department for many years had offered speakers to community groups on matters related to health, including cardiopulmonary resuscitation (CPR). From 1976 to 1978, the community relations department, at the direction of the community affairs committee of the board of directors, and, with the impetus of P.L. 93–641 (the National Health Planning and Resources Development Act of 1974), looked for new ways to initiate health education programs in the hospital and the community.

A practicing cardiologist at Mount Zion who has worked nationally for a number of years in several areas relating to emergency coronary care proposed that the community relations department develop a handy, wallet-sized card on which animated figures would move to depict the motions of CPR. He felt people could review the card periodically to recall their CPR training so their memory would be fresh if they had to use the method in an emergency.

The community relations department recognized the value of making such a card available to the public, both as an educational service and as an innovative public relations device. The resulting card, "The ABCs of CPR," was a natural extension of the hospital's community education program. The project had four goals:

1. To develop an animated, wallet-sized plastic card that, when tilted, would depict CPR in motion.
   A. The card was designed to be used primarily to recall proper CPR technique after the person had taken a class on the method.
   B. The card's secondary purpose was to motivate people to learn CPR.
2. To distribute the card as a free public service to Mount Zion constituents as a component of the hospital's community health education program.
3. To make the cards available to the mass public by selling them at the hospital's production cost, thus maintaining a break-even budget.
4. To enhance the hospital's image as an institution concerned with the public's emergency needs.

In February 1977, development of the "The ABCs of CPR" card began. The animated drawings on the front were developed by the hospital's medical artist. The text was composed by the physician and the community relations staff.

The front of the card displays three pictures that depict the motions required for the ABC (airway, breathing, and circulation) sequence of CPR. The images illustrate the head tilt for establishing an airway, the technique of pinching the nose and forming a mouth-to-mouth seal for breathing, and the movement of the hands to compress the chest. When the card is tilted, the pictures appear to merge to create the illusion of motion.

On the back of the card, "The ABCs of CPR" are listed, with instructions for each step. There also is an illustration of the proper pressure point and the position from which a carotid pulse may be obtained.

After the material was reviewed by the hospital's legal counsel, a disclaimer was added at the bottom indicating that the card was not a substitute for taking a class and learning the proper technique for performing CPR and related procedures for special cases.

Test trials of the final artwork were made on several persons to be sure the drawings and the explanation were understandable—even to someone who had not taken a CPR class. As a result of those trials, the numbers "1, 2, 3" were added on the botton front to identify the starting position from which to view the card.

The card was endorsed by the National Committee for Emergency Coronary Care, a group of seven eminent physicians who were pioneers in development of such care across the country.

The card was copyrighted so that Mount Zion could retain exclusive rights to its production and could exercise some control over how it was distributed.

A packaging folder was developed concurrently. The folder tells how to manipulate the card and identifies other conditions in addition to heart attack when CPR can be used. The attention-getting folder with its slogan "You May Save a Life with CPR!" provides an additional opportunity to identify Mount Zion Hospital and Medical Center.

Since the hospital had never carried out a public relations project of such mass appeal, it was not known what kind of response to expect. In many cases the responses indicated unexpected needs, such as the possibility of companies' ordering large quantities of cards if they could add their own logo. That accommodation was made to meet consumers' demands.

Several requests were received for CPR wall posters. In response, an animated wall poster (with the same information as the card, printed on both sides), 8½ inches by 19 inches, was developed. Plans were being made to sell the poster, which was regarded as a perfect item to place by swimming pools, tennis and racketball courts, golf clubs—any place where sporting events are held. The poster also can be a useful teaching aid to CPR instructors.

Because of the overwhelming interest in the English version of the card, it was decided to produce similar ones in Spanish, Chinese, and Hebrew. San Francisco has large Spanish- and Chinese-speaking populations and the card was seen as a new entree into those communities. The card was developed in Hebrew because of Mount Zion's traditional ties to the Jewish community.

Volunteers were found to translate the card into the various languages. These translations then were corroborated by several other individuals to assure accuracy. The next hurdle was to find typesetters in these languages, which was done.

To respond quickly as new aspects of the project were recognized, simple typed information sheets were utilized rather than brochures or slick marketing pieces. However, "The ABCs of CPR" card sells itself because it meets a need, and the inexpensive, straight-forward marketing approach has been successful.

"The ABCs of CPR" cards were distributed to the "Mount Zion family" several days before a new conference that introduced them to the public. Employees received cards in their paychecks. Cards also were sent to the medical staff, the board of directors, auxiliary and volunteers, donors, the board of directors of the Jewish Welfare Federation, and the boards of its constituent agencies.

Cards also were sent to the following other groups that had an interest in CPR: members of organizations who had attended CPR classes at Mount Zion; public officials at all levels—from the Mayor of San Francisco to the then HEW Secretary, Joseph Califano; physicians who attend continuing education courses at Mount Zion; new house staff officers and new employees; 900 persons who have had heart attacks; administrators of San Francisco hospitals and of Jewish hospitals across the country; and Mrs. Jimmy Carter for her family and the Cabinet wives.

"The ABCs of CPR" card was introduced at a news conference on November 10, 1977. The session was covered by the local ABC affiliate (Channel 7), the *San Francisco Chronicle, San Francisco Progress, Jewish Bulletin,* four local radio stations, and Physicians Radio Network. In addition, news releases were sent to 200 media outlets all across the country. The press kit included a news release and a sample card. A history of the development of CPR and a copy of a Gallup Poll indicating the number of persons who had taken CPR courses in the country were included to help editors understand the universal application of the method and of the card.

From the news conference coverage the community relations office received 5,000 requests for CPR cards from individuals and organizations. Predictably, inquiries came from CPR teachers, health care professionals, and paramedics. But many were unpredictable requests such as from the owner of a car wash and from the proprietor of a funeral parlor. Each had had heart attack victims at their business. This unexpectedly large immediate response attested to the need for the card.

A news release on "The ABCs of CPR" generated a two-paragraph item in the March 24, 1978, *CHA News* (weekly newsletter of the California

Hospital Association). From that mention, more than 150 inquiries were received from hospitals throughout California. Twenty-two of those medical facilities purchased more than 6,000 cards for their CPR programs.

In addition, articles were printed by the California Department of Health in its *Emergency Medical Services* newsletter. In April 1978 an article appeared in the *Mission District News* and in May 1978 in the *Ragan Report* in Milton Moskowitz's column "Socialissues."

A condensed version of the news release was sent in June 1978 to the hospital associations in the 49 other states and the District of Columbia for possible inclusion in their newsletters. Indications were that hospital associations in Georgia, Kansas, and Oregon used the item. Seventeen inquiries were received from hospitals in those states, with 610 cards sold.

The following articles and resulting orders for cards also were generated by the condensed release:

The Midnight Globe, August 8, 1978. Circulation 1.4 million, 2,000 requests for cards.
Family Weekly, August 20, 1978. Circulation 12 million, 25,000 cards ordered.
Occupational Hazards, December 1978. A total of 250 inquiries received that generated large orders from many corporations.
Better Homes and Gardens, January 1979. Circulation 23 million, 20,000 cards ordered.

To keep track of how many responses each publication attracted, they were asked to print their initials as part of the address to Mount Zion. This was not always done, however, so the responses resulting from the following publicity are unknown:

Army Reserve Magazine, July–August 1978.
Emergency, July 1978.
Fire Command, September 1978.
Police Times, October 1978.
Marketing Communications, October 1978.
Forum on Medicine, February 1979.
Petroleum Newsletter, April 1979.

The outpouring of interest, the inquiries, and the orders received for the card confirmed the definite need for such a reminder on how to implement the method.

Project Finances

"The ABCs of CPR" project was recovering most of its production costs (excluding staff time). The original price structure was 35¢ each for orders of 1 to 15 cards, 30¢ each for 16 to 49, and 25¢ each for 50 or more cards—plus postage. It was estimated that costs could be recovered on the initial order of 50,000 cards on the basis of distributing 10,000 cards free, selling 10,000 at 35¢, 10,000 at 30¢, and 20,000 at 25¢.

The prices were established after totaling all costs of the original 50,000-card order. These included printing the wrap-around folder, die cutting, folding, inserting, typesetting, messenger service, phone calls, artwork, postage, paper, envelopes, photocopying, and miscellaneous expenses. Total expenses were $16,000 for 50,000 cards.

Summary

In all, 225,000 cards had been distributed at the time this was written in 1980. The community relations office had sent more than 2,000 information kits to individuals or organizations across the country who had inquired about the card.

Orders came from individuals and groups all across the United States and Canada and initially were filled by volunteers and staff in the community relations department. An order sheet was developed listing the prices and how the card could be purchased. A special receipt form also was designed. Financial procedures were developed for cash control, recovering charges, and sales tax records.

The types of organizations that order cards include corporate safety programs, ski patrols, nursing classes, CPR teachers, military units, hospitals, doctors and dentists, airlines, school districts, the American Red Cross, hotels, farm bureaus, insurance companies, the Federal Aviation Administration, banks, advertising specialty companies, construction companies, and church groups.

Most of the individuals in these organizations already had taken a CPR course and wanted the card as a review device. Many were in the health or safety professions and indicated that "The ABCs of CPR" card provided an extremely useful review tool that was important in their work.

Blue Cross of Northern California ordered 50,000 cards to be distributed through its group health plans to persons who had taken CPR classes. The organization's logo and the words "distributed by Blue Cross of Northern California" were added to the back; these cards were printed in blue and black (instead of the original red and black) to match the color of its logo. Blue Cross developed its own folder and a radio announcement to publicize the card and promoted it in its employee newsletter. In addition, it published a full-page advertisement in a Sunday newspaper supplement and used an item in *Blue Cross News*.

Because of Blue Cross's interest, it was anticipated that other insurance companies or businesses might be interested in distributing the card with their own logo. To accommodate that possibility, an information sheet was developed that explained the option to add an organization's name and logo to the back of the card for orders of 5,000 and above. A price estimate was included.

Although some organizations did express interest, no orders were received besides that from Blue Cross because of the expense involved in individualizing the card. However, a considerably less expensive means has since been developed to add the logo to cards that have been printed already.

It was particularly gratifying that many of the individual requests for the card were from persons who said the publicity had motivated them to learn CPR. Because of the card, several groups in San Francisco were motivated to take CPR classes at Mount Zion.

Through the card, the Mount Zion name has reached audiences that would not have been touched by the institution's regular publications or communications.

Recognition of the educational importance of the card was received by the publication of "Enhancement of Recall of Cardiopulmonary Resuscitation (CPR): Use of a Moving Image Card to Review the Dynamics of CPR" in the May-June 1979 issue of the medical journal *Heart and Lung*. The project has been accepted widely and has received two national awards: the MacEachern Award in Hospital Public Relations and the Association of American Medical Colleges Award in Medical Education Public Relations.

OVERVIEW OF CASE 13

Issues to Consider

1. What is the competitive climate for Mount Zion Hospital and what are the major target markets it serves or may serve in the future?
2. Is there a set of specific objectives that might help guide the community relations department in coping with the environment in which the hospital finds itself?
3. How useful are the four project goals in relation to the needs of the organization?
4. What evaluation can be made of the "ABCs of CPR" project?

Discussion

1. Competition, Survival, and Future Markets

Mount Zion, like many other urban hospitals, is in a difficult environment with respect to long-term survival. The case provides several critical clues. For example, since 1977 the annual occupancy rate has declined 4 percent each year. At that rate, the rate may hover just above 60 percent in less than three years. The likelihood for reversing the trend is not high, given the overbedded situation that exists.

The high volume of ambulatory care service is and will continue to be an important factor. As noted, the Western Addition is an up-and-coming area. The nature of the population (those interested in renovating and upgrading the neighborhood) is most likely to be better served by outpatient care.

The hospital has attracted a sizable elderly market. The elderly account for 20 percent of the population in the city, whereas in the U.S., only 10 percent are over 65. Almost half Mount Zion's patients are over 65 and many services are oriented to that market. As described, reduced reimbursement for Medicare and Medi-Cal produces problems for the hospital, particularly in maintaining and expanding programs for the elderly.

Given the current and potential economic problems, the hospital needs to develop emphasis on the higher reimbursement levels that might be attained from the new businesses coming into the Western Addition and the young adult market that appears to be moving in.

2. Marketing Objectives

The question is: How does the community relations department interface with the needs of the hospital? Objectives established by the hospital's marketing director might include:

1. To maintain the current usage and awareness level of the elderly market segment.
2. To create awareness and services to serve the potential growth markets (industry and young families) that are developing in the Western Addition. The objective is to stop the decline in occupancy and/or increase the share of ambulatory usage.

3. Goals and Objectives

To assess the card project, its goals should be viewed in terms of how they helped accomplish the organization's desired objectives. Unfortunately, the four project goals stated (there may have been others but they are not given) are not tied to the organization's needs, they do not have any quantitative statement by which success can be measured, and no time frame is provided for the project.

Specifically, the first "goal" actually is a tactic for using the organization's resources. Part A (to recall CPR technique) and Part B (to motivate learning of CPR) are objectives but are not designed for any viable market the hospital wishes to serve. Indeed, it may reach a viable market—but no market was identified. The question is, "to motivate what people?" This is an example of being all things to all people. The second "goal" also is a tactic, not a strategy, except that it is stated in terms of the community education program, for which no objectives were cited in the case.

The third "goal" also is a tactic except that it has a measure of success built in—to break even. Selling anything at production cost does not make it available to the mass public. It may make it more appealing to some segments at the lower cost.

The fourth "goal"—image enhancement—comes the closest to a workable objective. However, the case provides no indication of what the current image is nor any evidence of image erosion. To make this a truly workable objective, a level of current image needs to be stated. Without it, there is no way of knowing whether the goal has been reached.

4. Evaluation

The project certainly has received wide acceptance. It does facilitate the needs of the important elderly market segment. Unfortunately, that market never was singled out nor were objectives set that could be measured.

All the needed financial data are not provided in the case but the approximate cost of the 225,000 cards distributed so far can be put at $72,000 ($16,000 expense ÷ 50,000 cards × 225,000 cards distributed = $72,000). While the selling price was not given for cards sold through the *CHA News* (6,000 cards), other associations (610 cards), the articles (47,000 cards from three articles), Blue Cross (50,000 cards), and the balance to others, an estimate can be made:

1. Number of cards given away free = 10,000/50,000 distributed = 20% free or 80% sold
2. Number of cards sold = 225,000 × 80% = 180,000 cards sold
3. Average income from each card sold:

   10,000 at 35¢ = $3,500
   10,000 at 30¢ = $3,000
   20,000 at 25¢ = $5,000
                   $11,500

   $11,500 ÷ 40,000 cards = 28.75¢/card
4. Estimated total income = 180,000 cards sold × 28.75¢/card = $51,750

Based on the information provided in the case, the estimated income of $51,750 is $20,250 less than the $72,000 estimated expenses. Evidently the third "goal" will not be met.

There is no established method to measure the improvement of Mount Zion's image, so there is no way the fourth goal can be assessed. The tactic as set forth in the second goal has been met. It appears that some of the institution's constituency has been reached, as well as the "Mount Zion family." The first tactic was accomplished by the production of the card, and the implied objective of recall or CPR has been aided by giving cards to former course graduates. There is an indication that the card motivated some persons to take the course at Mount Zion as well as elsewhere.

CASE 14. THE SAINT ELIZABETH FOUNDATION: FUND RAISING FOR A HOSPITAL

On February 5, 1976, the board of trustees for the Saint Elizabeth Foundation asked the executive director, Joan Simmons, to evaluate the organization's entire fund-raising program. The board felt that, even though the foundation was only three years old, its fund-raising efforts should have been more rewarding. It wanted to know what needed to be changed to provide quicker and greater financial aid. She was to report her findings and propose a revised approach to the purpose of the foundation at the next board meeting in three months.

The foundation was the fund-raising arm of Saint Elizabeth Hospital in Pittsburgh. It was a separate nonprofit corporation through which all monies donated to the hospital were directed. The foundation's existence had been marked by three economically depressed years. Consequently, fund raising had been difficult and slow.

The hospital carried out a major construction/replacement building project during that period. Poor weather and labor strikes had interrupted it for several months. Inflation took its toll on the bond issue that was let by a governmental unit to finance the project. The $33.5 million construction budget proved insufficient and some major equipment had to be deleted temporarily. The new building became operational six months later than budgeted. As a result, the hospital lost more than $1 million in revenue and developed a severe cash flow problem. Management had taken a 5 percent reduction in salary; hourly employees were reduced 5 percent in hours worked, where possible, and a cost reduction program was under way.

Hospital Background

Saint Elizabeth Hospital was opened in May 1932 by the Sisters of Faith of Pittsburgh. Its capacity increased from 250 to 522 beds through several building programs. Through the years the hospital grew more valuable to the Pittsburgh community in the services it provided. Because of the recent construction, there was a new, enlarged emergency room; larger and additional surgical suites; an enlarged mental health center; an ambulatory outpatient surgery center; and an expanded clinical practice center. There also were plans for a clinical practice building that would include offices for private physicians and dentists.

The hospital extended its services to the community through outreach programs. Four years earlier, in a contract with the local county health district, the hospital had agreed to provide medical clinic services to persons and families in a large, low-income section. Residents there had no access to basic health care facilities. A similar inner-city health center was planned for the near future, also to be operated by Saint Elizabeth. The outreach efforts included a mobile rescue paramedic training program, three satellite community mental health centers, a children's program for emotional growth, a county juvenile prevention unit, and a mental health aftercare program called Tasks for Independent Living. All of its programs had helped to make Saint Elizabeth Hospital a vital asset to the Pittsburgh community and worthy of the financial contributions needed to keep it solvent and growing.

The Foundation

The Saint Elizabeth foundation was incorporated in June 1973. Up to then, the fund-raising organization had been called the Fund Development Committee. It was a structural part of the hospital organization. All charitable monies were funneled through that committee and were accounted for on the hospital's financial reports. The idea to establish a foundation emerged in 1970 with a long-term development program (not to be confused with a short-term effort such as corporate, business, and individual solicitation for a building drive). The long-term program was to be continuing and include provisions for annual giving, for memorial and special occasion gifts, and for deferred gifts such as life insurance agreements, wills, bequests, and trusts.

As the beginning of the expansion project drew closer, it became imperative to establish a foundation for two major reasons:

1. When the hospital went into debt for the new facility, its cash was committed to debt repayment. However, gifts separated into a foundation were exempt from that requirement, and the foundation trustees, rather than the bondholders, had control over such funds.
2. Federal controls under the Phase II of the Economic Stabilization Program directed that before any hospital could increase charges for its services, it had to use up all its reserves, including securities. Therefore, it was to the hospital's advantage to form a separate foundation and remove all gift monies from its accounting records.

Other factors in deciding to establish the foundation were:

1. A separate account would be set up for the foundation; no gift monies would be mingled with other hospital funds.
2. Unrestricted gift funds would be carried over from one fiscal period to another rather than cleared from the books on June 30, which was the practice in the hopital's accounting system.

3. The hospital would get full reimbursement from Medicare rather than having the donations deducted from the amount that program normally would reimburse.
4. The deferred gift potential would be increased; a foundation organization could serve psychologically as a stronger base for seeking and receiving charitable gifts in the form of trust agreements and pooled life income contracts.
5. There would be increased gift potential from foundations because foundations give to foundations.
6. There would be a possibility of acquiring private foundations. Because of restrictive regulations in the 1969 Tax Reform Act, some private foundations were expected to fold within a few years. Since the assets of some of these entities might be transferred to charitable, nonprofit organizations, there was a possibility that a hospital-related foundation might attract some of them.

The principal functions of the foundation were:

1. To inform, educate, promote, and otherwise encourage gifts for the benefit of the hospital.
2. To receive, hold, invest, disburse, or otherwise handle gift funds in harmony with donors' wishes and in conformance with the purposes of the foundation and the hospital. The gifts could include cash, securities, annuities, trusts, life income agreements, bequests, real estate, or other property of value.
3. To receive or acquire property for management (the physicians' office building, other properties).

Establishing a foundation would place the institution in a better position to strengthen the confidence of prospective and previous donors so they would give even more serious consideration to providing financial support, particularly large gifts, to the hospital in the future.

Organization

The Saint Elizabeth Foundation was composed of a 15-member board of trustees (drawn from the hospital's governing board, the hospital staff, the medical staff, and the community at large), an executive director, a public relations associate, and an administrative secretary (Figure 8-1). The executive director and the administrative secretary were on the payroll of the hospital, which was reimbursed by the foundation for part of their wages. Their employee benefits came through the hospital. The executive director was employed full time by the foundation, but the administrative

Figure 8-1 The Saint Elizabeth Foundation Organization Chart

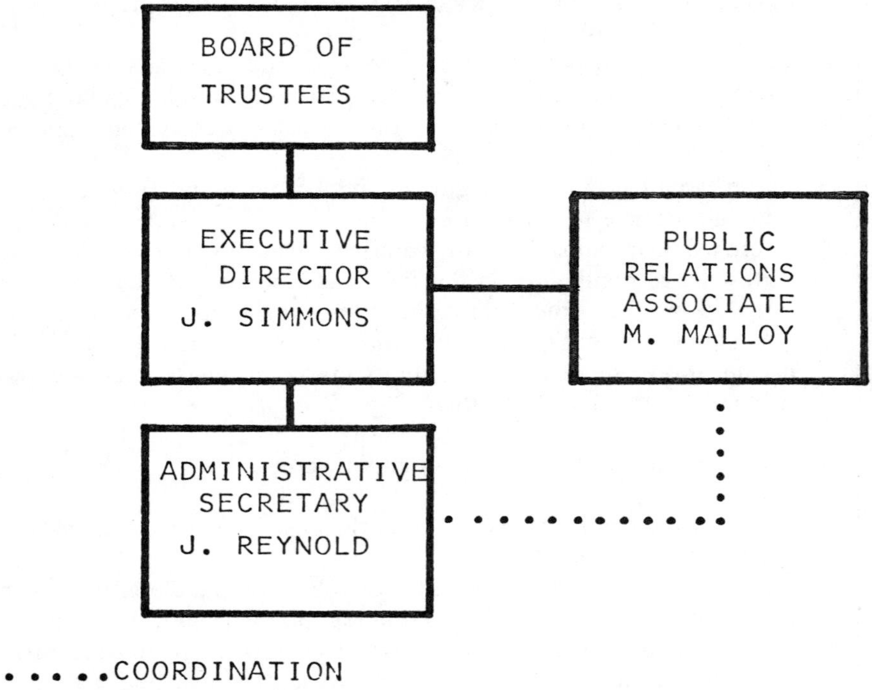

```
┌─────────────────┐
│  BOARD  OF      │
│  TRUSTEES       │
└────────┬────────┘
         │
┌────────┴────────┐        ┌─────────────────┐
│  EXECUTIVE      │        │   PUBLIC        │
│  DIRECTOR       │────────│   RELATIONS     │
│  J. SIMMONS     │        │   ASSOCIATE     │
│                 │        │   M. MALLOY     │
└────────┬────────┘        └─────────────────┘
         │                          ⋮
┌────────┴────────┐                 ⋮
│ ADMINISTRATIVE  │                 ⋮
│  SECRETARY      │ ⋯⋯⋯⋯⋯⋯⋯⋯
│  J. REYNOLD     │
└─────────────────┘
```

· · · · · COORDINATION

Source: St. Elizabeth Foundation records.

secretary's time was split between the foundation and the hospital public relations office. Exhibit 8-1 lists the duties of the administrative secretary.

The duties of the executive director were the most all-encompassing, as shown in Exhibit 8-2. She had the responsibility of handling the day-to-day operations of the foundation. She planned, organized, and administered all fund-raising activities, personally contacted all business and major private donors, ensured that all donations were acknowledged immediately and handled properly, prepared the annual reports, searched for philanthropic organizations from which to request donations and prepared all the correspondence involved, and originated the concepts involved in each publication before it went to the artist. So many administrative details required her attention that the contacting of prospective donors and the follow-up activities required in fund raising were neglected.

The board of trustees had six committees:

1. Executive Committee: consulted with and advised the chairman of the board on all matters pertaining to the affairs of the foundation.

Exhibit 8-1 Duties of the Administrative Secretary

RESPONSIBILITIES OF THE ADMINISTRATIVE SECRETARY OF THE
FOUNDATION—CLERICAL FUNCTIONS

1. Type general correspondence and materials relating to the foundation including meeting minutes, disbursement and fund transfer reports, fund balances and other reports for distribution.

2. Distribute monthly financial statements of the foundation account and other reports to the Board.

3. Type all publication and special printed materials copy including the foundation annual report, *Touch Hands*, case statement, equipment needs brochure, will brochure, etc.

4. Oversee all incoming donations and see that they are processed.

5. Type thank you/receipts for each donor.

6. Send advice letters to individuals being honored and to families of those being memorialized.

7. Acknowledge gifts made as a result of special projects (medical education mailing and Jody Wall committee).

8. Type weekly summary of all gifts received.

9. Maintain file on previous donors, recording background information on each donor.

10. Maintain a card file of recent donors, by gift category. This is used primarily in preparing donor lists published in *Touch Hands*.

11. Set up a tickler file on major donors. Be responsible for remembering them on their birthday, anniversary, etc. with a card from the chairman of the foundation board.

12. Maintain records on special income from projects such as the brick sale and note cards.

13 Maintain records on the *Wall of Life* (giving categories and donors).

14. Maintain records on physician pledges to Commemorative Fund and be responsible for sending out reminders of overdue payments.

15. Coordinate all foundation mailings with the mailing house.

16. Perform miscellaneous office procedures, including answering the phones, disbursing mail, etc.

RESPONSIBILITIES OF THE ADMINISTRATIVE SECRETARY OF THE
FOUNDATION—ASSISTANT FUNCTION

1. Provide assistance to the foundation executive director with special functions and projects including help on coordination and follow through.

2. Supervise production (work with art director, photographer, typesetter and printer) of printed materials to include case statement, foundation annual report, equipment needs brochure, will brochure, annual mailing, deferred giving newsletter, donor recognition and advice cards, gift envelopes, etc.

3. Assist in coordination of materials for the equipment needs brochure, foundation annual report, annual mailing, case statement, and other special brochures.

4. Handle design and production of refund wrapper special gift envelopes, similar brochures and programs, meeting mailers, Jody Wall committee mailers, etc.

5. Work with suppliers (printer, paper merchants and specialty printers) on bids for publications and printed materials.

6. Take minutes at foundation meetings and prepare for distribution.

7. Maintain accounting of monies received in foundation accounts. Review with totals prepared by accounting.

(continues)

Exhibit 8-1 continued

8. At the request of the executive director prepare comparative gift summaries by mailings, dollars given, donors by category, and funds by category.

9. Process disbursements and prepare report on disbursements from unrestricted or special purpose funds for the foundation board.

10. Do research on prime prospects which may involve trips to the court house, library and other resource places.

11. Assist the executive director in the design and ordering of plaques and other recognition items.

12. Assist with the formation and "staffing" of an organization of "Heart Care Alumni"—all former heart patients of Saint Elizabeth Hospital who have been discharged from the hospital's coronary care unit. The purpose is to stimulate financial support for this function of the hospital. This effort would include the identification of a volunteer core group, preparation and distribution of printed materials, conducting education meetings to which these alumni would be invited, and other related activities. (This was a planned new activity.)

13. Coordinate details on special events and meetings. Includes securing all visual aids and refreshments as needed.

14. Work with data processing in converting present mailing system to the computer and including donors.

15. Oversee all volunteer efforts and services in the department.

16. Attend administrative secretaries meeting and any other meeting that might increase knowledge in fund raising.

17. Attend one seminar per year to stimulate professional growth.

Source: St. Elizabeth Foundation records.

2. Disbursement Committee: authorized disbursement of money from any of the funds.
3. Finance/Investment Committee: invested, reinvested, and generally managed the assets of the foundation.
4. Legal/Accounting Committee: advised the board on changes in regulations and on legal matters.
5. Program/Project Committee: served as the nucleus for the entire board in planning, implementing, and administering fund-raising programs.
6. Donor Recognition Committee: handled special recognition activities for major donors.

Market Strategy

When Ms. Simmons became director of the Fund Development Committee in 1970, she began developing a mailing list. At that time the mailings were *Touch Hands* (the primary publication of the hospital through the years), the hospital Annual Report, and an annual solicitation mailed in December. The donor market was cultivated by mailings to individuals. If large corporate donations were solicited, the foundation had to register with the Chamber of Commerce to obtain permission to conduct a fund

Exhibit 8-2 Duties of the Executive Director

MANAGEMENT RESPONSIBILITIES ASSIGNED TO THE FOUNDATION
EXECUTIVE DIRECTOR

1. Provide general supervision of foundation activities.

2. Work with the hospital fiscal services department to maintain financial records, prepare audit information, and governmental reports for the foundation.

3. Provide staff assistance to the foundation board. Prepare and circulate agendas; approve disbursement requests; prepare new regulations and procedures as recommended by the foundation board; prepare special reports and do research as required; follow through on staff recommendations and board assignments.

4. Prepare and administer the foundation budget. Maintain budget control. Periodically review workload and statistics budget and revise each fiscal period.

5. Develop procedures for the operation of the department; develop and submit such procedures for inclusion in the Hospital Policy Manual and Cost Center Manual.

6. Establish foundation goals and time-table quarterly.

7. Develop a detailed written program of work for the foundation manual and implement.

8. Prepare a detailed printed statement on the case in favor of giving to Saint Elizabeth Hospital and the Saint Elizabeth Foundation.

9. Conduct weekly review of prospective donors to the hospital.

10. Make personal calls on potential donors (when possible with a member of the foundation board).

11. Plan a more detailed gift recognition program for donors, especially those who have given as a result of the commemorative brochure.

12. Follow through on restricted gifts such as landscaping to make sure donors' wishes are met—may include meetings with architect and prospective landscapers and donor. Follow through on gifts restricted for specified pieces of equipment.

13. Work with architect, necessary outside consultants, plaque manufacturers, etc. on development of the *Wall of Life* for the plaza area.

14. Work with donors on specific wording for plaques in new facility and on the *Wall of Life*.

15. Review all patient admissions adding selected former patients to the mailing list. Select easily identifiable previous donors and arrange for them to receive a flower from the president of the hospital.

16. Check daily newspapers for information about Pittsburgh area business leaders who are previous donors or who are prospective donors.

17. Provide conceptual assistance to the Hospital Auxiliary in planning fund raising projects and events. During the 1975-1976 year, special assistance to this organization as a consultant on the Autumn A'Faire.

18. Work with public relations director on opening of new facility. Initiate activities which honor donors such as a special luncheon or breakfast. Prepare a scrapbook for selected major donors of the event.

19. Develop concepts, write, and edit publications to include a case statement, equipment needs brochure, foundation annual report, annual mailing, will brochure, deferred giving newsletter, donor recognition and advice cards, gift envelopes, etc.

20. Determine printing specification for printed materials.

21. Investigate alternates on the annual mailing program and develop.

22. Develop and initiate more specific plans for a deferred giving program. To include preparation and production of a giving newsletter to be sent to previous donors. Distributed in March and August.

(continues)

Exhibit 8-2 continued

23. Prepare a special thank you mailing for donors at the beginning of the year to include a packet of gift envelopes.

24. Develop a special series of mailings for February and March—to be known as "Will" months each year.

25. Develop special mailings to foundations and local attorneys.

26. Work with department heads within the hospital on drafting grant proposals. Submit and follow through on these proposals.

27. Research the organizational structure of an associates group. Work with foundation board on establishing a special event this group could sponsor and do necessary staff work.

28. Research a special giving plan tailored for the Saint Elizabeth Foundation. An example is the Vincentury Plan.

29. Develop a special interest program in obtaining memorial gifts for the Saint Elizabeth Foundation by working with the area funeral homes. Program to include explanation to be used at the beginning of obituary column on how to make a memorial gift and a supply of gift envelopes.

30. Initiate a special donor recognition card to be used at the time of admission to the hospital.

31. Plan and execute special projects, presentations and events to include sale of calendar concept to other hospitals, sale of foundation merchandise such as x-ray prints and note cards; slide presentations, special meetings; special money making events such as an imaginary cruise, etc.

32. Plan and initiate special interest building programs which include health information forums, special seminars (estate planning) and a donor recognition day.

33. Attend educational and professional meetings.
   (a) Attend meetings of Pittsburgh Area Development Directors
   (b) Four meetings (one each quarter) of the Pennsylvania Association for Hospital Development held under the auspices of the Pennsylvania Hospital Association
   (c) Attend the annual meeting of the National Association for Hospital Development in Miami
   (d) Attend another national meeting which will assist in improving the general development performance

34. Attend meetings of the hospital department heads.

35. Attend special meetings of the Hospital Administrative Council.

RESPONSIBILITIES OF THE PUBLIC RELATIONS ASSOCIATE/FOUNDATION EXECUTIVE DIRECTOR

The public relations associate/foundation executive director is primarily responsible for developing and coordinating the preparation of *Touch Hands* and the hospital *Annual Report*.

The foundation administrative secretary is handling the production and coordination of these publications in consultation with the PR associate/foundation executive director so that her time is more available to donors and prospective donors.

1. Planning content and editing copy for *Touch Hands* magazine. Supervising an art director, artist, photographer, typesetter, and printer in the production and distribution of this publication. *Touch Hands* is published in August, November (special calender issue), February and May. (Public relations assistant is involved in planning and writing *Touch Hands*, excluding calendar issue.)

2. Planning concept, writing and editing copy for the hospital *Annual Report*. Supervising an art director, artist, photographer, typesetter and printer in the production and distribution of the report. The annual report is distributed at the annual meeting in September.

Exhibit 8-2 continued

> **3.** Determining printing specifications (paper and special treatments), working with suppliers (printers, paper merchants, specialty printers) on bids for *Touch Hands*, a special calendar issue and the hospital *Annual Report*.
>
> **4.** Prepare and administer portion of the public relations budget related to special printing projects which include *Touch Hands* and the *Annual Report*.
>
> **5.** Consult with the public relations director on special projects.
>
> *Source:* St. Elizabeth Foundation records.

drive in Pittsburgh for a certain period of time and toward a certain financial goal. That was not really what she had in mind for raising funds.

Ms. Simmons's philosophy about fund raising was that it was the end result of a long period of "friend raising." Donors made gifts to organizations about which they knew something. Involvement and participation of potential donors with the hospital and/or the foundation were essential to gift development. The long-range success of a program lay in turning noncontributors into contributors, the cultivation of new contributors into regular contributors, and the cultivation of regular contributors into everlasting contributors. Many friends in the community and a large percentage of former patients had the potential to make gifts to the foundation. They had to be kept informed about what was required to provide first-class services and facilities and about how important the hospital was to every person living in its service area so that the maximum gift potential could be realized. Small donors had to be encouraged to feel that they were valued supporters of a worthwhile cause.

During the previous four years Ms. Simmons's program for fund development had progressed through several stages:

1. Transforming the Fund Development Committee into the Saint Elizabeth Foundation, with its own annual report to the public.
2. Informing the public about the foundation through the quarterly magazine *Touch Hands*, the hospital *Annual Report*, the "refund wrapper" (a fund-raising gimmick wrapped around a refund check when a patient's bill was overpaid), letters, brochures, effective news media press relations, and good community relations.
3. Building a solid constituency of individuals, organizations (business, industry, charitable groups, foundations), and medical staff support; this was a continuing development—a never-ending solicitation for small donations.
4. Encouraging annual gifts from individuals and corporations by sending year-end mailings.
5. Encouraging memorial donations and gifts for particular occasions by including special envelopes in all mailings.

6. Encouraging major gifts by stating the hospital's needs for special equipment and furnishings and promising to commemorate donors by special recognition.
7. Establishing an associates' group, the Friends of Saint Elizabeth.
8. Promoting special projects such as the first annual Autumn A'Faire, which was organized to help draw public attention to the cause of Saint Elizabeth Hospital; it was a successful Gay 90s bazaar with entertainment, displays, and articles to buy.

The following fund-raising devices had not yet received any concentrated effort: a special giving plan tailored for Saint Elizabeth Foundation, deferred giving plans, and wills and bequests. One of these areas was to receive attention after the Friends of Saint Elizabeth program was operating smoothly.

The mailing list of 12,000 names was the foundation's primary market. It was segmented into foundations (1 percent), medical staff (4 percent), attorneys (4 percent), volunteers (6 percent), alumni (12 percent), employees (15 percent), former patients of the coronary care unit (15 percent), and miscellaneous community leaders and former patients (43 percent). The mailings to former patients were highly selective, based on information that would qualify them as good potential donors (location of residence, occupation, estimated income). The mailing list had been reduced recently from 14,000, with most of the names deleted from the miscellaneous group.

The foundation had no clear-cut financial goal. Its prime objective was to establish a solid, long-term development program, which meant starting small with a mailing list of good potential donors. During the initial stage, the board established a nebulous goal of $1 million to be achieved in 18 months (by December 31, 1974). According to Ms. Simmons, about 40 percent of that was attained. Part of the overall goal was to raise $200,000 from the physicians who used the services of the hospital, but after two and a half years the 116 doctors had pledged only $135,000. There was no concerted effort by the entire organization to achieve that goal. It was as if the board had said to the executive director: "There is the goal; *you* achieve it."

One problem was that the trustees were reluctant to solicit funds personally from peers in their respective business circles. They attended the quarterly board meetings and made suggestions but did none of the legwork involved in fund raising. In fact, it took a great deal of persuasion by the executive director to get some of the physicians on the board to permit use of their letterhead stationery in presenting the foundation objectives to the other doctors. When the foundation began, the trustees had been told that they would not be required to solicit funds. Newer trustees, however, were anxious to be active and not to be figureheads.

During the three years of the foundation's existence the executive director concentrated initially on building a strong mailing list, then branched out into activities (Autumn A'Faire and smaller events conducted through the volunteers). She sought direct donations through the mailings, then followed up with personal visits to major donors and important prospects. The concept of deferred giving was relatively new in the fund-raising field and she had not yet worked actively on it. She merely made appropriate literature available to anyone seeking it but made no effort to push that method.

The Friends of Saint Elizabeth project was about ready to be sent to the board of trustees and the hospital administration for approval. The Friends were classified by the amounts they donated: $100 annually, or $2,500 one time, or $5,000 as a deferred gift. In return they would receive special treatment at any time they were patients in the hospital. They would receive a hospital courtesy card, special linens, and special dietary and other services. Ms. Simmons proposed that the money received from the Friends be assigned to an endowment fund from which the principal could not be withdrawn for a certain period; only the interest could be used. She wanted a fund that would have an undiminishable long-term growth.

The foundation administered 26 funds into which donated monies were deposited. Donors could specify that their gifts be assigned to certain funds (called restricted funds) to be used only for purposes specified in their designation. Table 8-1 shows the total funds received for the fiscal years 1971 through 1975 and the balance of funds on hand. The sharp increase of 1975 over 1974 was derived primarily from the Commemorative Fund,

---

Table 8-1 Funds Received by the Foundation

Total funds collected for fiscal years:

1970-1971	$199,939
1971-1972	$271,492
1972-1973	$120,643
1973-1974	$175,519
1974-1975	$323,390

Balance of funds in the bank:

June 30, 1975	$572,522
December 31, 1975	$661,750

Major gifts for 1974-1975:

Philanthropic organizations	$36,224.22
Businesses	2,750.00
	$38,974.22

Source: St. Elizabeth Foundation records.

Table 8-2 Donor Responses to Mailings
           July 1, 1974 - June 30, 1975

Mailings	Number of Donors	Dollars Given
Alumni mailing	53	$ 586.00
Annual mailing	69	2,723.00
Annual report	24	1,120.00
Equipment needs brochure	0	
Foundation annual report	7	170.00
Funeral home	9	190.00
Medical education mailings	63	3,289.50
Refund wrapper	15	139.78
Touch Hands	109	4,997.42
	349	$ 13,215.70
Gifts not related to a mailing directly but in response to commemorative opportunities, etc.	446	286,044.30
	795	$299,260.00

Source: St. Elizabeth Foundation records.

which received $288,000 from many sources. Individuals donated funds to furnish individual rooms and provide new pieces of equipment in the new building and received special recognition for their gifts.

Table 8-2 lists the mailings conducted by the foundation in a year. The mailings informed prospective donors that literature was available on deferred giving plans (wills, life insurance, annuities). Table 8-3 shows the

Table 8-3 Donors by Category
           July 1, 1974 - June 30, 1975

Donor Categories	Number of Donors	Dollars Given
Alumni	41	361.00
Attorney	6	375.00
Major gifts	1	750.00
Coronary care patients	34	1,029.00
Employees	67	2,292.64
Medical staff	135	8,488.50
Major gifts	74	103,744.28
Miscellaneous	356	7,667.20
Major gifts	28	171,300.46
Volunteers	51	1,178.00
Major gifts	2	2,073.92
	795	$299,260.00

Source: St. Elizabeth Foundation records.

Table 8-4 Comparative Balance Sheet

	June 30	
	1975	1974
Assets		
Cash	$ 46,923	$ 656
Pledges receivable	94,088	
Investments	431,311	281,914
Accrued interest	2,225	5,468
Other	2,575	8,191
Total Assets	577,122	296,229
Liabilities		
Due to Saint Elizabeth Hospital	4,600	
Fund balances		
Restricted purpose fund balances	495,787	208,615
General purpose fund balances	76,735	87,614
Total fund balances	572,522	296,229
Total liabilities and fund balance	$577,122	$296,229

Source: St. Elizabeth Foundation records.

major gifts and the total funds collected during fiscal year 1974–1975. Tables 8-4 and 8-5 present the foundation's current balance sheet and income statement.

Awards

The foundation had been recognized as a progressive organization. It received the Award of Excellence for Total Development from the National Association for Hospital Development for 1974 and 1975. In 1975 the foundation publication *How Your Name Can Live On through a Gift to Life* received an award from the Beckett Paper Company and was exhibited in its display shown throughout the United States. At the 1975 National Association for Hospital Development, the magazine *Touch Hands* and the hospital *Annual Report* both received first place awards, the foundation *Annual Report* a second place, and a three-part fund-raising package (commemorative brochure, facts brochure, and the *Wall of Life* mailer) a first place.

The Future

Ms. Simmons felt that the foundation could grow faster and produce better results if she had a larger staff, greater involvement by the board

Table 8-5 Comparative Statement of Revenues and Expenses

	June 30	
	1975	1974
Revenues		
Support		
Contributions restricted for specific purposes	$294,774	$227,927*
Contributions for general purposes	,486	93,023
Investment income	24,093	18,614
Total revenues	323,353	339,564
Expenses		
Financed by restricted purpose funds	27,647	33,172
Financed by general purpose funds	19,413	10,163
Total expenses	47,060	43,335
Excess of support over expenses	$276,293	$296,229

Source: St. Elizabeth Foundation records.
* Contributions restricted for specific purposes in 1974 included $174,983 accumulated by Saint Elizabeth Hospital and transferred to the foundation.

of trustees, and more support from the hospital administration. She believed that with a staff of two assistant directors and two secretaries she could do everything she had in mind for developing an outstanding foundation. The assistant directors would handle the publications and special events and assist the director with deferred and major gifts, administrative work, and the compilation of statistics.

However, a substantial growth in the foundation would be determined by whether she could get satisfactory answers to the following questions: Would the foundation board of trustees and the hospital administration be willing to experiment with new marketing techniques? Would they also be willing to expand the foundation staff?

OVERVIEW OF CASE 14

Issues to Consider

1. Would the foundation have been better served if the hospital had undertaken a citywide drive in the early 1970s with emphasis on

corporate giving? Would this have helped establish St. Elizabeth's "need" in the minds of the residents of the service area?

2. Would a clearly defined dollar goal have been appropriate? Is there a need for a plan focusing on deferred giving?

3. Should the trustees have committed themselves to a participatory role upon establishment of the foundation? Is it possible to involve them in the activity at this date? What rationale would be used?

Discussion

1. Community Awareness

Often an institution's perception of community awareness is overstated. No positive opportunity should be lost to present and represent the current needs, plans, and future programs of the hospital since many prospective donors to the foundation might be available but perhaps unknown to the development department at any given time.

2. The Benefits of Goals

An established goal for corporate donations would be helpful since (1) it would establish a dollar goal for planning purposes; (2) it might induce the corporate community to contribute dollars not currently being donated elsewhere; (3) it might impress noncorporate givers that the business community also was supportive of the institution; (4) it would alert the larger community of the need for long-range support in order to continue first-rate health care; (5) it would prepare the groundwork for an "asking posture" for future activities; (6) it would provide media opportunities that in turn could highlight the hospital's services and thus generate more fund-raising possibilities.

Successful fund-raising drives for urban health care institutions are similar to successful programs in collegiate settings. In both, stated goals provide motivation, inspiration, and the opportunity to apportion the responsibility among volunteers and givers. No person likes to fall short of a personal responsibility for an overall goal. A foundation goal with specific dollar amounts should have been established with board commitment at the outset. Trustee involvement in goal formulation helps develop a sense of responsibility. A large foundation gift at the very outset could serve a positive psychological purpose.

The foundation trustees might espouse some of the things the hospital needs and invite a solicitation specifically for those items. This could be used as deferred or planned giving, and should be established as early as possible so that the entire philanthropic concept is imbedded in the minds of prospective donors, with a choice of the programs, trusts, pooled income funds, and so forth available for these types of contributions. To involve the young, affluent, prospective donor, it might be well to highlight the tax savings as well as the prestige of being a major contributor.

3. Trustees as Participants

All too often, highly placed citizens feel their personages and influence will be sufficient for trustee involvement with foundations. In the contemporary economic climate, the adage of "get, give, or get off" is appropriate. Participation on a peer-to-peer basis is something the staff cannot accomplish in the same way the trustees are requested and expected to do. The trustees must recognize their singular ability to solicit from friends, thus freeing staff members to solicit and plan in a way more suitable to their level. Trustees should be included as participatory workers in a foundation campaign at its outset, when a carefully detailed presentation of their individual responsibilities should be made.

4. Prestige and the Large Donor

The foundation was established to provide continuing support for the hospital irrespective of day-to-day situations. Thus, the trustees must be kept up to date on its services, projections, and so forth. Trustees may know of untapped resources. However, if the hospital's needs or plans are not known to the trustees, potential contributions may be lost. In other words, foundation trustees should have a working knowledge of the entire hospital's long-range plan(s).

If St. Elizabeth is not a specialty hospital, efforts must be directed to those who might be more interested in underwriting particular (specialty) services.

Chapter 9

Service Development

CASE 15. COLONIAL MANOR HOSPITAL: MARKETING OF OUTPATIENT SERVICES

In December 1975, Robert L. Kidd, chief administrative officer of the Colonial Manor Hospital of Florence, Ala., was reviewing its operations and drafting a development plan to be submitted to his administrative board. He felt several developments in the health care field both nationally and locally made it necessary that Colonial Manor intensify its marketing efforts in the future. He believed a systematic marketing approach with a specific plan would be essential to maintain its competitive position in the area and a satisfactory level of earnings as a private hospital. He also felt that the institution should develop both outpatient and inpatient services to utilize its capacity fully and increase overall earnings. First, he concentrated on developing outpatient utilization.

Background

Colonial Manor Hospital was built in 1965 as a nursing home, then converted to a 79-bed hospital. Humana, a national chain of investor-owned hospitals, purchased the facility in 1969 and added a 21-bed wing, bringing the bed count to 100. In 1975, the hospital operated at 89 percent occupancy and was in the process of expanding to 155 beds.

There are several hospitals in the vicinity of Florence and the Tricities of Tuscumbia, Sheffield, and Muscle Shoals (Figure 9-1). The Eliza Coffee Memorial Hospital in Florence is the largest, with 296 beds. Colbert County Hospital and Coffee Memorial were both undertaking expansion programs that would add a total of about 96 beds to their capacities. Coffee Memorial has a physical therapy wing affiliated with a crippled children's program. The hospital serves as a regional mental health center and is the primary community emergency center.

Figure 9-1 Geographic Location of Colonial Manor Hospital

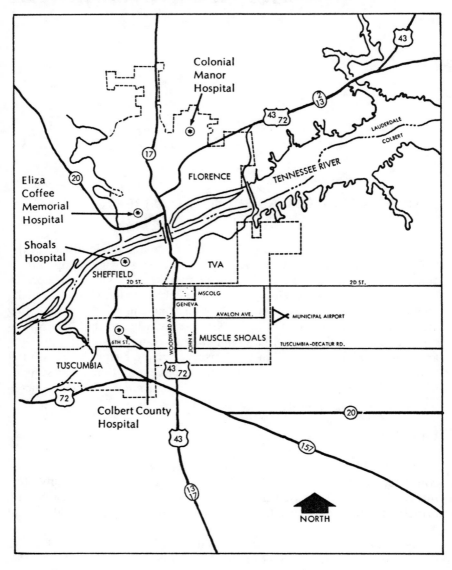

Florence is a community of about 36,200 (1975 estimate) and the county seat of Lauderdale County, population 70,500. The Tricities across the Tennessee River (Tuscumbia, Sheffield, and Muscle Shoals in Colbert County) had a total population of close to 70,000. Assuming a stable growth rate for this area, the populations for Florence and Lauderdale County were expected to be 38,500 and 72,900, respectively, by 1980. Analysis of the age distribution in Lauderdale and Colbert Counties in 1970 showed that 9.0 percent were 65 or older and the median was 28 compared to 27.1 for the state and 28.3 for the U.S. The birth and death rates for Lauderdale County were 15.4 and 8.9, respectively, which were lower than the national averages—17.5 and 9.5. It was considered a medium-income area with 17.4 percent of families with incomes less than $3,000 and 10.9 percent about $15,000. Median family income was $7,608, higher than the state figure of $7,263.

Florence serves as the trade and service center of northwest Alabama, southern Tennessee, and northeastern Mississippi. It also is an educational center for the region since it was the site of the University of North Alabama. It is considered the bedroom community for executives employed by industries south of the Tennessee River such as Reynolds Metal, the Tennessee Valley Authority, Union Carbide, Ford Motor Company, and textile and fertilizer plants.

Florence also is the center for health care for the whole region, including southern Tennessee and northeast Mississippi (Figure 9-2). The Colonial Manor medical staff had grown from 52 in 1969 to 78 in 1975 and represented many specialties that drew patients from the entire region. In 1975, a urologist and an internist joined the staff. Another physician expressed interest in coming to the area. The members of the medical staff of Colonial Manor and their activity status are listed in Table 9-1.

Colonial Manor performed most of the orthopedic work in the community because of the concentration of orthopedic surgeons on its staff. Pediatric work was increasing, especially with the addition of a specialist to the staff. Increased activity in this specialty was expected to continue with the impending arrival of the urologist, who wanted to concentrate on pediatric urology. Eleven physicians had offices in the professional building next to the hospital, and the hospital management was considering the construction of a second professional building nearby. Utilization statistics for fiscal 1974 and 1975 are shown in Table 9-2.

Environmental Analysis

Government-supported programs such as Medicare, Medicaid, crippled children, indigents, and others, pay hospitals on a cost basis. With new

Figure 9-2 Geographic Summary of Florence Hospital Admissions

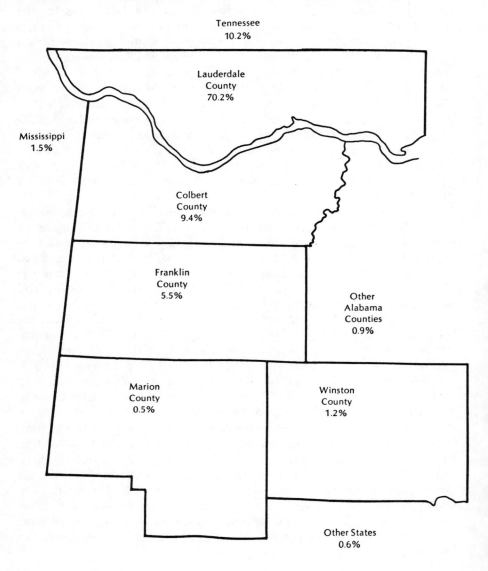

Table 9-1 Medical Staff at Colonial Manor Hospital in 1975

Specialty	Active	Associate	Courtesy
Urology	1	1	1
Pathology	1		1
Surgery	3	1	5
Radiology	1	2	4
Ophthalmology	1		3
Orthopedics	5		
General Medicine	4	4	7
Internal Medicine	1	1	5
Neurosurgery	2		
Anesthesiology	1		2
OB/GYN			3
EENT			1
OB			1
GYN			1
Psychiatry			1
Pediatrics			4
Dermatology			2
General Practice & General Surgery		2	6
ENT			
Total	20	11	47

regulations limiting the number of days a patient with a particular diagnosis could stay as an inpatient, hospitals had to start programs of marketing outpatient services. (Exhibit 9-1 outlines government regulations on inpatient costs.)

Hospitals faced another problem in that emergency room and outpatient services often resulted in increased bad debts. Most insurance companies did not cover outpatient services and others met only a percentage of the bill, leaving a balance for the patients to pay. Hospitals had to strive hard to collect these small balances, resulting in increased costs to them.

Colonial Manor Hospital also was investor-owned and liable for state and federal sales and property taxes. As such, it competed with city and county hospitals that did not have to pay taxes. Thus, its rates often were higher than those of competitors. On the other hand, Colonial Manor was located in a better neighborhood than the others and had the room to expand if necessary.

Other Services in the Immediate Area

Colonial Manor experienced keen competition mainly from Eliza Coffee Memorial, which was a city and county hospital. Coffee Memorial offered

Table 9-2 Utilization Data for Colonial Manor Hospital
Fiscal 1974 and 1975 (July 1–June 30)

	1974	1975
Admissions	3,925	3,960
Patient days	31,437	30,620
Average length of stay (number of days)	8.0	7.5
Medical patient days	8,323	8,898
Surgical patient days	6,250	5,916
Gynecology patient days	1,074	939
Urology patient days	1,136	1,193
Orthopedic patient days	14,654	12,778
Pediatric patient days	—	896

UTILIZATION BY DEPARTMENTS

Department	In-patient (1)	Out-patient (2)	Total (3)	Out-patient % (2 as % of 3)
Physical Therapy				
7/73 - 6/74	38,287	8,413	46,700	21.2
7/74 - 6/75	31,129	6,952	38,081	17.9
Respiratory Therapy				
9/73 - 6/74	11,123	24	11,147	0.2
7/74 - 6/75	13,525	2	13,527	—
Emergency Room Visits				
9/73 - 6/74	640	2,222	2,862	77.6
7/74 - 6/75	1,071	3,467	4,538	76.4
X-Ray Treatments				
7/73 - 6/74	7,161	2,141	9,302	23.0
7/74 - 6/75	7,955	2,913	10,868	26.8
Laboratory Tests				
7/73 - 6/74	83,652	2,940	86,592	3.4
7/74 - 6/75	95,152	2,984	98,136	3.0
Surgery				
7/73 - 6/74	1,828	19	1,847	1.0
7/74 - 6/75	2,111	40	2,151	1.8

Exhibit 9-1 Limits on Inpatient Costs by Government Regulations

On April 17, 1975, there was published in the Federal Register (40 FR 17190), a notice of Proposed Schedule of Limits on Hospital Inpatient General Routine Service Costs for Hospitals With Cost-Reporting Periods Beginning On or After July 1, 1975. Section 1861 (v) (1) of the Social Security Act, as amended, permits the Secretary of Health, Education, and Welfare to set prospective limits on direct or indirect overall incurred costs of specific items or services or groups of items or services furnished by a provider, to be recognized as reasonable based on estimates of the cost necessary in the efficient delivery of needed health services.

1. The bulk of the comments dealt with the lowering of the limits to the 80th percentile. A number of commenters asserted that the limits were lowered to the 80th percentile only as a cost-cutting device, without consideration of the financial impact on providers or the possible reduction in the quality of care. Other commenters suggested that the lower limits based on the 80th percentile, with the accompanying lowering of the interim payment rate, would imperil the cash flow position of many providers.

2. Comments were made that the effects of such factors as educational programs, patient mix, or scope of service on the hospital's inpatient general routine service cost were ignored in the revised classification system. These factors were not ignored, but were carefully considered before the revised classification system was issued. It is true that institutions which have educational programs may incur higher costs than institutions without educational programs. However, the classification variables in the new system cause teaching hospitals to be grouped together. The regulations (see 405.460 [f] [2]) provide that, where a provider can demonstrate that its costs exceed the applicable limit by reason of educational activities or by the special needs of the patients treated, an exception can be made to the application of the limit, to the extent that the added costs flow from approved educational activities, to the extent they are atypical (although reasonable) for providers in the comparison group, or flow from the provision of special needs of patients treated and are necessary in the delivery of needed health care.

3. A number of commenters appeared to be under the impression that the limits apply to *total* hospital inpatient costs per day. It should be understood that the Schedule of Limits presented herein applies only to the hospital inpatient general *routine* service costs, but does not apply to the costs of services furnished in special-care units or to the costs of ancillary services. *(continues)*

Exhibit 9-1 continued

4. Some parties expressed the view that they have a lower average length-of-stay than comparable hospitals, due to the more intense services that they provide, and this results in their having a higher routine service cost per day. They believe hospitals with shorter length-of-stays result from differences in case mix or from the provision of more intensive ancillary services. Since the published limits pertain to general routine service costs, the application of the limits does not more adversely affect hospitals with a lower average length of stay.

5. A number of parties commented that the classification system and Schedule of Limits do not distinguish between whether a hospital is an old or new one. Thus, a hospital with a new building and, therefore, with higher capital and interest costs, may have a higher routine cost per day than would other hospitals with older facilities.

Although a newer facility may have higher capital and interest costs than an older facility, a newer facility, generally, incorporates more advanced design concepts, which permit it to operate more efficiently than an older one and incur lower repair and maintenance costs. Thus, the different cost consequences of capital and interest costs, on one hand, and repair, maintenance, and operation of plant costs, on the other hand, are reasonably accounted for in the published limits.

the same number and types of services as Colonial Manor and had certain medical equipment that Colonial Manor used from time to time.

However, Colonial Manor was in the process of acquiring a computerized axial tomography (CAT) scanner. This would enable it to perform brain scans, liver scans, and other related tests, which not only would increase the inpatient load but also would attract outpatients.

Kidd felt that recruitment of five or six more doctors should enable the Colonial Manor to compete effectively even after Coffee Memorial expanded its bed capacity. He believed that patients went where doctors preferred to practice and worked toward a doctor-oriented policy rather than a patient-oriented one. He felt that if the hospital could please the doctor, it would please the patient in the process.

Action Plan to Increase Outpatient Service

Laboratory

The laboratory had been operating at a profit margin of 37.5 percent, with outpatient revenues in July 1975 making up 4.4 percent of its total revenues. To increase outpatient utilization, Kidd recommended that the laboratory:

1. Request that a laboratory consultant study the current situation and recommend action on automated equipment.
2. Pursue agreement with a pathologist on hematology work to be done in the hospital.
3. Assign a hospital representative to approach the nursing homes in the Tricities and surrounding areas about performing laboratory work and conducting employee physicals, infection control tests, and cultures for them.
4. Meet with physicians coming into the area to acquaint them with the laboratory facilities and procedures to encourage them to use the hospital, rather than acquiring their own equipment and personnel.

Radiology Department

The radiology department faced competition primarily from the doctors. There were four x-ray machines in the professional building adjacent to the hospital and most of the physicians had had their own equipment when they moved in. New physicians generally used the hospital radiology department.

The radiology department performs about 200 procedures a month through the emergency room. The hospital had an agreement with a nearby nursing home and a new one under construction to do their x-rays. The x-ray department also did some industrial employee physicals for those whose physicians had no equipment.

As a result of the hospital building program, the added number of patients was expected to increase the department workload by approximately a third, so radiology was being expanded accordingly.

Radiology operated at a profit margin of 15.3 percent, with outpatient revenues comprising 19.3 percent of the total in July 1975.

To increase outpatient utilization, Kidd recommended that the radiology department:

1. Pursue construction of a second professional building nearby to provide easier access to the hospital radiology department for physicians with offices there.
2. Approach physicians on a one-to-one basis regarding outpatient radiology work. New physicians should be encouraged to use the hospital rather than investing in their own equipment. Older doctors who already had their equipment should be encouraged not to replace it

when it no longer was usable. This should not be too difficult in light of increasing costs and possible state legislation requiring inspections and the use of x-ray technicians, not just nurses, to operate equipment.

Physical Therapy Department

The physical therapy department was performing the largest number of procedures in the county, largely because of the concentration of orthopedic surgeons on the medical staff. The Colonial Manor department carried out far more procedures than the separate physical therapy wing at Eliza Coffee Memorial. Local schools had their own equipment for therapy involving athletic injuries. Industries in the area sent their injured employees to Colonial Manor for their physical therapy needs.

The physical therapy department operated at a profit margin of 54.3 percent and outpatient revenues comprised 13.1 percent of total revenues.

To increase outpatient utilization, Kidd recommended that the physical therapy department:

1. Contact nursing homes in the area to determine the market for physical therapy for their patients.
2. Contact area industries to determine interest in individual executive physical fitness programs developed by the physical and respiratory therapists. These programs would be conducted with the cooperation of physicians who performed the annual physical examinations.
3. Work with the communications department to develop outpatient brochures for physical therapy describing services and treatments and serving as prewritten prescriptions for the patients.

Respiratory Therapy Department

In the past, outpatient respiratory therapy work had not been sought actively because it was felt that the hospital lacked adequate personnel to handle any additional load. There was no commercial respiratory therapy service in the area although some individuals did have their own home equipment. Nursing homes would be the prime place to begin offering respiratory therapy.

The respiratory therapy department operated in 1975 at a profit margin of 36.8 percent but outpatient revenues had not been recorded accurately so it was not possible to measure that percentage.

To increase outpatient utilization, Kidd recommended that the respiratory therapy department:

1. Contact nursing homes and extended care facilities to determine their present service suppliers.
2. Analyze the feasibility, in line with the capabilities of the department, of servicing nursing homes, of treating homebound patients, and of establishing a home equipment rental service.
3. Conduct clinics on maintenance and calibration of home equipment.
4. Work with the communications department to adopt standardized brochures describing the services, which also could serve as prewritten prescriptions and instructions for the patients.

Outpatient Surgery

Outpatient surgery at Colonial Manor was limited by the lack of space, especially for recovering surgery patients. In the building program, the surgical suite was being expanded and one operating room was being equipped for outpatient surgery, with a recovery area.

Physicians had a positive attitude toward outpatient surgery so such procedures probably would increase in the expanded facilities. The new urologist indicated that he would want to do some cystoscopies on an outpatient basis and the ear, nose, and throat specialists also would be able to use this capability. With the increasing concentration on malpractice liability, many of the procedures performed in doctors' offices might be moved to the hospital.

The high occupancy rate and the expected gain in the number of physicians were likely to increase the use of outpatient surgery at Colonial Manor.

To increase outpatient surgery, Kidd recommended that Colonial Manor:

1. Develop an organized program for outpatient surgery, including scheduling personnel, procedures to follow, and a separate charge structure. This would be discussed first with physicians.
2. Make a formal presentation to the medical staff on the potential of outpatient surgery, the benefits of the hospital setting over the office for minor procedures, and the program just developed.

Central Supply

There was no place in the area to buy medical supplies such as slings, collars, dressings, braces, tennis elbow bands, etc., on an outpatient basis. A separate outpatient services department could sell these items, including fitting by an emergency room nurse or attendant.

To increase outpatient utilization, Kidd recommended that Colonial Manor:

1. Intensify efforts to obtain commitments from one or two more physicians for space in a new professional building in order to receive executive committee approval to proceed with this project. Another professional building near the hospital would provide needed office space for physicians being recruited by Colonial Manor and a built-in market for the hospital laboratory and x-ray departments. Since Florence is a regional health center, a second professional building could help make Colonial Manor the major facility.
2. Review the regional laboratory concept and follow up on obtaining automated equipment, especially automated hematology devices, since the competing lab did not have them. Given the size of the hospital and its high occupancy rate, the lab would be able to generate enough inpatient and outpatient utilization to justify some automation. If the lab was not automated, outpatients might utilize the services at the competing lab.
3. Develop a total outpatient surgery program, including setting up a separate charge structure because there was no other outpatient surgery program in Florence. With the hospital high occupancy rates, the concentration of health care specialties in Florence, the increase in the number of physicians in the area, and the growing emphasis on utilization of outpatient services, this program could be highly successful.
4. Encourage groups such as Weight Watchers, Future Nurses, childbirth classes, and so forth, to hold meetings in the hospital.
5. Sponsor public service clinics for such categories as diabetes, cancer, hypertension, obesity, and venereal disease; and provide pulmonary function tests.
6. Participate in Career Week by having the director of nurses and other department heads make presentations to area schools.
7. Maintain contact with area industries and contact any new ones to determine their health service needs. Consider issuing cards to industry employees with their insurance information that would allow them to be admitted without a cash deposit. Work with staff physicians to develop an "Executive Physical" package.

OVERVIEW OF CASE 15

Issues to Consider

1. How serious are the overall marketing problems facing the Colonial Manor Hospital management?
2. What evaluation can be made of the target market identified by Kidd? What additional analysis is needed?

3. What product, price, promotion, and distribution recommendations should Kidd make to the hospital's administrative board?

Discussion

1. Utilization and Marketing

There is evidence in the case to show that with a few exceptions, utilization lagged below capacity in the 1974–1975 period. The statistics indicate a decline in several outpatient categories, especially as a percentage of total patients. For example, the number of physical therapy outpatients declined by 17.4 percent, and the outpatient percent of total patients dropped from 21 percent to 18 percent. On the other hand, outpatient x-ray treatments increased 36 percent and outpatient emergency room visits 56 percent in the year.

There are large imbalances in the inpatient and outpatient composition for each department, and Kidd should investigate them in terms of the services provided by the hospital and remedial measures that could be undertaken to improve the proportion of the business that is on an outpatient basis. An evaluation is needed of the reasons for the physical therapy decline, the rapid growth in the emergency room and x-ray treatment departments, and the static position of the laboratory tests department on outpatient services at the same time that inpatient utilization was growing by 14 percent.

A wide variety of alternative methods is available to evaluate the strengths and weaknesses of the outpatient services and facilities of the various departments. For instance, information is needed on who is utilizing the services offered by each department, in what magnitude, and for what reasons. Kidd correctly recognizes the critical role of the physicians in marketing hospital services to the ultimate consumers—the patients. There is no indication, however, as to the nature and dimensions of physicians' behavior in terms of motivations to choose a particular hospital, the choice criteria they might use, the hospital attributes that would be significant in their selection and continued patronage, and so on. These types of information will provide significant input for developing a comprehensive marketing strategy for the hospital. In the absence of such knowledge, there is no firm basis for evaluating the various efforts Kidd has outlined.

2. Target Market Evaluation

Kidd seems to assume that by attracting new physicians into the proposed professional building, additional demand for hospital services can be stimulated. However, almost two-thirds of the doctors practicing at Colonial Manor are in the "courtesy physician" category rather than active or associate (Table 9-1, supra). This seems to imply that considerable promotional effort is needed to encourage physicians already practicing in the area to make greater use of the hospital.

Thus, there seem to be two distinct groups of physicians whose patronage needs to be cultivated—those already practicing in the area and those who need to be recruited to the region. Kidd can undertake a cost-benefit analysis of the past activities of these two segments to help indicate the priorities and the relative emphasis to be placed on each segment. The present promotional approach does not take into account the differences between the two.

Another distinct segment of the market for hospital services is the institutional element, including nursing homes and other facilities needing health care services. To obtain business from this segment, a different marketing strategy may be required. Nursing homes, businesses, and other institutional customers buy the various hospital services on a bulk basis, so attracting them may require establishing special rates. The plan outlined by Kidd takes a general approach, with emphasis on contacting these institutional customers. To succeed in this, however, more systematic information must be gathered and analyzed regarding their special needs, how they are serviced now, and what gaps exist (if any). Such information will provide an appropriate basis for developing suitable marketing strategies for this segment.

In summary, while Kidd seems to recognize the various segments of the market for the different hospital services, his marketing approach is too generic. In its present form, it does not take into account the differences among the segments and the significance of these differences for an effective marketing strategy.

3. Recommendations

The expansion from 100 to 155 beds will result in a severe drop in the occupancy rate unless the number of patient days is increased substantially. The hospital is thinking of adding a number of new services to stimulate additional business. It is fair to assume that there is a limit on the capital available for new equipment. Thus, some priorities must be set on what equipment to buy. This will require some marketing research, namely, asking the nursing homes, businesses, specialists, and general practitioners in the area what services they would like that are not available now.

It may turn out, for example, that even though the competing laboratory does not have hematology testing equipment, this device will not produce sufficient revenue to pay for itself. Once equipment costs are known, it should be relatively simple to compute a break-even point for the number of tests that would have to be performed per year to pay back the cost of the machine over a reasonable period of time. Instead, it may turn out that other equipment, which may not be nearly as sophisticated and expensive, may produce revenues much greater than the break-even level and thus be a much more attractive capital expenditure.

Serious consideration should be given to the adoption of different rate structures for the various services by taking into account both the demand and supply factors. In hospitals, services typically are cost-based without consideration of demand. The cost-volume relationships usually are not analyzed systematically in arriving at pricing strategies.

Kidd's recommendations can be evaluated on a department-by-department basis. Only 4.4 percent of the laboratory revenues are from outpatient services, indicating considerable growth opportunity in this department. Before a hospital representative is sent to a nursing home, some research should be done to find out what the facility is doing now, how much it is paying for services, what Colonial Manor could do to obtain a higher proportion of this market, and so forth. The same is true for the new physician segment of the market. It may be that the profit margin is so high for these services that all doctors prefer to set up their own laboratories for most testing procedures. It would not make much sense to have a representative calling on doctors if there is not much potential for success.

The contribution margin on radiology is very low, only 15.3 percent of revenues. Kidd should analyze cost and price sensitivity of various buyers of these services to determine whether this margin can be increased through cost reduction or a raise in prices. If not, the low margin may be an attractive selling point to promote to new and older physicians to encourage them to use Colonial Manor's services instead of buying or replacing their own equipment. Given the rising cost of x-ray equipment and the increasing legislation on inspection of technicians, the radiology department appears to offer substantial potential for greater sales and profits.

Physical therapy offers the highest profit margin percentage of all departments, making increased sales in this area a very attractive objective. The five orthopedic surgeons and the heavy outpatient volume suggest that Colonial Manor has great expertise in this field and should be able to offer more and better services than any of the competition. Kidd's idea of contacting nursing homes and industries appears sound. He should try to determine what services they are using now, from what hospitals, and at what cost. The high profit margin might enable him to offer these services at a bulk rate and still have plenty of margin for profit. The brochure should be developed only after this research has been conducted.

The respiratory therapy and outpatient surgery departments have extremely low outpatient volume. This undoubtedly results from a lack of personnel and space in the past but the expansion program should change this. Outpatient surgery appears to offer a great deal of potential, especially given the increased attention to skyrocketing medical costs. Instead of making a formal presentation to the medical staff members on the potential benefits of outpatient surgery, Kidd should ascertain why they are not doing more such operations and what would be needed to enable the doctors to increase their use of this service.

CASE 16. GOOD SAMARITAN HOSPITAL (B): A MARKETING APPROACH TO NEW SERVICE DEVELOPMENT

Glen Blackwell, assistant administrator in charge of Good Samaritan Hospital's marketing and development program, studied the information he had requested concerning the institution's computerized electrocardiogram (ECG) system. William C. Norris, M.D., the director of the cardiovascular department, had produced the information on short notice and Blackwell was impressed with the unit's efficiency. He was continually on the alert for ways to increase utilization of a department. In looking over Dr. Norris's report, Blackwell was convinced he had discovered a truly marketable service with a high probability of success.

Good Samaritan Hospital Background

Good Samaritan Hospital was established in 1874 by a group of church women to minister to the sick and infirm among the newcomers and immigrants to Toledo who had no homes and/or families. After 104 years of growth and expansion, Good Samaritan was the largest metropolitan hospital in northwestern Ohio. It maintained 732 beds, numerous outpatient clinics and services, and a staff of 620 physicians and 750 nurses to provide medical and health care to the Toledo metropolitan area and surrounding communities.

Good Samaritan's Computerized ECG

In 1976, Good Samaritan installed a computerized ECG system that had proved highly satisfactory. With this system, an ECG is taken at the patient's bedside and the reading is relayed to the computer, where it is recorded and interpreted. An unconfirmed reading can be reported to the patient's bedside in 20 to 50 seconds. The ECG is considered "unconfirmed" since it has been read only by the computer. A cardiologist then "overreads" or interprets the ECG and feeds any necessary changes in the unconfirmed report back into the computer. This "confirmed" report is recorded and stored on a computer disc that can be referred to quickly if necessary. The computer proved to be a reliable interpreter of normal ECGs, with a calculated accuracy of 98.8 percent. The remaining 1.2 percent of the readings varied slightly in borderline situations.

Need for Market Analysis

Blackwell and Dr. Norris lunched together to discuss the situation in greater detail. Blackwell learned there would be little difficulty in expanding the ECG facilities to include sharing the system with outside institutions. Later, he met with Dr. Randolph, a well-known member of the marketing faculty at the local university, to work out details for an internship program for the marketing department. He told Dr. Randolph, "I have discovered a unit in the hospital that has a fabulous market potential that so far is virtually untapped. It is a can't-miss proposition if I ever have seen one."

"Two years ago, the cardiovascular department installed a computerized ECG system," Blackwell began. "At that time the computer's manufacturer referred to us three potential users who were interested in sharing a system like this. A hospital in Michigan taps our system by using its own portable ECG output carts. It then receives the unconfirmed reports and its own physicians overread them. Family Physicians, a group practice, also uses its own carts for unconfirmed reports that are then interpreted by a Toledo Hospital cardiologist and sent back. The Family Practice Center near Good Samaritan also receives unconfirmed readings on its own carts.

"So, the market is there for the service. All we need is to contact hospitals and clinics in the area to see which ones are interested."

"Now wait a minute, Glen," Dr. Randolph interrupted. "You know that if at all possible, even on promising projects, it still is advantageous to survey the market first. On past projects you have always wanted to get additional information first so you could conduct a thorough situation analysis."

"Do you think that is necessary in this instance?" Blackwell asked. "After all, the computer is here already, so it should not cost much extra to expand its utilization."

"Let's look at it this way," Dr. Randolph reasoned. "Right now you know that three other institutions have been sufficiently interested to become sharers. Other than that, you have no way of knowing the degree of interest any other parties might have. Do you have any idea how knowledgeable others are about the system? Do they understand the benefits of the system or do they have any misconceptions?"

"I'm not sure," Blackwell conceded.

"What about your pricing structure?" Dr. Randolph continued. "What would you charge sharing institutions?"

"I suppose we would just use the present rate structure," Blackwell said, "although I'm not certain whether it would have to be modified."

"It would seem to me that some research could help determine the optimal pricing pattern," Dr. Randolph said. "It would give some idea of the price elasticity for the ECG service. I also noticed that you were limiting your potential market to hospitals and clinics. It would seem to me that some types of specialists also might be interested in a service of this nature."

"I must concede defeat," Blackwell said. "I guess I was getting a bit too hasty and was overlooking some things."

"It's not that bad," Dr. Randolph said. "In fact it would seem likely that this is a good area to expand into. But let's be certain and play our best hand instead of preparing a rough-shod proposal. I would be glad to help you prepare a research survey to enable you to determine whether a potential exists and to prepare the optimal marketing strategy for the computerized ECG. If you could arrange a meeting with the director of that department we probably could find information that will short-cut our informal investigation and we can expedite any field research required."

Blackwell quickly assented.

Analysis of the Situation

At the meeting to analyze the ECG situation in greater detail, Dr. Norris agreed to serve as the resource person from his cardiovascular department so Blackwell was positive they would be supplied with accurate, up-to-date information. He had discovered early in his work as marketing director that departmental heads almost always were eager to help in any way to expand their units' utilization. Sometimes, after studying proposals and doing research, they discovered that the potential to justify expansion did not exist.

Blackwell explained to Dr. Norris that Dr. Randolph was planning to help ascertain the market potential for the computerized ECG. He asked Dr. Norris to explain how the system had been working on a shared basis.

"We have had very few problems with the shared systems," Dr. Norris said. "Long distance telephone lines are used to transmit an ECG. The only difficulty is the computer's tendency to terminate transmission if there is too much static or extraneous noise on the lines, or if a patient moves during a reading so as to invalidate the reading. Sharing institutions have been able to retransmit these ECGs along with ones that were not sent properly without being charged for them. The system also is designed so that transmissions are prioritized automatically so that the most urgent are processed first, with the others called up as the computer becomes available."

"Could you give me some idea what you are currently charging the sharing institutions?" Dr. Randolph asked. "It would help me to know how much you charge for the cart rental, computer fees, and the overread option for starters."

"Perhaps it would help you to know how much the carts cost per year also," Dr. Norris replied. "The purchase price per unit is approximately $13,800 and is depreciated over a five-year period. Each one has its own service contract, which costs $1,860 a year. So far the sharing institutions have purchased their own carts but we estimate that if we choose to expand the sharing system that we could offer carts for rent or lease as an option to the sharers. We have estimated that the rental would be around $450 per month."

"As far as the price per reading goes," he continued, "we currently charge $3.50 for the computer fee if the sharing institution performs between 100 and 200 ECGs per month. The overread option is $4.15 per reading. However, the sharing institutions must feel they are priced too high since some choose to overread their own. Some physicians do not even consider the overread necessary since the computer generally is recognized as being more accurate than ECGs performed without its aid. But the main choice regarding the overread seems to be whether our local certified cardiologist should do it or whether the sharing institution should have a resident physician to do it. Our cardiologist is available 24 hours a day, which is a definite advantage. Incidentally, he is very well known and respected in the medical community in northwestern Ohio and we feel this is a major benefit of our program."

"You mentioned that some physicians do not consider the overread option to be a necessity," Dr. Randolph said. "Have you any idea how many physicians do use it and to what extent?"

"We are unsure of that," Dr. Norris replied, "except for the general understanding that some use it very little and some use it a lot. It all depends on the individual preferences of the physician."

"How aware would you say physicians and hospitals are concerning the benefits of the computerized ECG?" Dr. Randolph asked.

"We are aware of two hospitals that have installed computerized ECGs, but so far this is a new concept in the medical field."

"Then it is altogether possible that sharing institutions might be unaware of the benefits from the computerized ECGs or might even have misconceptions concerning the system," Dr. Randolph commented.

"Yes, that is quite possible," Dr. Norris responded.

"What, then, would you consider to be the prime advantages of the computerized ECG that a potential sharer might be unaware of?" Dr. Randolph asked.

"The computerized ECG is definitely a more efficient means of reading and interpreting ECGs," Dr. Norris said. "For one reason, it reduces the time required by the physician to read the ECG and it allows almost instantaneous recording of the results. Immediate emergency bedside readings are available around the clock and that has to be a definite advantage. Also, the computerized report can prevent early morning cancellations of surgery because of ECG findings since an interpretation by computer is available the day prior to surgery."

"What do you think some possible misconceptions might be?" Dr. Randolph asked.

"There are always those who fear equipment failure, but that is very rare with this type of program," Dr. Norris replied. "Also, some feel that computerized ECGs are more expensive, when in actuality the efficiency of the system can reduce the cost. There could be some who do not realize that calculations of intervals and cardiac rates and configurations are done more accurately by computers. I think one area of concern might be where physicians feel that comparisons of prior ECGs are best left to the physician rather than to computers. There are always some who feel that computers are too impersonal and too likely to make mistakes."

"What type of specialists would be the most likely to be interested in using this computerized ECG?" Dr. Randolph asked.

"The most frequent users are three types of specialists," Dr. Norris replied, "those in internal medicine, family practice, and, of course, cardiology."

Blackwell then asked Dr. Randolph, "What specifically are you going to attempt to do about the computerized ECG program?"

"Initially, it would be desirable to survey the potential users of this system, preferably by mail, to hold down the cost. I plan to prepare a questionnaire to send out to the physicians Dr. Norris indicated, along with the hospitals and clinics it northwestern Ohio and southeastern Michigan," Dr. Randolph explained. "It could help us to find out how many would be interested in renting carts at the proposed rental price and current computer fee. It also would be useful to know how interest patterns change as the price of the computer fee is increased or decreased, so that price elasticity can be projected.

"We also could gather information indicating the present knowledge of the potential market for computerized ECGs, along with possible misconceptions. We could discover how many physicians are using the overread option and how essential they feel that function is. This could aid in determining an appropriate price for this feature.

"Finally, we could gain some idea about present ECG and computerized ECG usage patterns. We could find out how many ECGs physicians are taking weekly and how many of these are interpreted by computer. It would be beneficial to discover how reliable physicians feel the computer is in interpreting ECGs. From this information we will be more certain about the market potential and be able to adapt a marketing strategy to capture that market."

"We can get the names and addresses of the physicians and hospital administrators from the local medical academy as soon as you know which specialties you want to include," Blackwell said. "Also, I think it would be prudent to develop a detailed statement of the objectives of this study as well as a preliminary draft of a questionnaire so we can get Dr. Norris's comments on it. There may be some medical terminology we should use and he can give you a specialist's reaction to your questionnaire."

Dr. Randolph agreed.

OVERVIEW OF CASE 16

Issues to Consider

1. Should a market survey be conducted? How is the cost-effectiveness of a survey evaluated?
2. How should Blackwell approach the pricing of the computer-assisted ECG?
3. What options are available to Blackwell to increase the response rate of a survey of physicians?

Discussion

1. The Survey and Its Cost Effectiveness

Before the research is initiated, the hospital should specify the objectives of the computerized ECG study. The study should include a definition of the target market. It also should provide information that would allow Good Samaritan Hospital to relate to these potential users in a more efficient manner than would be possible without the use of primary marketing research. The type of information gathered should include current usage levels, pricing preferences and information, and concerns and perceived benefits, along with demographics.

In this case, an obvious question arose: When is it advantageous (or not) to conduct a market survey before introducing a hospital service? Blackwell was positive the computerized ECG was needed but lacked information on its feasibility and practicality. Under these circumstances, an unbiased or trained person can help identify difficulties that may have been overlooked.

As a general rule, it is a good idea to conduct a survey to define the target market(s) and the qualities that are pertinent to the product or service being offered. However, if there is considerable evidence that the service meets a market need, if the cost of research cannot be justified (that is, costs are exceeded by the potential profit), or if the survey will alert a competitor and cause the competitive edge to be lost, then a survey may not be justified. In these circumstances, time and money spent in research and development could be jeopardized.

It also is possible that there may be times when a market already is clearly defined and the extent of its knowledge can be determined easily. The needed information may be available already. In such an instance, gathering additional data might be redundant. Care should be taken to make sure the information is pertinent and parallel to what is needed.

In rare circumstances a person may have thorough knowledge of a market and also have the gift of sufficient insight concerning what it needs that no further research is essential. However, this usually is not the case and some field research generally is justified.

On a relatively new concept such as the computer-assisted ECG, it would seem logical that in most instances the benefits of a market survey would outweigh the costs as well as negate the time delay in marketing the service. These benefits would accrue since the hospital would be more certain of a market. It could gain insights as to where the market is located and how knowledgeable it is about the service. Information can be gained that will prove useful in pricing the service at the optimal level for both Good Samaritan and the users. In addition, information can be gathered to serve as a basis for the marketing plan, including the promotional literature, educational services for physicians, etc. In summation, a market survey will provide Good Samaritan with the information necessary to formulate the optimal marketing strategy. Decisions will be made in an orderly fashion and will provide support to back them up as a result of a well-conceived and well-executed market survey.

2. Pricing

As the current computer fee is $3.50 per reading and the cost of owning or leasing a cart is about $450 a month, these assumptions should be stated in the questionnaire. Several approaches to pricing are feasible, some based on cost and others on demand analysis.

The $450 cost per month is a fixed figure that will decline per reading as utilization increases. However, the computer fee is a variable cost that fluctuates in proportion to the number of readings. Furthermore, for Good Samaritan, this computer fee is a contribution to the already sunk cost of the computer itself. It is possible, then, that $3.50 is not the optimal price to charge. Usually, the demand for hospital services is considered to be inelastic with regard to price since the benefits outweigh the cost. The importance of the cost to the patient also usually is minimal since third party payers foot a substantial portion of most bills. However, if the concept is to gain acceptance, physicians must be convinced that the computer is a better and less expensive way of providing ECG services, so the pricing issue is important.

A survey question that quoted the computer fee at both higher and lower rates, with the physician responding to the likelihood of using the service at the different costs, could provide insight on an optimal pricing strategy. This question should state that the physician assumes 100 to 200 readings per month, since at lower usage patterns the rate is likely to be higher while at higher utilization there is a possibility of quantity discounts. Further, charging what the traffic will bear undoubtedly is unethical and inappropriate. Although not stated in the case, consideration also must be given to the price that competitors charge. Even more importantly, the price should be competitive with the fee charged by a physician for both the initial reading and the overreading. If too much more than this is charged, the service may not be used.

3. Mail Surveys

In mail surveys, a frequent problem is the difficulty of obtaining a high response rate to ensure that the results can be projected accurately.

There are techniques for increasing the response rate. Postpaid return envelopes is one of the more obvious. The physician also can be sent a preannouncement that a survey is forthcoming. A gift or monetary reward may be sent for the physician's participation. For example, an Indian head penny, a Continental dollar pendant, playing cards, a tie clasp, etc., may be used. Research indicates that the receptionist typically screens the physician's mail, so cooperation there is essential as the doctor otherwise may not receive the questionnaire. A follow-up letter can be sent to thank the physician for filling out the survey and a reminder can be sent to those who do not respond. Personally written postscripts also may increase the rate of response.

Usually a response rate of 20 to 40 percent can be expected for a mail survey of physicians. The mail survey has the advantage of being inexpensive, yet without a sufficient response the results are not very meaningful. Therefore, the foregoing techniques should be used to raise the rate of response. The replies to the initial mailing also should be compared to those received from the follow-up request to discern any significant differences in response patterns. (A sample survey is provided in Exhibit 9-2.)

Exhibit 9-2 Sample Questionnaire for an ECG Survey

1. As you may know computers are being used in the interpretation of ECGs. Have you had any experience with computer interpreted ECGs on your patients?

 ___Yes   ___No   (1.

2. If you could own or lease a cart for $300 a month and the charge for a computer interpretation was $3 50, how interested would you be in obtaining these computer assist ECGs?

 ___ Extremely interested   ___ Slightly interested
 ___ Moderately interested   ___ Not interested   (2)

3. How likely would you be to use the service if the fee was the following?

Fee Without Overread (Assume 100-200 Readings per Month)	Strong Possibility (8 in 10 or Higher)	Good Possibility (6 in 10)	Slight Possibility (3 in 10 or less)	
	(1)	(2)	(3)	
$3 74	_____	_____	_____	(3)
3 50	_____	_____	_____	(4)
3 25	_____	_____	_____	(5)
3 00	_____	_____	_____	(6)

4. Some computer assist ECG programs have their ECGs overread by resident physicians. Others use a local certified cardiologist known to physicians in the area served. How important to you would it be to have a cardiologist in Northwestern Ohio available to over-read the computer assist ECGs. based on your criteria for overreading?

 _____ Absolutely essential   (7)
 _____ Desirable but not essential
 _____ Makes no difference
 _____ Resident physician reading preferred

(continues)

Exhibit 9-2 continued

5 If a local certified cardiologist were to read the ECGs, how much more would it be worth to you to have his service, assuming that the resident-read ECG would cost $3.50 per ECG?

—$5.00 ($1.50 more)   —$6.00 ($2.50 more)
—$5.50 ($2.00 more)   —$6.50 ($3.00 more)
                                       Expect both to
                                       be the same.
                                                                        (5)

6 Of the last 100 ECGs you had taken on your patients, about how many overreads did you request?

—None   —30-49%
—1-19%   —50% or more
—20-29%
                                                                        (6)

7 Some physicians believe that computers can do a more reliable job of evaluating axis and specific interval readings than the typical physician. Others disagree. How do you feel about this?

—Strong agree
—Agree   —Disagree
—Undecided   —Strongly Disagree   (7)

8 From your personal experience as well as those of your colleagues, of 100 ECGs read by a computer, how many would you expect to be interpreted accurately?

—All of them
—90-99%   —Less than 70%
—70-89%   —No opinion
                                                                        (8)

9 Many statements have been made concerning computer-assist ECG programs. Would you please tell us if you agree or disagree with the following, or don't you have an opinion?

	Agree	Disagree	No Opinion	
a. The efficiency of hospital and physician office personnel is enhanced by these programs.				(12)
b. Immediate emergency bedside readings are feasible in a computer assist program around the clock				(13)
c. Since ECGs interpreted by computers can be available the day prior to surgery they can thereby prevent early morning surgery cancellation due to ECGs findings				(14)
d. Comparison with prior ECGs is an important physician function and should not be done by computers				(15)
e. ECG reading time of physicians is reduced by these programs				(16)
f. Equipment problems are rare with this type of program				(17)
g. Calculations of intervals and cardiac rates and configurations can be done more accurately by computer than by physicians.				(18)
h. ECG interpretations can be placed on a patient's chart almost immediately after recording with a computer assist program				(19)
i. The efficiency of these programs can reduce the cost of unit ECGs				(20)

CASE 17. MOUNT CARMEL MERCY HOSPITAL AND MEDICAL CENTER: A SERVICE ELIMINATION DECISION*

Mount Carmel Mercy Hospital and Medical Center was established in 1939. It is owned and operated by the Sisters of Mercy of the Province of Detroit. When it opened in 1939, it had 325 beds and 125 bassinets, with 208 employees. Through expansion programs over the years, the facility had increased to 557 beds.

As of July 1972, Mount Carmel Mercy Hospital had 1,700 employees, a medical staff of 375 physicians, and a house staff of 125 physicians. During the fiscal year 1971–1972 it had 19,098 admissions, 12,432 readmissions, 39,151 emergency room visits, 16,131 ambulatory health center visits, 29,759 diagnostic service visits, an average daily census of 483, and an average length of stay of 9.3 days. Mount Carmel's operating income was $24.2 million, its assets $22.4 million. Tables 9-3 and 9-4 present income state-

---

* Some of the data have been modified in minor ways for clarity of presentation. The reader should note that in 1972 the area-wide health planning system was in place and the National Health Planning and Resources Development Act of 1974 with its Health Systems Agency planning system was not yet enacted.

Table 9-3 Income Statement

(Year Ending June 30)

	1972		1971
Patient Revenue		$24,141,531	$21,569,657
Other Revenue (net)		59,609	81,213
		24,201,140	21,650,870
Less Expenses			
Salaries and wages	$14,829,442		$13,374,411
Supplies	3,503,032		3,101,157
Employee benefits	1,446,984		1,283,950
Repairs and maintenance	1,143,350		1,055,927
Depreciation	602,257		582,664
All others	1,922,926		1,608,053
Total Expenses		23,447,991	21,006,162
Excess of Income Over Expenses		753,149	644,708
Reductions from Income for Mount Carmel's Charitable Community Services		376,137	334,953
Net Excess Available for Expansion of Services		377,012	309,755

Source: Mount Carmel Mercy Hospital and Medical Center, 1972 Annual Report.

Table 9-4 Balance Sheet

(Year Ending June 30)

	1972		1971	
Current Assets				
Cash..............................	$ 133,255		$ 666,901	
Patient accounts receivable (net)..........................	3,347,804		3,519,272	
Other accounts receivable.....	37,883		30,180	
Inventories and prepaid expense.........................	447,290		505,521	
Total Current Assets.........................		$ 3,966,232		$ 4,721,874
Other Assets				
Investment (at cost)	489,283		-0-	
Building fund savings account	554,726		273,530	
Unamortized debt expense....	150,403		65,000	
Total Other Assets..........................		1,194,412		338,530
Fixed Assets				
Land, buildings, and equipment.............................	17,589,357		15,479,818	
Less accumulated depreciation	7,007,200		6,431,394	
	10,582,157		9,048,424	
Construction in progress.......	6,655,962		1,186,810	
Total Fixed Assets		17,238,119		10,235,234
Totals......................................		22,398,763		15,295,638
Current Liabilities				
Accounts payable...............	1,052,448		1,248,024	
Accrued salaries	501,822		371,857	
Accrued vacation/sick pay.....	791,112		719,892	
Other payables..................	770,028		107,152	
Medicare and Blue Cross advances......................	535,410		943,200	
Mortgage payable-current	105,697		90,000	
Total Current Liabilities......................		3,756,617		3,480,125
Long-Term Liability				
Mortgage payable...............	920,000		1,010,000	
Notes payable...................	4,836,085		500,000	
Total Long-Term Liability....................		5,756,085		1,510,000
Capital				
Balance at June 30.............................		12,886,161		10,305,513
Totals		22,398,763		15,295,638

Source: Mount Carmel Mercy Hospital and Medical Center, *1972 Annual Report.*

ments and balance sheets for the 1971 and 1972 fiscal years. Construction plans for fiscal 1972–1973 included a parking deck for 750 cars and a new $3 million professional office building that would be erected on the Mount Carmel grounds. In terms of size, Mount Carmel was one of the largest hospitals in the United States. Of the 44 hospitals in Detroit, only three were larger.

Mount Carmel Mercy Hospital was a nonprofit, nongovernmental community hospital devoted to the objectives of (1) providing a wide range of high-quality patient care services to the community and (2) participating in the education of physicians and other health care professionals.

Relative to physician training, there were 125 interns and residents. As a teaching hospital, Mount Carmel had training programs in nursing service, pharmacy, dietary, medical records, radiology, anesthesia, respiratory care, pathology, physical medicine and rehabilitation, and physician assistant.

Committed to providing quality care to all who sought it, regardless of race, creed, or ability to pay, Mount Carmel had continuously provided the community with a wide range of services. Among its medical service departments were: surgery, internal medicine, obstetrics and gynecology, pediatrics, laboratory, radiology, general practice, and physical medicine. Figure 9-3 is an organization chart of Mount Carmel. Table 9-5 presents data on patients discharged, total patient days, and average stay by type of service during the 1971 and 1972 fiscal years.

In August 1972, Mount Carmel faced a major decision. The number of deliveries had declined from a high of 6,733 in 1958 to a low of 2,610 in 1971. As a result, the obstetrical department of 70 beds had an occupancy rate of only 46 percent. At issue was whether the department should be closed and the service be provided by other facilities in the area or reduced in terms of number of beds.

The Hospital Industry

Hospitals in the United States are classified in various ways. The most common is by ownership: (1) federal, (2) state and local, (3) nongovernmental nonprofit (sometimes called community general or voluntary hospitals), and (4) nongovernmental for-profit. Others are by type of stay (long stay and short stay) and type of service (general, medical and surgical, psychiatric, tuberculosis, and so forth). In 1972, 6,046 of the nation's 7,061 hospitals were short-stay, general hospitals. Fifty percent of the total consisted of nongovernmental nonprofit (community general) hospitals that accounted for 41 percent of the total beds. Table 9-6 presents a breakdown of hospitals by type for 1972.

Another interesting characteristic is that most of the nation's hospitals are relatively small (Table 9-7). Of the total 7,061 in 1972, 639 hospitals or 9.0 percent had more than 500 beds; 267 or 3.7 percent had 400 to 499 beds; 436 or 6.2 percent, 300 to 399; 734 or 10.4 percent, 200 to 299; and 1,433 or 20.1 percent, 100 to 199. The remaining 3,552 hospitals, or 50.3 percent, had fewer than 100 beds. Thus, in terms of size, more than half of the nation's hospitals had fewer than 100 beds and only 9 percent more than 500.

In terms of activity, Table 9-8 presents data on the hospital industry nationally for the period 1962–1972, including the number of hospitals, total beds, admissions, occupancy rates, outpatient visits, births, and number of employees.

Four major trends developed during that period. Admissions increased from 26 million in 1962 to 33 million in 1972. The occupancy rate—the average number of beds being utilized—declined while outpatient visits rose substantially from 99 million to 218 million. In addition, the number of births declined by 16 percent from the high of 3.8 million in 1962 to 3.2 million.

The Hospital Quadrangle

In 1968, four hospitals in the northwest metropolitan section of Detroit formed the Metropolitan Northwest Detroit Hospitals, Inc. Generally known as the Quadrangle, the four members were: Mount Carmel Mercy Hospital and Medical Center, Grace Hospital, N.W., Sinai Hospital, and Providence Hospital. (Providence is in the adjoining suburb of Southfield; however, all four hospitals are within four miles of each other.) Table 9-9 presents the bed size, occupancy rate, number of annual admissions, total expenses, payroll, and number of personnel of each of the four Quadrangle members.

The Quadrangle's objectives were to (1) seek to maintain and/or improve the quality of patient care provided by its members, (2) seek ways to reduce the total cost of hospital care in the northwest section of Detroit, and (3) provide a forum to channel cooperative efforts of the four hospitals in constructive directions. With the trends of (1) increased demand for administrative accountability by the public and government, (2) the rapidly rising level of hospital care cost, and (3) structural changes in health care delivery, the four hospitals sought ways to respond positively. One consideration was sharing professional services.

A unique characteristic of nongovernmental, nonprofit hospitals in comparison to industrial organizations was that charges to and payments to hospital providers by third party payers such as Blue Cross, the federal government, and private insurance companies were based on reasonable

Figure 9-3 Mount Carmel Mercy Hospital and Medical Center
Organization Chart (1972)

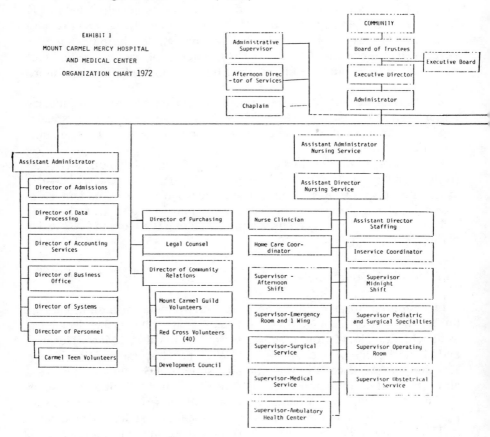

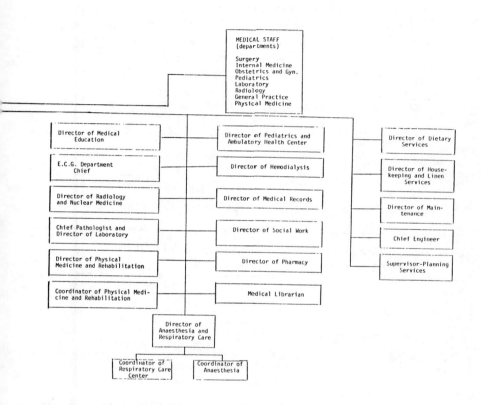

Source: Internal records of Mount Carmel Hospital and Medical Center, Detroit.

Table 9-5 Patients Discharged, Total Days, and Average Stay by Type of Service

Fiscal Years 1971 and 1972

	Patients Discharged		Total Days		Average Stay in Days	
	1971	1972	1971	1972	1971	1972
Department of						
Medicine	6,383	6,946	74,716	80,890	11.7	11.7
Surgery	9,940	9,330	90,239	83,668	9.1	9.0
OB	3,514	2,847	15,716	12,918	4.5	4.5
GYN	1,379	1,346	9,425	9,421	6.8	7.0
Pediatrics and						
Adolescent Medicine	2,984	3,012	13,791	15,024	4.6	5.0
General Practice	666	661	6,723	8,556	10.1	12.9
Totals	24,866	24,142	210,883	210,477	(Avg.) 8.5	(Avg.) 8.7

Source: Mount Carmel Mercy Hospital and Medical Center, *1972 Annual Report.*

Table 9-6 Classification of Hospitals by Type, Total Beds, and Percentage, 1972

Total		Federal		State/ Local		Nongovernmental Nonprofit		Nongovernmental For-Profit	
Hospitals	Beds*	Hospitals	Beds*	Hospitals	Beds*	Hospitals	Beds*	Hospitals	Beds*
7,061	1,550	401	143	2,300	699	3,515	639	845	65
100%	100%	5.6%	9.2%	32.6%	45.0%	50.0%	41.2%	12.0%	4.1%

* Bed totals are in thousands.
Source: Data based on: *Hospital Statistics, 1972*, American Hospital Association, pp. 20–21.

Table 9-7 Hospitals in U.S. by Number of Beds

Hospital Size (Beds)	No. in This Category	Percent of Total
More than 500	639	9.0
400–499	267	3.7
300–399	436	6.2
200–299	734	10.4
100–199	1,433	20.1
Fewer than 100	3,522	50.3
Totals	7,061	99.7*

* Total does not add because of rounding.
Source: Data based on: *Hospital Statistics, 1972*, American Hospital Association.

Table 9-8 Data on United States Hospitals, Selected Years

Year	Number of Hospitals	Number of Beds (in thousands)	Admissions (in thousands)	Average Daily Census (in thousands)	Occupancy (percent)	Number of Outpatient Visits (in thousands)	Births	Number of Personnel (in thousands)	Total Hospital Expenses (in millions)
1962	7,028	1,689	26,531	1,407	83.3	99,382	3,857,626	1,763	$6,735
1967	7,172	1,671	29,361	1,380	82.6	148,229	3,283,711	2,203	10,461
1972	7,061	1,550	33,265	1,209	78.0	219,182	3,231,875	2,671	19,530

Source: Data based on: *Hospital Statistics, 1972*, American Hospital Association, p. 19.

Table 9-9 Detroit Quadrangle Hospitals

12-Month Period Ending September 30, 1971

	Number of Beds	Annual Admissions	Average Daily Census	Average Occupancy Rate	Total Expenses (in thousands)	Total Payroll (in thousands)	Number of Personnel
Mount Carmel Mercy Hospital and Medical Center	557	19,846	495	88.9	$21,006	$11,804	1,527
Grace Hospital, N.W.	418	14,450	373	87.6	15,600	NA	1,250
Providence Hospital	400	15,270	358	89.5	16,057	9,288	1,090
Sinai Hospital	478	17,189	435	95.2	21,305	10,956	1,347
Totals	1,853	66,755	1,661	90.3	73,968	32,048*	5,214

* Total is for three hospitals, Grace omitted.

Source: Data based on: *Hospital Guide Issue, 1972,* American Hospital Association, p. 111 and 117.

costs incurred. Consequently, a specific facility had little incentive to reduce costs and services so long as they were comparable to those of others in the area.

In a geographic area where there was an excess of hospital beds—that is, facilities were being underutilized—the fixed costs of empty beds had to be spread over those that were filled. Consequently, while the costs for any individual facility might be in line with those in its area, the total for care provided to the community was higher.

As a result, the Quadrangle sought potential service consolidations. The impact would be the reduction of the total number of beds allocated to a specific service in all four facilities and the increased occupancy rate in those that would maintain the service. It was felt that sharing and consolidating some professional services would (1) provide better care and (2) reduce the costs of hospital care for the community as a whole.

The chairman of the steering committee of the Detroit Hospital Quadrangle was Dr. Thomas R. O'Donovan, administrator of Mount Carmel Mercy Hospital and Medical Center. He described to the casewriter the Quadrangle's philosophy of sharing services as follows:

> By exploring the sharing of professional services, such as obstetrics and pediatrics, neighboring hospitals can better utilize their current available space. They may even save money by avoiding the construction of expensive facility additions for other high demand services by reclassifying the beds in the closed service. To make the sharing of services work requires teamwork and cooperation. Historically, hospitals have been "stand-alone" facilities with each offering a totality of services. Heretofore, there has been little need or incentive to work together to accomplish patient care objectives. The question is, can cooperation work or does institutional chauvinism prevail?

The Quadrangle was formed to explore these problems and attempt to instill a sense of interhospital cooperation.

Administrative Philosophy

In elaborating on his administrative philosophy, Dr. O'Donovan stated:

> I am a firm believer in Management by Objectives and the development of capable staff to administer the day-to-day operations at Mount Carmel. I feel that Mount Carmel is an innovative hospital. I am quite aware of the fact that the Executive Director

and I have the responsibility for managing an organization that will enable physicians to treat their patients. However, it is my hope that this hospital may serve as a model for others. We are a nonprofit hospital dedicated to providing quality care and teaching. In that respect, our ultimate responsibility is to the community both in terms of offering a wide range of services and providing quality care at reasonable costs.

Some of the things we have attempted to do in the last seven years are (1) be cost effective, (2) be responsive to the needs of the community, and (3) maintain our tradition of a high level of care to all who seek it. As one of the largest hospitals in Detroit, and the nation, for that matter, Mount Carmel must serve in the role of one of the institutional leaders. Among the internal changes we have introduced are (1) the development of a comprehensive wage and salary structure and (2) the overseeing of various expansion programs. Among the various external activities in which I have had a part are serving as the National Educational Director of the American Academy of Medical Administrators and actively participating in area committees formed for the purpose of initiating cooperative efforts among area hospitals. The Detroit Hospital Quadrangle is one example.

In the 1972 fiscal year, several specific service areas have required my attention. The first was the dramatic increase in the utilization of our emergency room. For example, the utilization frequency rose from 27,705 in 1969 to 39,151 in 1972. As a result, early this year construction to double the size of our emergency room was begun in order to accommodate this service area shift needed by the community.

However, we are experiencing another shift in service utilization, specifically, in Obstetrics and Gynecology (OB-GYN) where there has been a decline in the number of deliveries. During the 1971 fiscal year 2,610 babies were delivered, while only 2,152 were delivered in the 1972 fiscal year. That represents the lowest number of babies delivered since 1942 and a 68 percent decline from our peak number of deliveries of 6,733 in 1958. (Table 9-10 shows the number of deliveries at Mount Carmel for the fiscal years 1940–1972.) Since our 70-bed Obstetrical Department now has an occupancy rate of 46 percent in the 1972 fiscal year, my im-

Table 9-10 Total Deliveries at Mount Carmel Hospital, 1940–1972

Fiscal Year	Deliveries	Fiscal Year	Deliveries
		1956	6,418
1940	234	1957	6,615
1941	1,581	1958	6,733
1942	2,558	1959	6,106
1943	4,296	1960	5,790
1944	4,270	1961	5,123
1945	3,610	1962	4,505
1946	3,665	1963	4,190
1947	4,501	1964	4,019
1948	4,726	1965	3,966
1949	4,565	1966	3,620
1950	4,773	1967	3,480
1951	5,485	1968	3,036
1952	6,113	1969	2,884
1953	6,463	1970	2,766
1954	5,865	1971	2,610
1955	6,299	1972	2,152

Source: Internal records of Mount Carmel Mercy Hospital and Medical Center.

mediate concern is whether to continue, modify (in terms of beds allocated), or discontinue this service.

Sharing OB

In keeping with the Quadrangle's objective of sharing services, the alternative of consolidating the obstetrical department within one or several of the other member hospitals was being considered. Three of the four hospitals had experienced a low occupancy rate during 1971. Table 9-11 shows the number of OB beds, average daily census, percent of occupancy, and length of stay for the Quadrangle hospitals.

When evaluating the advisability of maintaining or phasing out the obstetrical service, Dr. O'Donovan made the following points:

> We have to evaluate many factors in order to make a decision. Mount Carmel, being a 557-bed hospital and having had an active Obstetrical Department since it was founded in 1939, has many reasons to continue this department. Even though many smaller hospitals with small OB units have closed throughout the country, never before in history has a unit as large as ours (70 beds) been closed.

Table 9-11 Quadrangle OB Data, Fiscal Year 1971

	Mount Carmel	Grace N.W.	Sinai	Providence
No. of OB Beds Available for Delivered OBs	70	67	53	50
Average Daily Census OBs Delivered	39	38	46	35
Percent of Occupancy OBs Delivered	56	57	87	70
OBs Delivered	2,610	2,646	3,336	2,623
Inpatient Days OBs Delivered	14,145	13,971	16,796	12,880
Average Length of Stay, OBs Delivered	5.4	5.3	5.0	4.9
Total Births (including SBs)	2,640	2,671	3,384	2,656

* Average.
Source: Internal records of Mount Carmel Mercy Hospital and Medical Center.

The OB service is one of the services we provide in order to fulfill our community responsibility. However, we also have another responsibility which consists of cooperating with areawide planning agencies and the Quadrangle. Relative to the latter, the Quadrangle has the purpose of sharing services in order (1) to avoid duplication of facilities and services, (2) to help decrease costs to the community as a whole and (3) to improve the quality of patient care.

Advantages of Phasing Out OB

Dr. O'Donovan said the reasons favoring Mount Carmel Mercy Hospital's closing its obstetrical department were:

1. *Declining Occupancy.* The 70-bed unit at Mount Carmel Mercy Hospital has had a steadily declining census due to the declining birth rate. The birth-rate data point toward a continued downward decline in the years ahead. At this time in 1972 the average occupancy of the obstetrical department was 46 percent. This means that over 38 of the 70 beds were vacant on any given day. Generally, when a hospital has an occupancy rate in obstetrics of less than 70 percent, this results in an unfavorable financial position for the hospital.

Mount Carmel has lost over $350,000 per year in its obstetrical department in the last few years even though our room charges are $67 a day for a ward, $72 a day for a semiprivate room, $48 a day for the nursery, and $170 for use of the delivery room. Generally, many hospitals tend to suffer financial losses in their obstetrical department, regardless of their level of occupancy, because of the up-and-down nature of the level of occupancy. It is difficult to predict the peaks and valleys of births that will take place in any given hospital. It is not easy to temporarily layoff OB nurses when the census is down for a few days at a time.

Even with declining occupancy, one of our options would be to continue the service on a reduced scale, specifically, establishing a unit of perhaps 35 to 40 beds. This would result in a unit that would have a sufficient number of beds to maintain an 80 percent to 90 percent occupancy rate, unless, of course, the birth rate continued to slide in the years ahead.

It is also important to note that if the hospital gave up OB, the present 70 OB beds could be devoted immediately, without any remodeling necessary, to medical/surgical beds. This would increase the occupancy from the present 46 percent for the 70 beds to over 90 percent since this has been the general level of occupancy in the medical/surgical area at Mount Carmel in recent years. Demand for medical/surgical beds is expected to be high in the years ahead. In fact, there is a large waiting list, and the Urgent and Emergency List is quite extensive. Thus, reassignment of these OB beds to medical/surgical would tend to serve the community more by taking care of the patients that are waiting at home for beds, and, of course, it would serve the internists, surgeons, and general practitioners of the hospital medical staff very well.

2. *Remodeling Required.* In order to continue its obstetrical department, a major program of remodeling would be necessary as required by the Michigan Department of Public Health. The architect's estimate for these changes is $1.3 million. The hospital would face a major challenge in obtaining the $1.3 million. A further issue here is that the Economic Stabilization Program of the Federal Government is in full swing and there is a question as to whether or not Mount Carmel can increase its costs to the point of being able to obtain a price exception. On the other hand, the required funds could possibly be obtained by debt financing.

3. *A Furtherance of the Spirit of Sharing Services.* The prime purpose of the Quadrangle is to share services. Deletion of the obstetrical program of our hospital and merging it within the Quadrangle would be an extremely important act of teamwork. For example, Providence Hospital had an occupancy rate of 70 percent in 1971 based on 50 beds, and Grace Hospital, N.W. had an occupancy of 57 percent based on 67 beds. If the majority of our OB-GYN physicians delivered their patients at Providence or Grace, this would increase their hospital's occupancy and also reduce their costs/bed. In addition, a larger concentration of patients and house staff would result in better patient care and improvements in their teaching programs.

4. *Decreased Costs to the Community.* The final advantage of phasing out our Obstetrics Department would be the reduction of the number of OB beds in the area. Consequently, those members of the Quadrangle retaining OB beds would experience higher occupancy rates, and the total costs to the community would be decreased by reason of eliminating the costs associated with empty beds.

Disadvantages of Phasing Out OB

Among the reasons for not phasing out the Obstetrical Department, Dr. O'Donovan listed the following:

1. *Disadvantaged Patients.* One of the major reasons for not phasing out the Obstetrical Department is the fact that over 700 of the births last year at Mount Carmel were made by low-income patients. We have a contract with the Detroit Maternal Infant Care Program. It is a federally financed program administered by the state in which low-income mothers are given prenatal care, the delivery, and postnatal care of the child.

The question is whether or not we can obtain community support for a phase-out decision. If these disadvantaged mothers were turned away because it was not possible for them to be delivered at Providence or at some other hospital with a reasonable level of convenience and without a reduction in the level of care, the community would certainly react negatively. Much thought has to be given to our community service responsibility in this area.

2. *Are There Sufficient Beds Available in the Area?* Another important consideration is whether the other Quadrangle hospitals could absorb our patient load. This matter has to be examined very carefully.

3. *Staff Privileges*. Provided that an adequate number of beds are available at Providence, Grace N.W., and Sinai Hospitals, it is extremely important that all Mount Carmel OB-GYN physicians be given additional staff privileges at some or all of those hospitals to take care of their OB patients. One consideration is that the vast majority of the OB-GYN doctors at Mount Carmel be extended privileges at Grace and Providence Hospitals. Most of the OB-GYN doctors at Mount Carmel will probably accept this arrangement, although they would have preferred that the facilities at Mount Carmel be continued. The reason for this is that they would have to make rounds at two hospitals, if they did their GYN at Mount Carmel and their OB at Providence and/or Grace.

4. *Present OB Personnel*. A major question is what to do with the 110 employees presently working in our OB-GYN department. They include nurses, LPNs and nurses' aides. Some could be hired at Providence (perhaps about 10 percent), and the remaining number could be retrained through inservice programs and reassigned to medical/surgical, pediatrics, emergency, or the intensive care units.

5. *Image*. Another problem facing Mount Carmel is that a major hospital with over 500 beds tends to retain a much better image if it has a well-rounded program. Retention of the obstetrical department would maintain this strong image.

6. *Potential Loss of GYN Surgery*. It is most important for a general hospital to retain a well-rounded program. Even if OB is lost, it is still important to retain GYN. There are many who would predict that a hospital that loses its OB service would tend to lose its GYN service within a few years because of the tendency of the OB-GYN doctors to want to do their OB and GYN work at the same hospital.

If, in fact, a loss of GYN did occur at Mount Carmel in the future, this would affect the teaching program of medical education. Not only would the house staff in other clinical areas not have the OB department for experience, but they would also lose the GYN surgery. This would make it quite likely for the residency review boards to discontinue approval of residencies in radiology, medicine, and general surgery, if a sufficient range of clinical material was not available at the hospital.

Mount Carmel could, of course, promote GYN surgery as much as possible by extending favorable boarding times and assigning beds to the GYN physicians who moved to Providence and/or to the other two Quadrangle hospitals. It is also important for a hospital to have GYN residents cover our GYN clinic on a rotation basis.

7. *Lack of Acceptance on the Part of the Medical Staff.* This has been alluded to before, but it is an important disadvantage for a hospital to lose its OB department when the physicians do not accept that decision of the board of trustees. There have been cases in the United States in which a hospital has given up an obstetrical department and the medical staff has sued the hospital to prevent this from happening. This creates all kinds of conflict, and it certainly points out the great importance to any hospital that attempts to share services that medical staff involvement at each and every step of the way is necessary.

Since the Michigan Department of Public Health had ordered that physical renovation of the Obstetrics Department begin by January 1, 1973, Dr. O'Donovan had to (1) evaluate the alternatives available to Mount Carmel, (2) propose a course of action to the board, and (3) develop the implementation plan within the next six months.

OVERVIEW OF CASE 17

Issues to Consider

1. What are the options available to Mount Carmel Mercy Hospital and Medical Center as it reviews its obstetrics ward operation?
2. What are the advantages and disadvantages of closing the obstetrics ward?
3. What process should a health care provider follow in evaluating a possible service elimination?

Discussion

1. The Options Available

As the health care industry has grown, so has Mount Carmel. From 1939 to 1972, it expanded from 325 beds to 557, 70 of which are designated for obstetrics. The trend in obstetric departments across the nation is toward decreasing utilization with a resultant overabundance of such beds. Mount Carmel has experienced this same phenomenon. The occupancy rate in its obstetrics department in 1972 was 46 percent. It has been determined that, to be efficient, utilization of the ward should be at 85 percent. Mount Carmel's obstetrics department is far below that level and, to attain it, would need a daily census of 59.5 compared to the average 32.2 beds that were occupied daily in 1972. The key issue is whether the required increase in utilization is possible or even realistic given past trends and future demographic predictions.

The administrator reports that the declining utilization trend has become a problem for Mount Carmel and requires attention. To add to the dilemma, the Michigan Department of Public Health has mandated that the hospital remodel its obstetrics department. The estimated cost of remodeling to meet the standard specifications is $1.3 million. The administrator now must evaluate the following options to resolve the situation:

1. eliminate obstetrics at Mount Carmel and assign its 70 beds to the medical/surgical departments
2. modify the obstetric department to reduce the number of beds to 30
3. invest the $1.3 million in order to continue to provide an OB department of 70 beds and hope for increased occupancy

2. Advantages and Disadvantages

The administrator realistically stated the advantages and disadvantages of phasing out the OB department. The arguments for phasing out include:

1. Declining Occupancy: The national trend is a declining birth rate, resulting in a decrease in the occupancy rate in OB departments. Mount Carmel reports it has lost more than $350,000 a year in its Obstetrical Department in the last few years. A key question is: How long can a hospital be expected to maintain a department that is unable to support itself financially?
2. Converting OB Beds to Medical/Surgical Beds: The administrator says that if the hospital gave up OB, those 70 beds could be devoted immediately, without remodeling, to medical/surgical use. He be-

lieves this would increase the occupancy from the present 46 percent for those 70 beds to more than 90 pecent since that has been the general level of medical/surgical occupancy in recent years. He predicts that "Demand for medical/surgical beds is expected to be high in the years ahead."

3. Remodeling Required: The Michigan Department of Public Health has mandated that the OB ward be remodeled if it is to continue operation. The cost is expected to be $1.3 million.

4. A Furtherance of the Spirit of Sharing Services: By eliminating its own OB department and referring patients to the three other Quadrangle hospitals, Mount Carmel will be demonstrating "teamwork." The administrator suggests that bringing up the OB census levels in the other hospitals will result in "better patient care and improvements in teaching programs."

5. Decreased Costs to the Community: The decreased costs referred to are those associated with maintaining empty beds.

The disadvantages of phasing out the OB ward at Mount Carmel were stated by the administrator as follows:

1. Disadvantaged Patients: Mount Carmel has a community responsibility to low-income patients in the Detroit area. The hospital has a contract with the Detroit Maternal Infant Care Program to provide prenatal care, delivery, and postnatal care. Unless these individuals can be cared for by the three other Quadrangle hospitals "with a reasonable level of convenience and without reduction in the level of care, the community would certainly react negatively."

2. Are There Sufficient Beds Available in the Area? It has not been determined whether the other Quadrangle hospitals could accommodate all of Mount Carmel's OB patient load. This must be determined before a decision is made.

3. Staff Privileges: Staff privileges for Mount Carmel's OB-GYN physicians will need to be extended to the three others if its OB department is eliminated.

4. Present OB Personnel: If the OB ward is eliminated, the staff of 110 (not including physicians) must be retrained, transferred to other departments, or let go.

5. Image: The Mount Carmel image may be altered if it does not offer an obstetric department because it no longer will have a well-rounded program.

6. Potential Loss of GYN Surgery: Once a hospital eliminates its OB department, it is just a matter of time before it drops its GYN service

because physicians prefer to have both OB and GYN at the same hospital.

7. Lack of Acceptance on the Part of the Medical Staff: Unless the medical staff supports the board decision to eliminate a service, there may be difficulties not only with the hospital structure but also legally. The legal history documents numerous cases of medical staffs opposing the hospital.

3. The Evaluation Process

The administrator has been concerned with consumers' accessibility to medical services, hospital image, internal and external marketing, and market share. What has not been addressed is the methodology for determining when to eliminate a service. A Health Care Service Elimination Model can be divided into seven stages:

Stage 1: Environmental Assessment includes an internal and external inventory, evaluation of community interest and involvement, and examination of trends.

Stage 2: Elimination Criteria consider the nature of the service, its usage, trend of usage, its contribution as an input to other services, etc.

Stage 3: Performance Ratio Analysis gives formulas for a cost accounting analysis of the service. This also provides objective input into the decision-making process.

Stage 4: Elimination Decision.

Stage 5: Elimination Plan.

Stage 6: Implementation.

Stage 7: Review and Evaluation.

The model addresses the issue of internal barriers to service elimination (example: the extent the service is equated with the organization and the retraining of staff) and external barriers (physician attitudes, patterns of community behavior, and federal, state and local funding). Most importantly, the process of monitoring the life of a health care service should be continuous.

The administrator's most valuable tools when deciding on the future of a service are (1) using a Health Care Service Elimination Model to monitor the status of the service and (2) using health care marketing principles to understand consumers' needs, the facility's image, service competition, and market share. In the case the author does not define the service market and the target market nor are the geographic, psychographic, and demographic elements of the target market given. The current utilizers are not analyzed and plotted geographically. It is essential to analyze past utilization, determine present occupancy, and estimate future needs. To obtain this information, the administrator can: (1) perform a needs assessment of the service market, (2) conduct focus groups with members of the community, (3) conduct focus groups or survey the referring physicians, and (4) conduct a market audit. The administrator who has a conceptual picture of the market's changing needs will have vital ammunition to aid in making a decision. Questions that will arise include: What are the needs of the people being served? Is there a duplication of services of equivalent quality in delivery and accessibility?

In this case, readers might tend to favor eliminating the OB ward. However, essential information that is not provided includes: price, distribution, personal contact, advertising, publicity, and sales promotion.

If it be assumed that the best interest of the hospital and the community is to eliminate the obstetric department the Mount Carmel administrator now is in a position to:

1. demarket the OB ward at Mount Carmel
   a. to the community (external marketing)
   b. to the physicians and staff (internal marketing)
2. market the three other Quadrangle OB departments
   a. to the community
   b. to the physicians
3. market the conversion of OB beds to surgical beds
   a. to the community
   b. to the physicians and staff

To accomplish the many outcomes of the decision, once it has been made by the board of trustees, it is essential to develop a marketing strategy and implementation plan. The marketing strategy should include the principles of demarketing a service and its market both internally and externally.

Development of a Marketing Plan: Assembling the CAPS

The marketing process enables health service organizations to develop a plan to guide relationships with patients and other publics. A marketing plan describes chosen markets, the timing and quantity of financial and human resources allocated to each market segment, while forecasting the expected results. The cases in this section examine the marketing strategies of a free-standing medical emergency center, a hospital, a hospice, a rural primary care center, and a health maintenance organization.

All organizations pursue marketing in order to plan, transact, and facilitate voluntary exchanges with the targeted populations. The marketing plans of the organizations covered in this section include minimal efforts (Central Alabama Primary Care, Inc. and Toco Hills Medical Emergency Center) as well as more formal presentations (Community Health Plan). Minimal efforts in market planning often occur when the health care facility has a real or perceived mandate to serve the entire community. In such an instance, the marketing plan should be general, featuring a broad range of services, limited communications efforts, and cost-based pricing. However, very few markets are homogeneous, sharing perceived service needs and preferences. The approach in most cases is to focus attention on specific market segments in the hopes of becoming the provider of choice for populations whose needs, attitudes, and preferences are most consistent with the resources and capabilities of the facility.

A marketing plan involves defining target populations, along with orchestrating the services, communication efforts, access/availability strategy, and price decisions for each market segment. These factors are all variables of the marketing plan, which should be responsive to the health status of markets served and their service objectives. Also, the plan should be supported by consumer research on changing needs, attitudes, expectations, preferences, and satisfaction levels of market segments. Community Health Plan, described in Case 22, illustrates the major components included in

271

a well-defined marketing plan. This community plan identifies the market to be served, enrollment goals, services to be offered, communications programming, distribution decisions, pricing procedures, and policies necessary to achieve these goals.

How does a health care organization develop a marketing plan? For many organizations, the point of initiation may be to invite a consultant to review the marketing environment. Central Alabama Primary Care, Inc., Case 19, sought such a review. The consultants' report, as described in the case, exemplifies typical results to be expected from such an exercise. The report highlights the need for market-based data provided by consumer research to support the marketing plan.

A second approach to development of a marketing plan is to conduct a marketing audit which assists management in evaluating the populations, services, marketing programs, and the plan's effectiveness. As defined by Kotler, a marketing audit is:

> . . . an independent examination of the entire marketing effort of an organization covering objectives, programs, implementation, organization and control, for the purpose of determining what is being done and recommending what should be done in the future.[1]

The marketing audit provides a *base line* for development of a marketing plan. The first time a marketing audit is administered, management should expect that many questions cannot be answered adequately with available data. As shown in Case 18, depicting the Toco Hills Medical Emergency Center, management may need to conduct post-audit research before a marketing plan is fully developed and implemented.

Marketing plans may vary substantially in content and detail. However, successful plans share the philosophy that consumers buy solutions not products; they purchase results, not services. The responsive organization systematically and continuously measures the pulse of the market and develops strategies which satisfy the perceived needs of consumers in an efficient manner.

---

[1] Philip Kotler, *Marketing for Nonprofit Organizations* (Englewood Cliffs, N.J.: Prentice-Hall, Inc., 1975), p. 56.

Chapter 10

The Marketing Audit

CASE 18. TOCO HILLS MEDICAL EMERGENCY CENTER: A MARKETING AUDIT FOR A HEALTH SERVICES ORGANIZATION

Ms. Elizabeth Shine, assistant director, Toco Hills Medical Emergency Center, had just arranged to meet the next day with four graduate students at Emory University. The four students had just finished an analysis of the marketing function at Toco Hills Medical Emergency Center (hereafter referred to as Toco Hills MEC). They were enrolled in "Marketing for Health Services Organizations," an elective course offered by the Master of Community Health Program and taught by a member of the marketing faculty. The marketing analysis was conducted by a technique called a marketing audit.[1]

Origin and Growth of Toco Hills MEC

The Toco Hills Medical Emergency Center was founded in Northeast Atlanta by Drs. Fred Cowan and Selwyn Hartley in May 1978. Its purpose was to provide high-quality emergency medical care to the community at large. Its owners viewed it as an emergency room without a hospital. They believed that private enterprise could do a better job than public hospitals of treating the kinds of problems people take to an emergency room. Both physicians had extensive training and experience in emergency medicine: Dr. Hartley still was associated with Clayton General Hospital's emergency room; until recently, Dr. Cowan had been head of the emergency room at Southwest Hospital. The Toco Hills Medical Emergency Center was formed as a corporation, Medical Emergency Centers, Inc., with Drs. Cowan and Hartley the stockholders and codirectors. They had spent more than a year and a half exploring the possibility of a free-standing emergency center before contracting to establish one. To determine the desired services and equipment for such a center, they called upon their own experiences and visited similar centers around the country.

The Toco Hills MEC is in a spacious, 40,000-square-foot, free-standing building in a large shopping center with ample parking space. The building previously had been an auto supply store. The businesses in the shopping center include: sporting goods, books/stationery, clothing, shoes, a health spa, Army/Navy, pet supplies, furniture, liquor, a French restaurant and two fast-food restaurants, and a small complex of medical/dental offices. The physical setting of the Toco Hills MEC was attractive, with high ceilings and bright colors. The waiting room had ample seating in comfortable, capacious leather chairs. Magazines were available for both adults and children. The receptionists, nurses, and technicians were friendly, helpful, and courteous during each visit of an audit group of graduate students from Emory University. One nurse "moonlighting" at the center on weekends expressed a desire to work full time because of her respect for Dr. Cowan as a physician as well as the nature of the work.

The center was open seven days a week, 365 days a year, from 8 A.M. to midnight. Almost all patients were walk-ins with only about one out of 100 arriving by ambulance. Volume had increased since it opened. During the first few months, some 700 patients a month were treated. By October 1978, the figure had reached 900. There was no information as to why this increase had occurred.

The layout provided physical space for increased patient volume. In March 1979, average utilization was 30 to 50 patients per 16-hour period, or 2 to 3 per hour. If all space were used, close to 150 patients per day (about nine patients per hour) could be seen; however, staff size would need to be increased.

Personnel

The staff consisted of the following:

1 physician per shift (total M.D.s: 2 physician coowners plus 4 part time)
1 R.N. per shift (total R.N.s: 4 full time, plus 2 part time)
1 technician (laboratory and x-ray) per shift (total technicians)
1 receptionist per shift (total receptionists)
1 radiologist (part time)
1 business manager
1 laboratory supervisor (also serving as purchasing agent)
assistant director
accountant and lawyer available on request.

The assistant director was Ms. Elizabeth Shine, Dr. Cowan's wife. A psychiatric social worker, she was a consultant on marriage and family problems. Her services were not part of the emergency center, although referrals were made to her. However, she maintained a private practice at the center.

Staff meetings were held every two weeks to discuss problems and propose solutions. The personnel turnover rate was low. One laboratory technician and one nurse were asked to leave because the quality of their work was not up to the standard set by the directors/owners. If patient volume continued to grow, an additional physician would be hired. Dr. Cowan intended to seek one with extensive emergency room experience (family practice or surgery). A recent medical graduate was preferable because such a person was likely to have the kind of experience necessary for emergency medicine. There were no plans for hiring physician assistants or nurse practitioners. Dr. Cowan's view was that such professionals must be able to function independently of the physician in a practice like theirs. If the physician had to review daily the activities of a P.A. or N.P., little economy would result.

Market and Market Segments

Dr. Cowan regarded all members of the community as potential patients. The directors/owners believed the center would attract the following market segments: single persons; newcomers to Atlanta, many of whom lived in apartments in the center's area; and visitors staying in local motels. Although their records had not been analyzed, patients were known to reside in a large geographic area surrounding the center (Figure 10-1). Most seemed to come from the immediate area (Toco Hills, Emory, Druid Hills, Center for Disease Control, Clairmont Road, Buford Highway, Decatur, or Stone Mountain). It appeared that those who came from outside the immediate area did so because the Toco Hills Center was closer than DeKalb General Hospital, which had the nearest hospital emergency room, and had a shorter waiting period.

Dr. Cowan believed the center served an area that was quite stable, with little anticipated change in age, income, or occupation. The decrease in the school-age population already had been under way before the center opened. Pediatric patients had not been major users of the center so a continued decline in that population group would not have adverse effects. Dr. Cowan also speculated that most parents had a private physician for their children and relied on the emergency room in the hospital with which their doctor was associated. In general, after nine months of operation, Dr. Cowan had observed no real difference between the original target markets and those actually using the center.

Figure 10-1 Location of Toco Hills MEC and Surrounding Areas

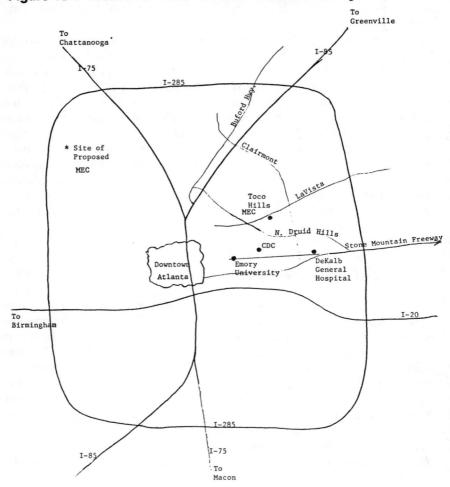

Competitors

The Toco Hills MEC had no directly comparable competitors in Georgia. The concept of a free-standing emergency medical center was new and growing around the country, with examples in Rhode Island, Kansas, Texas, and Arizona; in all, there were about 30 in the U.S. The owners of the center anticipated that others of its type would open in Atlanta. In fact, they had been approached for information by two physicians who intended to open one in Northwest Atlanta, about 12 miles from the Toco Hills MEC.

Hospital emergency rooms and private physicians were regarded as the main competitors. Some private physicians viewed the center as a potential threat to their practices, particularly if their patients were to visit the center for minor problems such as colds, earache, symptoms of flu, etc.

The convenience of having an emergency center open until midnight, including weekends, was a feature private physicians could not match. It was important to Drs. Cowan and Hartley that these physicians not become antagonistic to the center; therefore, they were careful to discourage patients of such doctors from using the center for primary care. They did not encourage patients to drop in for physicals or multiphasic tests. Few physicians referred patients to the center. For those who did, Drs. Cowan and Hartley reassured them that their patients would return to their care after receiving emergency services. The After Care Instructions given to center patients clearly spelled out that only emergency medical treatment had been given and that it was not intended to be a substitute for complete medical care. The patient was advised to see a private physician or the follow-up doctor (the M.D. who treated the patient at the center) for any new or remaining problems.

The only operating license required for the Toco Hills Medical Emergency Center was a business license, the same as that needed for a private physician's office. When the center incorporated, the owners asked the North Central Health Systems Agency (HSA) if review would be necessary. Since the HSA had no familiarity with this new kind of facility, it said no review would be required.

Products and Services

The medical services offered by the center were not unique. It was the manner in which they were given that was innovative. The characteristics that set the Toco Hills MEC apart from a hospital emergency room were: short waiting periods, lower costs, more personal patient/staff interaction, and attractive physical environment.

From the private physician's point of view, the center's competitive threat to the individual practitioner might be: hours of service, no appointment necessary (drop-in), and ample parking space. Patients seeking nonemergency primary care would have to weigh the importance of these conveniences against the somewhat higher cost of services at Toco Hills as compared to a physician office visit.

The center had a capability to treat up to 9 patients at a time, with 12 beds. The space was laid out as follows:

3 general examination cubicles separated by sliding curtains
1 ob/gyn examination room with door
1 ear, nose, throat/dental examination room with door
4 trauma areas with trauma stretcher (including one area with complete cardiac care equipment except for inserting pacemaker)
1 orthopedic room for casting
1 x-ray room
1 laboratory area
1 large nurses' station and large supply area
1 central supply area
1 waiting room area
2 private offices

The facilities and equipment were similar to those of a hospital emergency room, with corridors wide enough to move beds from one area to another. Technical facilities were entirely adequate, according to Dr. Cowan. Most laboratory work was done at the center, although some tests were sent to the National Health Laboratories in Washington, D.C. If volume increased sufficiently to warrant the expenditure, Drs. Cowan and Hartley considered buying ultrasound equipment for diagnosis of acute problems and blood gas equipment for diagnosis of acid-base problems. The use of ultrasound equipment would require a full-time radiologist. Present equipment did not allow for full diagnosis of surgical problems or head trauma. Such cases were referred to specialists. If a fracture was not displaced, it could be set at the center; if it was displaced, the patient was referred to an orthopedist. The physicians at the Toco Hills MEC did not go into hospitals to treat patients. Patients who required hospitalization were referred to their own physicians; if they had none, they were referred to a specialist.

The types of problems most commonly seen at the center were fractures and lacerations. Medical problems outweighed the surgical. X-ray equipment was used the most, blood chemistry the least. The DeKalb County Health Department referred clients to the center for vaccinations.

Major decisions on current services and future expansion were made by both partners informally. Dr. Cowan could not recall any services that had been discontinued. The first phase of expansion planned was in the area of employment physical examinations—industrial, executive, and preemployment. Physicals were done for the General Electric Credit Corporation, Prudential Medicare, Georgia Pacific, and Southern Bell Training.

The center did not own an ambulance service; however, Central DeKalb Ambulance Service used garage space at the center. Atlanta area ambulance services did not take patients to the center unless they specifically requested it. Dr. Cowan explained that many Atlanta-area emergency medical technicians were trained at DeKalb General Hospital so it was their practice to take patients there.

Fees and Payments

The Toco Hills MEC was less expensive than a hospital emergency room but more expensive than a private physician. The center's overhead was higher than that of a private physician's office since it operated 16 hours a day. The Center charged no emergency room fee. Its physician's fee was $25, compared to a hospital emergency room minimum of $15 plus and M.D. fee of $15 to $20. A throat culture at Toco Hills was $5 ($10 in a hospital emergency room) and a blood count with complete differential was $9 ($15 in a hospital). X-rays cost 15 to 20 percent less than if done at a hospital. Most laboratory work was done immediately at the center; hospitals charged an extra fee. In any cost comparison, the length of waiting time must be considered. At the center, the average turnaround time (entry, waiting period, exit) was 40 minutes while in a hospital emergency room the wait could be four hours or longer.

Since its opening, the center had increased some of its fees because, as a result of low volume, the original levels were not covering overhead costs. In a hospital, the emergency room usually loses money. Other units of the hospital (inpatient) make up the difference and add to profits. At Toco Hills, any increases in the price of supplies or utilities caused fees to rise. It was planned to keep the $25 physician fee while increasing the prices on specialized laboratory tests. Drs. Cowan and Hartley hoped to realize a profit in another six months.

Patients were requested to pay at the time services were provided. This could be done with cash, check, or major credit card. The Toco Hills MEC would not accept Medicare, Medicaid, or any other kind of third party payment. Patients were given a copy of their treatment record and could file for reimbursement themselves. However, Dr. Cowan made it clear that the center would handle any acute or life-threatening problem without demanding immediate payment. For patients who could not afford to pay in full at the time they were seen, a payment schedule was established. Fees were the same for everyone. The center received 90 percent of all payments due, a percentage higher than in hospital emergency rooms.

Promotion

By March 1979, the center was functioning smoothly. Therefore, more attention could be given to advertising and promotion. The owners were acutely conscious of the bias against advertising in the medical community and therefore promoted the center in a conservative manner. When it opened in May 1978, there was local television and newspaper coverage of this new form of emergency care. Later, a TV spot was filmed and a slide show prepared for use at club and organization meetings. The owners had identified parent-teacher associations as a primary target for promotion and intended to seek permission from parents to have their children taken to the Toco Hills MEC if they were injured during school hours.

The most aggressive promotional activity was the distribution of the center's first brochure (Figure 10-2). It was to be distributed in shopping centers, pharmacies, hotels/motels, places of employment, and apartment houses catering to single persons and newcomers to the city. The effectiveness of the brochure had not been evaluated.

Neither had there been a systematic evaluation of the center's image. Dr. Cowan felt that its reputation and image were quite good, based on the fact that 15 to 20 percent of its patients returned for services.

Ms. Shine, the assistant director, was convinced that the center had made considerable progress in the ten months since it had opened. She knew, however, that there were always better ways to do things and welcomed an analysis of its marketing operation by the four graduate students (Exhibit 10-1).

NOTE

1. For a description of a marketing audit, see Philip Kotler, *Marketing for Nonprofit Organizations* (Englewood Cliffs, N.J.: Prentice-Hall, Inc., 1975), pp. 55–75.

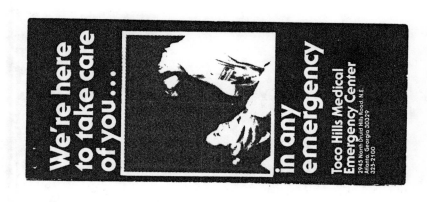

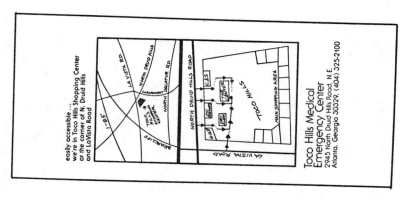

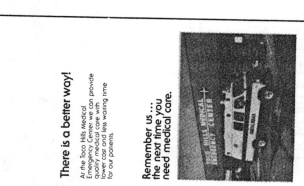

Figure 10-2 Folder Promoting Toco Hills MEC

Figure 10-2 continued

We are concerned about: rising medical costs... impersonal patient care... long waiting periods in busy hospital emergency rooms... There is a better way!

The Toco Hills Medical Emergency Center is an emergency room without a hospital attached. We know that illness or injury creates not just physical pain, but fear as well. If you do not have a doctor, or you need the services of an emergency room, your problems seem even worse. The Center is designed to fill the need for high quality, available medical care.

We provide:
- A complete medical staff including **physician, registered nurse** and **technician** always on duty.
- **Convenient hours** ... the Center is open **every day of the year** (including weekends and holidays) from **8:00 a.m. to midnight.** No appointments are necessary.
- A pleasant quiet reception room and dedicated staff that genuinely cares about you.
- **All laboratory and x-ray facilities** necessary to assess medical problems from a simple case of flu to any major emergency that might arise.

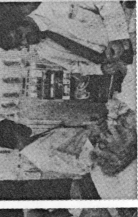
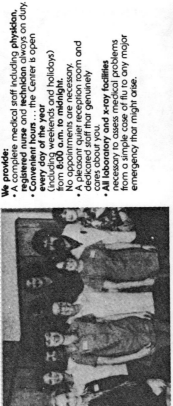
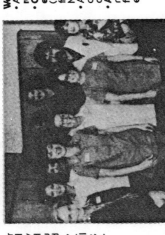
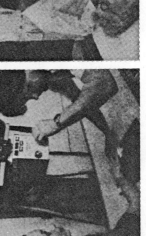
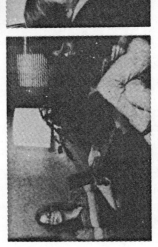

Source: Toco Hills Medical Emergency Center, Atlanta.

Exhibit 10-1 Evaluation Report by Graduate Students

TOCO HILLS MEDICAL EMERGENCY CENTER: A MARKET AUDIT

RECOMMENDATIONS

The marketing of any health care organization is a difficult and challenging responsibility. Unlike other products and services, the object here is not to "create" a demand for emergency care, but to inform potential consumers of the existence of the facility, the services offered, and the quality of care available in the event of an emergency.

Setting of Objectives

Statements of basic strategy and purpose can set the direction for any organization, health type or otherwise. The directors of the Toco Hills MEC have established general goals, but clear-cut objectives should be outlined. They must be specific, reality oriented, time specified, and should call for achievement, evaluations, and verification. Use of objectives will provide employees (including the owners) with a sharper definition of their roles. No formal decision-making criteria appear to have been established for the addition or deletion of services. It may be that the Center has not been in operation long enough, the patient volume growth large enough to warrant this kind of evaluation. As the Center approaches its first year of operation, it is suggested that meetings be scheduled on a regular basis in order to discuss all aspects of operation of the Center, including an objective evaluation of services.

Data Gathering: Prospective

Decisions regarding use of current services, age range of patient population, geographic areas served, most common diagnoses, must be made on the basis of objective information. A sharper definition of the Center's desired market segments and more precise data with which to evaluate these segments are needed. Knowledge of the patient population and where they come from will allow Drs. Cowan and Hartley to determine which markets have been reached and which may be responding to promotional activities. Information obtained at the time of admission is one simple way to gather data. A section at the bottom of the admission form, for example, could request the following information with a carbon copy which could be detached for data-gathering purposes:

(continues)

Exhibit 10-1 continued

(use zip code)
- Patient is coming   home   (   )
  from: work   (   )
                       other   (   )

- Time of patient visit (hour and day)
- Time of patient departure (hour)
- Patient age
- Patient marital status
- Reason for emergency visit
- Is this a follow-up visit?
- Is this a first visit?
- How did you hear of the MEC? Brochure (   ); Word of mouth
  (   ); Friend (   ); Saw the sign (   ); Other (   ).

Information of this type then can be transferred to a master control form
or programmed into a computer.

Data Gathering: Retrospective

A community survey should be designed to determine consumer
awareness. Questions could include the following:

- Have you heard of the Toco Hills Medical Emergency Center?
  (If "yes") How did you hear of it?
  Personal or family use (   ); Word of mouth (   ); Friend (   ) or
  acquaintance (   ); Saw brochure (   ); Other (   ).
- What kind of facility is it?
- Have you or any member of your family used the Center?
  (If "yes") Under what circumstances?
  (If "yes") Were you satisfied with the services you received?
  (If "yes") Would you use the Center again?
- Now that we've told you about the Center, would you use it in
  an emergency?
  (If "no") Why not?
- Where do you go in a medical emergency?
- Do you have a family physician?
- How long have you lived in Atlanta? At this address?

Exhibit 10–1 continued

The value of a survey such as that suggested above would be to: (1) learn if consumers understand the services being offered; (2) inform consumers unaware of the Center that a new community service has been established; and (3) gain information on the experience of those consumers who have used the Center.

Attracting New Markets

An intensive effort should be made to inform the community of the existence of the Toco Hills MEC and the services it offers:

1. To increase Center "visibility," an Open House might be held. The community would be invited to tour the Center. Perhaps a service such as the checking of blood pressure would be provided free of charge. Potential consumers would have an opportunity to meet the staff. Early in April, WSB-TV is sponsoring a health fair for the public. Health facilities in Atlanta are invited to participate in the fair by offering some service. In order to gain visibility in the community the Toco Hills MEC might participate in this activity.

2. Athletic injuries will increase as spring approaches and more members of the community take part in a variety of physical activities. The availability of the Center during the weekend is a positive factor to emphasize in its promotion to this group. Market research may indicate where athletes spend their time in the community. The Center could then focus on leaving promotional materials in these locations, such as the European Health Spa, the Golf and Tennis Center, Hickok's in the Toco Hill Shopping Center, and the newly opened Sporting House in Executive Park. Consideration should also be given to designing a brochure, perhaps abbreviated, directed primarily to this market segment. Contact should be established with the YMCA/Decatur which schedules its athletic games for children on Saturdays.

3. The pediatric population served by the Center is small. Where this market is concerned, parents want to establish a relationship with a physician, and must be reassured that their children will receive quality care. To establish such confidence, the Center could offer a free community service in order that parents have an opportunity to visit the Center and meet the staff. One such service might be an evening meeting for the community in which the physician owners give a short, informative talk on poisons and antidotes. As an added promotional tool, the Center would give to all who

(continues)

Exhibit 10-1 continued

attend a chart listing the most common poisons and antidotes. The telephone number of the poison control center, the police, and the Toco Hills MEC would be included on the chart.

4. As a health care facility, the Toco Hills MEC might take an active role in promoting first aid and CPR classes. The Red Cross and Heart Association sponsor the instructors. If low evening volume allows space for these kinds of activities, it would provide a good opportunity to bring potential consumers into the Center, as well as providing a community service. Any fees charged would be nominal in order to cover additional costs to the Center.

5. With increased national attention on fitness and prevention, the Toco Hills MEC could provide space for programs in nutrition and weight reduction. As an added service, members of a weight reduction group could have their weight monitored at the Center, their "drop-in" hours restricted to those times of lowest patient volume.

6. As private physician suspicion and wariness dissipate, the Center should identify those physicians most likely to refer their patients to the Center during weekends, evenings, or vacations.

Promotional Tools

Well-designed brochures are an excellent sales tool. In order to be effective, they should be attractive, easy to understand, with the salient information simply worded and easily found at first glance. Since the first brochure of the Toco Hills MEC is just now being distributed, it is too early to determine its effectiveness. When the next brochure is designed, it might be tested for its effectiveness (design, clarity, and message) among several consumer groups. To increase its value to the consumer, a tear-off card might be incorporated into the brochure— a card small enough to fit into a wallet to be used for identification or medical alert, also including the number of the Toco Hills MEC, ambulance service, or police. A tear-off might be of the type which could be pasted onto a telephone or bulletin board.

OVERVIEW OF CASE 18

Issues to Consider

1. What problems and opportunities confront the Toco Hills MEC as it approaches a profitable level of operations? What market segments should it focus on?
2. What promotional efforts should it undertake to reach its target markets?
3. How can the audit team's recommendations be evaluated?

Discussion

1. Problems and Opportunities

A rather formidable list of problems and opportunities can be developed for Toco Hills Medical Emergency Center. The center faces problems in market definition, segment delineation, development of promotional tools, and development of a service mix that will meet the needs of the selected market segments. The biggest problem in March 1979 was that it attempted to be all things to all people.

The center had several attractive opportunities. The immediate area was heavily populated and appeared to be underserved for emergency medical services. The facility was accessible and featured competent staff and modern equipment. The major opportunity lay in the area of focusing on and attracting narrowly defined market segments for which the center's services were appropriate. Such targets included, but were not limited to, schools at all age levels; businesses, particularly major employers; apartment complexes; and new residents whether transient or permanent.

2. Research and Promotion

Once the market segments were defined, the center might develop a promotional mix. The graduate students' audit recommended both retrospective research (previous customers) to determine reasons for using the Toco Hills MEC and prospective research (potential clients) to determine awareness, medical care needs, and present arrangements for use of medical services. The results of such research might suggest which services are most valued and what must be done to increase awareness and trial of the center.

The center already had developed a promotional brochure but had given little thought to its distribution. The audit suggested a review of the brochure by past and prospective clients that might lead to the development of more effective materials. The key is that the Toco Hills MEC did not know how patients selected it. It is entirely possible, for instance, that the center was used as a primary care facility by young professionals who had no family physician. This segment, if substantial, could be sought through appeals different from those used to solicit emergencies.

3. Evaluation of Recommendations

An evaluation should be made of the recommendations by the audit team. One useful way is to order the suggestions according to importance, then consider the costs of implementation and the benefits to be expected for the more important ones. Such analysis forces consideration of the constraints the center faces as it struggles to become profitable.

CASE 19. CENTRAL ALABAMA PRIMARY CARE, INC.*: PROBLEMS IN RURAL CLINICS

The Rev. Thompson, chairman of Central Alabama Primary Care, Inc. (CAPC), had spent an hour reviewing its operation with Les Kay, its new director, preparatory to a board meeting. Kay was discouraged and said the past two months had been the most frustrating in his life. He thought perhaps he had made a serious mistake in accepting the position. While his classmates from the university's hospital administration graduate program were settling down in new jobs as assistant administrators, he was presiding over three small rural health clinics that many persons—the more vocal ones, anyway—considered medically unnecessary and a waste of public funds.

Kay had taken the project director's job at the low point of CAPC's three-year existence. He had grown up in rural Alabama and, as he told the board of directors during his job interview, saw this as his chance to make a real difference in the lives of country people. Now he was not so sure he had the skills needed for the job. Things started going sour two weeks after he began work when the nurse practitioner in the Walton County Clinic quit in a bitter salary dispute. She said she had been promised a raise by the previous administration. None of the board members Kay queried were aware of the arrangement and he had asked her to wait until the panel could approve a personnel policy manual and compensation plan. Now the clinic had been closed for six weeks.

The paperwork was onerous. The project officer from Atlanta had been a great help but many an evening and Saturday had gone into drafting the policy and procedures manuals, the transportation plan, the patient care plan, and even the emergency evacuation plans for the three small clinics. Kay wondered why these problems were not discussed in graduate school.

Even the board of directors had become a problem. All members had appeared so enthusiastic and supportive when he was hired but now several treated him coolly. He felt he had done his best to involve them in making decisions, providing detailed financial projections, and, from what he could tell, meeting more frequently these two months than they had in the last two years. He could understand the feelings of the Walton County people since the clinic was closed, but he felt they should understand that recruiting a nurse practitioner for this part of the state was no small problem.

Now the board had to come to grips with the most difficult problem facing CAPC: low utilization. Despite an obvious shortage of health care in the region, few people used the clinics on a regular basis. The Rev. Mr.

---

* Central Alabama Primary Care, Inc. is a fictitious organization. The case represents a composite of thirteen rural primary care centers studied by the authors.

Thompson remembered that the Health Systems Agency director had told him a few weeks earlier: "This project got through our review committee by one vote and unless you can turn it around, I don't think they'll approve it next year."

History of Central Alabama Primary Care, Inc.

Central Alabama Primary Care Corporation was organized in late 1976 by Medical Center Hospital, a 300-bed facility in Center City (pop. 38,000), the county seat of Coulter County (pop. 47,000).

Over the preceding several years, Medical Center's emergency department had served a steadily increasing number of nonemergency patients, many of them unable to pay the basic $35 emergency room charge. The hospital's three-member emergency physician group asked the administration to remedy the situation, contending that the glut of nonemergency patients impaired their ability to treat severely ill or injured persons.

A review of emergency department records indicated that a large proportion of the nonemergency patients came from the three small rural counties adjoining Coulter County (Figure 10-3). Of the three, Sanders County (pop. 18,000) had the best health care resources: a 60-bed hospital and four general practice physicians. However, they were located in the southern part of the county, 60 miles from Medical Center Hospital. Dover County (pop. 15,000) had very limited health care resources: a 30-bed hospital that remained open only because of local pride and a single 68-year-old physician who practiced only part time. Walton County (pop. 13,000) had no medical care. Its hospital had closed in the early 1960s and there had been no physician for nearly ten years.

After several months of study and meetings, the hospital submitted an application to the Robert Hood Swanson Foundation under a demonstration grant program designed to test new ways of providing health care to rural communities. The application called for establishment of nurse practitioner clinics in each of the three counties that would be supervised by physicians from Coulter County. A community advisory council would be organized in each county as a source of policy guidance to Medical Center Hospital, which would manage the project.

When the hospital medical staff reviewed the application, many physicians objected to the nurse practitioner concept but the administrator urged them to accept the project as an experiment, citing these potential benefits:

1. reducing the load on the hospital emergency department
2. generating referrals to speciality physicians on the Medical Center staff (which might also improve hospital occupancy)
3. enhancing the Medical Center's image as a regional health resource

Figure 10-3 Catchment Area Profile: Central Alabama Primary Care, Inc.

Coulter County

300-bed hospital (Center City)
52 physicians (Center City)
Industry: Fairfax Steel employs 4,000 workers who commute from surrounding counties.

Sanders County

60-bed hospital (Ames)
4 physicians (Ames)
1 Nurse Practitioner Clinic (Princeton)
Industry: several small manufacturing plants in Ames. Textile mills in Princeton and Parkerville.

Dover County

30-bed hospital (Rock City)
1 part-time physician (Rock City)
1 Nurse Practitioner Clinic (Rock City)
Industry: Sewing mill in Rock City, farming (soy beans, cotton, cattle)

Walton County

1 Nurse Practitioner Clinic (Flatridge)
Industry: farming, especially chickens, pigs, cattle

Note: Small communities in Coulter, Dover, and Walton Counties not shown.

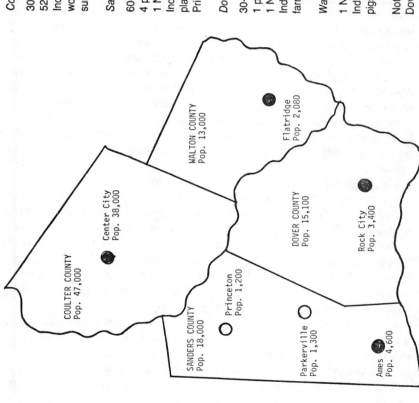

COULTER COUNTY
Pop. 47,000

Center City
Pop. 38,000

WALTON COUNTY
Pop. 13,000

Flatridge
Pop. 2,080

SANDERS COUNTY
Pop. 18,000

Princeton
Pop. 1,200

Parkerville
Pop. 1,300

DOVER COUNTY
Pop. 15,100

Rock City
Pop. 3,400

Ames
Pop. 4,600

After the three emergency physicians agreed to serve as preceptors, the grant application was approved by a narrow margin.

Several months later the Swanson Foundation approved a three-year grant of $200,000 a year with a July 1, 1977, starting date. The first clinic opened March 1, 1978, in Walton County using the long-vacant physician's office as a site. A nurse practitioner was recruited from the university's new family nurse practitioner training program. After a brief initial surge of interest, the patient load stabilized at six to eight visits per day.

The Dover County Clinic opened August 1, 1978, in a former grocery store that was renovated by the county commission. The nurse practitioner lived in the community and formerly had worked for the state health department in a regional family planning program. Utilization increased gradually, peaking at some 12 visits per day. The county's sole physician had been invited to serve as preceptor but refused to have anything to do with ". . . that half-baked nurse who thinks she's a doctor."

Sanders County had the most trouble getting started. Because there were four physicians in the county seat, that location was ruled out immediately and the community advisory committee had to choose between Princeton and Parkerville. For as long as anyone could remember, these towns had been bitter rivals whose football games sometimes ended in fistfights. Each town wanted its own clinic and some suggested the only alternative would be a clinic built halfway between and mutually inconvenient to both communities.

Under pressure to meet deadlines in the Swanson Foundation grant, the hospital administration selected Princeton as the clinic site while giving vague indications to Parkerville that a future clinic would be located in that town. Flushed with victory, the Princeton community went to work building a clinic from the ground up. There was a fund-raising event almost every week sponsored by Ruritan, the Volunteer Fire Department, or the Booster Club. Men spent their weekends setting concrete block, sheet rocking, and painting. A grand opening was held in May 1979, complete with ribbon cutting performed by a U.S. Senator.

Unlike the two other clinics, the Sanders County Clinic was staffed by a National Health Service Corps nurse practitioner who had received her training in the U.S. Army. Initial utilization was excellent, with as many as 24 encounters a day, but soon tapered off to a level of 10 to 12 daily. All were from the Princeton area, although many Princeton residents continued to make the long drive to Central City for routine health care.

In February 1980, representatives of the Swanson Foundation made a site visit to review the project. Funding was scheduled to end on June 30 and Medical Center Hospital had requested a one-year extension so the clinics could have time to achieve financial self-sufficiency. In a meeting with the hospital's medical staff, foundation representatives were told that, "People don't want to see nurses, they want doctors." The foundation soon wrote back that continuation funding would not be provided. Central Alabama Primary Care appeared doomed.

Walton County members of the community advisory council organized an emergency meeting of the three clinics, which took place in March in the Medical Center Hospital conference room. For the first two hours, chaos prevailed while participants tried to assign blame for the program's "failure." Then a representative from the Health Systems Agency described the Rural Health Initiative (RHI) program and suggested that an application still could be submitted, despite an April 15 deadline. The hospital administrator said Medical Center no longer wished to be involved with the project but would help develop the new grant application and would even help recruit a new project director.

In early June the Health Systems Agency received unofficial word that Central Alabama Primary Care would be approved for funding under the RHI program effective July 1, although the official grant award might be made later. Kay reported for work on July 1.

The Marketing Study

Kay had requested time at a board meeting to discuss marketing as a tool that could be useful to CAPC. While generally skeptical, the board had agreed to his request. He explained that he had taken a course titled "Marketing for Health Services Organization" that convinced him health care providers could benefit from improved attention to the attitudes, perceptions, and preferences of clients and potential clients. He passed out a summary prepared by his professor, A.B. Coe, and there was a lively discussion about the propriety of marketing the clinics' services. The board finally agreed to authorize funds for a marketing study of Central Alabama Primary Care.

Kay called his former marketing professor to locate someone who could perform the study. Much to his surprise, Professor Coe said he had grown up in rural Georgia and would like very much to do the review. The professor spent three days visiting the clinics, talking with staff, patients, and board members, and meeting with the administrator and some of the physicians at Medical Center Hospital. Two weeks later his report arrived (Exhibit 10-2). Kay mailed copies to each board member before the meeting. Professor Coe also agreed to be present and answer questions.

Exhibit 10-2 Professor's Report on CAPC Marketing

TO: Board of Directors
           Central Alabama Primary Care Corporation

FROM: Professor A. B. Coe
           Department of Marketing, State University

SUBJECT: Marketing Review of Central Alabama Primary Care Cor-
           poration

I was pleased to have the opportunity to visit with many of you last week during my brief review of your program. During my three days in the area, I was able to talk with over thirty people including your staff, clients, elected officials, and many of you. In general, I found that Central Alabama Primary Care Corporation and its clinics are seen as important resources for the communities they serve but there are misconceptions and problems which limit their effectiveness. Mr. Kay tells me he has discussed the marketing perspective with you so I will focus on my principal findings and recommendations. I look forward to meeting with you to discuss this report.

Strengths of CAPC

The program has, in a relatively short period of time, established itself in the service area as having the following attributes:

1. high-quality care
2. competent and courteous staff
3. modern equipment
4. accessible locations
5. reasonable charges

It thus appears that CAPC has a favorable image with regular clients and this is a solid base for further development. However, there are several weaknesses which are also quite evident.

Weaknesses of CAPC

CAPC has as its objective "the delivery of quality health care to rural communities, irrespective of ability to pay for care." However, the ability of the center to meet this objective is hampered by:

Exhibit 10-2 continued

1. lack of overall planning
2. lack of market-based data
3. lack of detailed objectives to support the overall objective
4. lack of strategies for implementing objectives

In general, the program is managed on a day-to-day basis. Little is known about the needs of the service area *as perceived by clients and potential clients*. There are no objectives concerning the types and amounts of services to be rendered, nor concerning the projected outcomes in terms of improved health status. This summary judgment is supported by the following findings, conclusions, and recommendations.

Market Definition

CAPC has no market definition, other than along county boundaries. It is tacitly understood that rural people have somewhat unique needs and encounter patterns, but no strategies are based on this understanding. A market orientation requires that principal segments be identified, their needs defined, and strategies developed for meeting the unique needs of each segment. Much of the data on market definition now exists in patient records and the utilization history. Some of the questions you must answer include:

1. How do you define your important market segments?
2. Why do they use your services?
3. What sources of information do they use?
4. Why do members of your important segments *not* use your services?

These questions can be answered by research, using your clinic records as a base. Also, simple consumer attitude surveys can help tell why your market uses or does *not* use your services.

Competition

Most of the board members feel that CAPC has little or no competition. However, from a client perspective, any method of maintaining or restoring health can be viewed as a competitor for the clinics. Therefore, your immediate competitors are:

(continues)

Exhibit 10-2 continued

1. self-care of health problems
2. out-migration to other areas where health care is available
3. no care of health problems

However, remember that you have four physicians in Sanders County and one in Dover County. There are also health departments in each county and they appear to offer some of the same services as your clinics—immunization, family planning, maternal and child health care. While your clinics offer most of the same services as a family doctor, little collaboration has been attempted with other formal providers of health care. Some of the questions you need to answer are:

1. What other health services are available in the area?
2. How do other services compare to ours (quality, cost, availability, etc.)?
3. How can we collaborate with other health providers?

Image

All of the staff and board members believe that the clinics have a positive image in the community but there are no data to support this contention. Also, it must be made clear that your image can vary substantially by segment and service. The fact is you do not know your program's image and the only people you talk to about the image are patients or friends of the clinics. These people are not likely to tell you what you do not want to hear and negative statements are probably discounted as "isolated situations."

The physical appearance of a health care center can be very important in creating an image in the public mind. All of you have visited the Sanders County Clinic in Princeton and know how much effort went into making a modern and attractive building. I noticed that one of the other clinics is dimly lit with incandescent bulbs and there was a hand-lettered sign in the window giving clinic hours. I think you'll find that a little money spent on proper lighting, professionally painted signs, and attractive color schemes will pay off in terms of your public image. By the way, two of the clinics had Coke machines in the waiting room. How does that affect your image as a health care provider?

Exhibit 10-2 continued

It is not enough to have excellent services at reasonable cost. The public must *know* what you have and know it without misconception. Also, the public must know the Center as more than "bricks and mortar." Health care is a very personal experience. The public must believe that you have warm, caring professional staff who are efficient and concerned about the client's health. If there is no image, you must create one. If there is a negative, misconceived image, you must correct it. If there is a negative but accurate image, you must do what it takes to remove the negative, even if it requires a change in personnel or procedures. The following questions must be answered:

1. What is our image by segment?
2. Who does not know about us?
3. What can be done to heighten awareness and knowledge?
4. What can be done to correct misimpressions?
5. What can be done to eliminate correct, but negative, impressions?

These questions require the continuous solicitation of feedback from clients plus periodic surveys of samples from principal segments. While action depends on findings, you must be prepared to take prompt and substantial action to develop a positive image where none exists, to correct misimpressions, and to correct negative factors (and to effectively communicate the changes).

While the clinics offer a mix of services, it is critical to understand that clients *buy results, not services*: they buy benefits such as restored health (or elimination of discomfort). You must realize that the client perceives your services more broadly than the moment of contact with the nurse practitioner. The customer thinks of "augmented service" which includes such seemingly inconspicuous items as travel time, waiting time, perceived empathy, filling out forms, voice inflections, professionalism, and many more. You can provide top quality service and still be perceived as a second-rate facility based on the amount of attention given to the other components of "augmented service" as perceived by the client.

Presently, the decisions on what services to add or delete appear to be made by the clinics' staff and board of directors. The marketing approach would be to determine what your principal market segments *believe* is needed. The following questions about services need to be asked:

(continues)

Exhibit 10-2 continued

1. What is the perception of principal market segments concerning the "augmented service?"
2. What can be done to enhance the "augmented service?"
3. Before adding a service, do you examine the market's perception of the need for this service?
4. Before eliminating a service, do you examine the *reasons* for low utilization or high costs per encounter?

These questions require surveys of past and present clients and potential clients. Furthermore, they must be ongoing since perceptions change over time.

Access and Availability

The Walton County and Dover County Clinics are located in the main shopping areas of the county seats. The Sanders County Clinic is located in one of the smaller communities, Princeton. All of the clinics have the same posted operating hours: Monday through Friday, 9:00 A.M. to 5:00 P.M., except Wednesday when they are closed in the afternoon.

I wonder if you have looked into the possibility of opening the clinics on Saturday as a way to improve utilization. Several people I spoke with said that Saturday is a day when people come to town to do their shopping. You could close the clinics on Monday, if necessary, so your staff has a five-day workweek.

When I was visiting the Sanders County Clinic, a sign on the door said that the clinic would be closed the following Thursday and Friday. By way of explanation, the nurse practitioner said she had to go to a National Health Service Corps meeting in Atlanta. I am wondering how often the clinics are closed "unexpectedly" like this and what effect this has on your accessibility . . . and how about your image?

To improve accessibility, have you considered going to your clients in selected cases, instead of having them come to you? For example, I learned that there are programs where elderly people are served lunch every day in each county. Perhaps you can develop an outreach program and arrange to schedule your services at a church, school, or similar location.

The common thread in access and availability issues is to know your market and its time and place needs. While surveys may be helpful, it may be possible to gain such input from each principal market segment in small group meetings.

Exhibit 10-2 continued

Promotion

Promotion can be viewed as any attempt to communicate a message or impression to a potential customer. CAPC has no objectives about what message to communicate, nor is the effectiveness of communication efforts measured. There is a brochure but its distribution has been haphazard. There has been no attempt to measure public reaction or impact on utilization. Other information devices such as calendars, wallet cards, telephone stickers, and mailouts have not been developed.

Public relations is also conducted in a haphazard manner. Some of the staff members have spoken to civic groups and schools on request but there has been no attempt to identify groups who need to know about the clinics and who might communicate the message to others. Groups such as Future Farmers of America, Parent-Teacher Associations, 4-H Clubs, Wednesday night prayer meetings, or civic clubs should be considered. You could invite groups to tour the clinics or even hold meetings there after hours.

An important component of promotion is atmospherics, defined as the clients' perception of the atmosphere in which services are rendered. Factors such as exterior signs, condition of the building, appearance of waiting rooms, cleanliness of the facility, attractiveness of staff uniforms, can convey a message that is favorable or unfavorable to your clients.

The solicitation of customer feedback also communicates an important message to your clients: you must care what they think, a message which suggests the client is important. Feedback should not only be solicited formally, but it should be simple, easy, and anonymous (unless the client wishes to make his/her identity known). Postage paid post cards addressed to the administrator is one simple way to solicit feedback. Another way is as a stuffer in bills sent to the client. A third way is random, periodic surveys by mail or by phone.

A special problem area in promotion is the recruitment of professional staff. The Center should identify the type of staff who are most desired and who would be happy at the Center. Then, the Center should develop contact with the possible sources of the desired medical staff and nurture relationships with the sources.

The common thread to the promotion problems is the identification of objectives and the measurement of results. The first part must be done by staff after review of *data* on image, awareness, and needs of principal markets. The second step requires that the Center evaluate how each message was transmitted and perceived.

(continues)

Exhibit 10-2 continued

Cost

Pricing decisions have been reviewed annually based in an attempt to recover expenses, with an additional increment for capital improvements. Cost decisions are closely related to utilization projections, since many costs are fixed. Ideally, prices should be based on *projected utilization*, in support of a *plan* to achieve desired level and timing of utilization.

A basic purpose of marketing is to *manage demand*. The Center experiences peaks and valleys in demand. Fall is a peak period as is each Wednesday morning. The Center should examine ways to *smooth demand*, so that peak periods are diminished and low periods are enhanced. To do this, attempts should be made to schedule people with routine checkups into low periods. Attempts should be made to arrange hours and services to fit the demand patterns. These steps can help to spread costs more effectively, while allowing for increased total utilization.

Cost can be used to stimulate demand for needed services as well. This is an extremely sensitive area since it is not advisable to encourage clients to purchase unnecessary services. However, a *free* first visit, or *free* (or lower cost) preventive diagnostics such as blood pressure or breast exams, can effectively bring new clients to the Center. The results of such activity, if properly promoted and scheduled, can be an enhanced image and an increased client base.

The review and recommendations presented in this brief report are intended to help the Center to increase its effectiveness in delivering quality health care to its service area. The perspective in this review is that the client and potential client must be considered in all decisions made at the Center. Who is the target client? What are his/her *perceived* needs? What does he/she think of the Center? How can we communicate more effectively? How can we meet perceived needs more efficiently? If these questions become a central part of the management philosophy at the Center, you will achieve your overall objective.

I look forward to meeting with you at the next board meeting.

Chapter 11

Marketing Planning

CASE 20. UNIVERSITY MEDICAL CENTER: PLANNING WITH MARKETING IN MIND

Background

James Carson, M.D., had been a faculty member at the University Medical Center for 15 years until three months ago, when he was appointed its vice president. A man in his late 50s, Dr. Carson had a nationwide reputation as a physician but now was intent upon providing sound management and direction to the Medical Center.

The University Medical Center was composed of the Schools of Medicine, Nursing and Allied Health, the Associated University Physicians (the private practice organization of the Medical School faculty) and the University Hospital. The hospital was a 528-bed facility offering both inpatient and outpatient services in all medical and surgical specialties as well as in many sub- and super-subspecialties. The hospital had 149,000 patient days and 108,000 outpatient visits per year. It conducted a complete residency training program for 230 physicians each year. The University Medical Center was a part of the larger university that was owned and operated by the state.

The Current Situation

Inpatient Care

Since taking office, Dr. Carson had been studying the overall situation of the Medical Center to determine the variables that affect management in such a complex service institution. He called upon his administrative assistant, Mrs. Barbara Johnson, to act as his sounding board as he attempted to further define the problems facing the center.

301

"I always knew this was a rural area, but to recognize that the whole eastern portion of the state represented by our health service area has only 550,000 people and is classified as a Nonstandard Metropolitan Statistical Area is really important," Dr. Carson began. "These people are scattered over 8,500 square miles. The really curious aspect of the demographics is that it is estimated that the population will grow only about 1 percent per year, according to the Health Systems Agency (HSA), yet our number of beds has grown in the last several years from just 389 to 528 and the faculty (medical staff) is beating down my door demanding another 160-bed addition. It seems obvious that the growth in beds is not related directly to the growth in population."

"That's true," Mrs. Johnson said, "but don't you believe that the phenomenon is due primarily to the role of the University Medical Center in the area, that is, being a referral, tertiary care center, especially for inpatient services? We're providing the most sophisticated and advanced techniques, procedures, and diagnostic and treatment modalities available in our area. There is no other hospital like us serving this area."

"That's a good point," Dr. Carson said, "and we must use that argument when we go to the HSA for new beds. The Medical School faculty has been adamant in its demands for new beds over the last several years. While we have been able to pick up additional general acute care beds, we can no longer ignore the need for more and better designed intensive care unit beds. We also must recognize the need by services such as internal medicine, which is running near capacity in its allocated beds."

"I can understand the faculty demand for additional beds," she commented, "but the overall statistical report on the utilization of our beds shows that we are running only about a 77 percent occupancy rate. While you are absolutely correct that services such as internal medicine frequently have occupancy rates of 95 percent, others, such as obstetrics, are consistently at about 50 percent."

"That indeed is what the statistical reports indicate," Dr. Carson replied. "But those kinds of services often need to have an excess number of beds so they can meet peak demand requirements. Nevertheless, we still need more intensive care unit beds in an area appropriately designed for such service as well as additional beds to relieve services that are running consistently high occupancy rates. But understand this, the new dean, the new assistant vice president, and I fully intend to provide leadership and direction to set this institution back on a path of controlled but appropriate growth. Beds are but one need. We have many others to face simultaneously. After all, we are an educational and research organization as well as a provider of patient care."

Shortly after Dr. Carson's appointment, he had named a new Medical School dean and created a new position of assistant vice president whose main responsibilities were to guide the administrative aspects of the hospital and of the Medical School faculty private practices. Reporting to the assistant vice president were the director of the Medical Center Hospital and the administrator of the Associated University Physicians (the title of the private practice conducted by the Medical School faculty members).

All department chairmen in both the clinical and basic sciences reported to the dean of the Medical School. In turn, the deans of the Medical School, the Nursing School, and the School of Allied Health, as well as the assistant vice president, reported to the vice president of the Medical Center.

Organizational Relationships

"Let me talk about some of the major problems which I think we are going to have to face as we set the direction for the next 20 years of the University Medical Center," Dr. Carson said. "Perhaps the most perplexing and discomforting situation revolves around our relationship with the rest of the university. Even though I am on a vice presidential level with other senior administrative officers in the university, at times I feel trapped by this organizational structure.

"For instance, despite our efforts to receive capital funds for vitally needed building programs in the Medical Center, our request to the university for such funds becomes mixed in with other requests from throughout the university and thus becomes diluted amidst all the requests. And then, of course, the state further dilutes the issue as it considers capital outlay requests for all state agencies—of which it will only approve a handful. We are dealing with people and human lives here in the Medical Center. We generate revenues for our patient care efforts, unlike most other programs in the university. Yet we have as difficult a time getting capital monies from the university and the state as does any other school in the university whose major function is to provide education and perform research."

Financial Relationships

"The finances of this institution are perplexing," Dr. Carson continued. "The fact that my chief financial adviser in the Medical Center reports simultaneously both to me and to the vice president for finance also bothers me, not to mention the fact that there is no such thing as retained earnings in our hospital because the monies that we don't spend at the end of the year revert to the state. Furthermore, we are different from a lot of hospitals since we are required to provide care to the indigent and are funded to do so by the state.

"Don't misunderstand, I think it is only appropriate that we provide care to the indigent since we are a state-funded public institution. But we are faced with a governor who ran on a platform of no tax increases. Well, I voted for him and I guess as a taxpayer I agree with that strategy, but this financial belt tightening by the state administration is certainly putting the crunch on us."

Certificate of Need and Long-Range Planning

"There is another whole area of concern that we haven't even addressed yet," Mrs. Johnson interposed. "You referred to it briefly when you mentioned the HSA. We must recognize that any capital expenditure we want to make in excess of $150,000 or that will add a new service or new beds to the hospital, will have to get approval not only by the university and the state to spend the funds but also by the HSA in the form of a certificate of need.

"I can tell you that these guys are playing for keeps. They are very concerned about containing costs and assuring that consumers are getting their dollars' worth out of the health care system. And of course HEW keeps telling us the system is rampant with waste and generally uncontrolled. As you pointed out, the state is not exactly overflowing with capital funds for building projects, especially by hospitals whose costs are rising dramatically. The state and the HSA are both painfully aware that by the old Hill-Burton standards of 4.5 beds per thousand population, our health service is overbedded by some 200 beds."

"But they have got to realize that we are a referral, tertiary care center that is getting patients from all over our area, indeed, from all over the state," Dr. Carson stressed.

"Very true," Mrs. Johnson said, "but where exactly are they coming from and what are their diagnoses? How has the length of stay changed over the last ten years and why are, or better yet, why aren't physicians referring their patients to us? With the HSA planning law's stress on consumer participation, what sort of services do the people of our area think we should be providing them? And don't forget what you said earlier about the fact that our population is growing at only about 1 percent per year yet we are on the verge of requesting a 30 percent increase in the number of beds."

The Environment for Primary Care and Competition

"We face many curious problems with regards to this Medical Center," Mrs. Johnson continued. "As you say we are a referral, tertiary care center but we are providing a full range of services to the people of our area. Certainly here in town we provide primary and secondary care services. Sure, some of them go across town to Community Hospital but a lot of them, especially the poor, come here. So we are not providing strictly referral and tertiary care services. Indeed, the new ambulatory care center we are opening next month is an indication of a recognition by the University Medical Center of the community's need for primary care services as well as the need to train primary care practitioners. And our community, in the case of primary care, certainly doesn't extend too far beyond the four-county area. People simply don't travel that far to get primary care.

"We can't forget the possible effect on our emergency room if Community Hospital opens the emergency room it is planning. With only about 29,500 visits to our ER, the displacement of services from there to the Community Hospital ER could be dramatic.

"This goes back, to some degree, to the 'town and gown' problem that we certainly face and that probably confronts any university-based hospital such as this. We are always the 'big guys in town,' indeed, in the region, and perhaps don't pay enough attention to what is going on in our front yard. Perhaps the people are looking for more personal service when they have to use the ER."

"What you say may be true," Dr. Carson said, "but we must remember we are serving an entire area and indeed have a responsibility to the entire state to provide both educational and health care services. We have got to be much broader in our perspectives."

"In the very broadest sense that is true," Mrs. Johnson agreed, "but sometimes we have to look at specific geographical areas and at the particular problems inherent to them. Take, for instance, the ambulatory care center. Outpatient services are consistently being stressed as an alternative to more costly inpatient care. Furthermore, we need to attract these ambulatory patients to our center so we can maintain an active and high-quality teaching program.

"Yet this is a beautiful area of the country and private practitioners, many of whom are graduating from our own medical school and finishing out residency programs here at the University Hospital, are settling into private practice in this area. In essence, they are competing with us for ambulatory patients. There probably are more private practitioners per capita in our area than anywhere else in the state. The point is that all of these kinds of factors will be considered by both the state and the HSA when we apply for a certificate of need."

The Effect of Technology

"It also is important to recognize that we are a technological leader in the health care field and certainly we have been able to respond to needs such as the availability of a CT (computerized tomography) scanner, sophisticated cardiac catheterization equipment, and so forth," Mrs. Johnson noted. "But even in certificate-of-need applications for technological advancements we have been placed under increasing scrutiny by the HSA about the need for sophisticated and very expensive equipment. After all, within the last two years we have committed nearly $5 million in lease payments for equipment we will use over the next five years. That is an awful lot of money that the HSA has reviewed for certificates of need. My frank opinion is that the HSA is getting a little concerned that we seem to be rolling past it one certificate-of-need application after another for increasingly expensive equipment. There doesn't seem to be any reason to it, no orderly plan of development behind it."

Dr. Carson agreed that she had some interesting points worthy of further consideration. He asked her to draw up an outline of the factors they had discussed so they could be analyzed with the other members of executive management. He also asked her to set up a meeting that would include all of the deans, the assistant vice president, and the University Medical Center comptroller and send them all a copy of her outline.

A Plan of Action

Two weeks later Dr. Carson opened his meeting by referring to his conversation with Mrs. Johnson. He recognized that the executive management team faced a complex matrix of factors that affected its decisions. The meeting discussed the outline, after which several suggestions were presented for Dr. Carson's consideration.

Alternative Approaches to Planning

The assistant vice president suggested that management historically had been concerned with the operations of existing systems and had not paid sufficient attention to long-range and strategic planning efforts. One result had been a patchwork building program and constant "fire fighting" by line management. Therefore, there was a need to hire a planning staff whose major concern would be to assure documentation of existing and anticipated programs, translate those programs into facilities needs, and monitor and coordinate their implementation. A coherent long-range plan also was needed to guide the actions of management as the Medical Center moved forward into the 1980s.

The assistant vice president's suggestion was to hire a senior level planner, possibly even at the assistant vice president level, whose sole responsibility would be for planning. In addition, sufficient staff should be made available to this new position to perform a myriad of tasks, including certificate-of-need preparation, monitoring of existing renovation and construction programs, program development, etc. Some of the staff members should be management engineers and systems analysts as well as program planners preferably at the master's level.

In addition, the assistant vice president strongly recommended that an outside consultant be brought in to develop a master plan, both in programmatic and facilities terms, for the University Medical Center. The executive emphasized the need to go outside for this consultant help because of the vast amount of work that must go into such a document and because the existing management team, even bolstered by the additional planning staff, could not produce such a plan expeditiously.

At this point Mrs. Johnson suggested that perhaps the executive management group should consider a marketing approach to planning and control. Such an approach would allow management to consider, from a long-range perspective, the external and internal forces that helped shape the center's direction while carrying this concept over into the implementation of such plans.

"Such an approach," Mrs. Johnson said, "could consist of market researchers, who would study both internal markets such as the medical staff and external markets such as the patients. Further, staff could aid our financial people with pricing decisions and we certainly can use some positive promotion of the Medical Center and our new programs. Because this type of effort would cut across all levels of the existing management structure, I should think this group would report to Dr. Carson."

The dean of the School of Allied Health suggested that a representative group be established as a long-range planning committee to develop a program that should be the guiding force behind the decisions and actions of the management team. Such an approach would ensure that all areas in the Medical Center were represented in long-range planning and would allow them to monitor the implementation of such plans as they were brought on line.

The dean proposed that such a group be composed of major clinical and basic science department chairmen, all of the executive management team, and any staff necessary to carry out the policies and directives of such a committee. He suggested it also could include the assistant vice president's proposals. The dean recommended that such a group meet regularly with people from throughout the Medical Center to coordinate the implementation of new programs. He urged that Dr. Carson chair such a committee.

Within a week of the meeting, Dr. Carson circulated a memorandum on this (Exhibit 11-1) among the members of executive management.

OVERVIEW OF CASE 20

Issues to Consider

1. What are the relevance and need for extending the marketing concept into a not-for-profit service industry, particularly as a managerial process involving planning, operations, and control?
2. What are the differences between a selling or promotion approach and a true marketing approach? Is marketing in the health care setting simply stimulating demand for services through promotion efforts or is it a process that can guide the development of goals, objectives, strategies and tactics for a health care delivery system?
3. What are the market segments that a hospital typically faces and why is there a need to develop strategies for those different segments?

Discussion

1. Need for a Marketing Concept

Dr. Carson, newly appointed vice president (CEO) of the University Medical Center, has inherited a troubled system of planning, operations, and control. This academic health center is a complex, state-operated facility composed of a medical school, a nursing school, a school of allied health, and a major referral hospital. The Medical Center has a history of weak administrative control, a concentration of power in the Medical School faculty, virtually no long-range planning, and an increasingly complex environment where external constraints continue to infringe upon management prerogatives.

This environment includes not only elements outside the university proper but also those of the larger university setting within which the Medical Center is nested. In the past, major issues have been dealt with in a "fire fighting" mode. Dr. Carson apparently is aware of the situation he has inherited. He has met with his senior line and staff officers and has drafted a management program aimed at implementing a long-range planning process and providing mechanisms by which administrative controls can be brought to bear on the University Medical Center.

Exhibit 11-1 Memorandum

UNIVERSITY MEDICAL CENTER

Manchester, Wyoming 91933

Office of the Vice President

MEMORANDUM

TO: Assistant Vice President
       Dean, School of Medicine
       Dean, School of Nursing
       Dean, School of Allied Health
       University Medical Center Comptroller
       Administrative Assistant

FROM: James D. Carson, M.D.
       Vice President

RE: Management Plan

Again, let me thank each of you for your input at our meeting of last week regarding the myriad of issues which face the Medical Center. I have considered your advice at great length and have decided that the following course of action should be implemented with the Medical Center management structure to address the issues which we discussed:

1.   I will initiate the paper work to establish five new positions within my office including a new position of Assistant Vice President for Planning. This new position will report directly to me and will be supported by four planners whose talents will be a mix of management engineering, systems analysis and program planning. I am also considering the possibility of hiring an architect into one of these staff positions to provide the expertise such a person could bring to our planning effort. The new Assistant Vice President for Planning will have line responsibility for this newly developed Planning Department, a subdivision of which will be a Management Systems Analysis Section. The Management Systems Analysis Section will work closely with the University Auditors in considering existing operating systems and working to improve the overall functioning of the Medical Center.

(continues)

Exhibit 11-1 continued

2. Prior to our Management Meeting one month from this date I would like each of you to prepare a list of suggested members for a Long Range Planning Committee to be constituted by a representative group of people from throughout the Medical Center. At a minimum this group will include all members of Executive Management and will be staffed by my administrative assistant, who will be executive secretary, and the members of the Planning Department. The charge to the Long Range Planning Committee will be to develop and maintain a long range plan for the Medical Center. This group will, however, be advisory to the Vice President for the Medical Center.

3. In an effort to expedite the efforts of the Long Range Planning Committee I will ask the Assistant Vice President to begin the process of determining what will be required in a Master Plan to be drawn up by outside consultants, and then to seek out prospective groups who would be able to perform this study for us.

4. The marketing approach suggested by Mrs. Johnson has some excellent potential for our utilization. I am therefore instructing that Mr. Edgar Schultz, Director of Public Relations for the University Medical Center, become a regular member and attendee of Executive Management meetings and that he follow through and publicize ongoing activities and development plans of the Medical Center as appropriate. I will also instruct Mr. Schultz to develop a marketing strategy for the Medical Center for our consideration at next month's management meeting.

Thank you for your attention to this most important matter. I think we have started off on the right foot in terms of providing management direction for the University Medical Center.

Specifically, Dr. Carson proposes to establish a new position of assistant vice president for planning. This is an attempt to consolidate all the planning efforts under one senior staff member. In addition, he will formulate a long-range planning committee composed of representatives from throughout the Medical Center. An outside consultant will be brought in to prepare a master plan. Lastly, Dr. Carson attempts to approach a marketing format by including the public relations director in all executive management meetings and by requesting that individual to develop a marketing strategy for the center.

The marketing approach had been suggested by a staff member. Dr. Carson has failed to appreciate the effects a full marketing program could have on his attempts to develop a sound management plan. The management plan he proposes is, in many ways, a patchwork approach to dealing with issues of planning, operations, and control.

An alternative approach would be to develop a marketing strategy. By utilizing the marketing axiom of product, place, price, and promotion, Dr. Carson could begin to consolidate his management efforts and achieve the complementary goals of good planning, smooth operations, and sound control. As with any large organization, there is a definite need to define its mission and the products or services it is to provide. In a large academic institution there are competing goals of education, patient care, and research. A planning approach would demand that strategies be developed in all three major areas and that the concentration of resources be divided among them in some fashion.

The issue of place refers primarily to what services will be offered and what segment of the market will be approached and served. In an institution as complex as a larger referral tertiary care center, the concept of market segments covers virtually the entire span of primary, secondary, and tertiary services.

The considerations of product or services and place are conducive to market research techniques that in essence amount to the same sort of planning research that can lead hospital executives to dissolve their long-range plans. Marketing research techniques can lead hospitals to discover services that the community needs but that are not being provided or are inadequate as well as identify existing services that are not utilized or are being offered inappropriately.

The pricing issue is not addressed specifically in this case because of the complex nature of the reimbursement system in the health care industry. The industry is characterized by a cost recovering (retrospective cost reimbursement) system as opposed to a consumer demand perspective. Therefore, pricing strategies established vis-à-vis third party carriers are not necessarily oriented toward consumer demand.

Finally, the promotion side of marketing, which so many hospital executives confuse with marketing per se, is a relatively well-accepted function of management in health care institutions. A major mistake that hospital executives tend to make, however, is equating marketing strictly with promotion.

2. Promotion and Marketing Differences

Specifically dealing with the difference between promotion and a true marketing approach, the case points out that Dr. Carson makes this common error of equating the two. For marketing to be implemented successfully in health care institutions requires that the highest levels of management understand what the subject represents and make an effort to apply its principles appropriately. Without a complete understanding of those principles, at least in concept, executives run the risk of misinterpreting and poorly evaluating the efforts of marketing personnel they hire.

With a broader approach to the vision of marketing—that is, to include the planning function as part of the responsibilities of the staff member designated with marketing responsibilities—will lead to more productive relationships between the chief executive officer and the marketing staff member and the results achieved by that individual. Indeed, this staff member in searching for information to carry out the marketing research activities, may well lead the CEO to identify problems regarding operations (the availability or nonavailability of services and their appropriateness) and the existence of control systems that generate sufficient data for management.

These control data are used by operational line officers as well as staff personnel carrying out the planning/marketing function. Obviously, without this internally generated information, any planning, marketing, or operational control effort will be hampered severely.

3. Market Segments

The issue of complex market segments is displayed dramatically in the University Medical Center. This institution, by virtue of its educational programs and its large size, provides a full range of services from primary care through the most sophisticated and most highly technological programs available in medicine today. As a result, management faces a situation where competing demands for resources arise from all sides. The marketing strategy, be it a long-range plan or strategy decisions on allocation of resources, tends to be politicized and/or randomly distributed.

With the development of a sound marketing plan and the research into the market segments that a hospital serves, management is provided with a working document that will permit assessment of the relative value of investing time, personnel effort, and financial resources in the provision of services by segment. Decisions of this sort revert back to considerations of the hospital's mission and the balancing of its various needs based on that mission statement.

The University Medical Center faces a situation where it is looked to by the residents of the surrounding region as their tertiary care center. On the other hand, the educational program and many local residents look toward the center as a source of primary care. For the Medical School, it is the prime source of teaching material; for many of the people of the community, it is the primary source of routine care. The hospital also faces demands for secondary and tertiary care, responsibilities that cannot be ignored in an institution of this size with its many valuable resources.

An important issue to evolve out of consideration of market segments is the fact that for hospital management, the physicians as a group constitute a market segment of their own. The fact that physicians act as agents for patients in the sense of demanding goods and services for those individuals is a fact that should not be lost upon hospital management. This segment can be broken down further to reflect primary care practitioners vs. specialists, and allows a more rational framework for consideration of needs of those segments. Consideration of all of these segments can lead to the development of strategies and provide a plan for the allocation of resources that eventually are turned into operational components of the hospital.

CASE 21. MINNEAPOLIS MEDICAL CENTER: PLANNING AND MARKETING HOSPICE CARE FOR THE TERMINALLY ILL

The Minneapolis Medical Center (MMC) is a large, multiservice medical center in the Minneapolis-St. Paul metropolitan area in Minnesota. In the summer of 1979, the Center's Cancer Committee decided it should implement a more integrated program of care for end-stage cancer and other terminally ill patients. To accomplish this goal, Howard Bell was hired as Coordinator for Hospice Care on October 1, 1979. Hospice care is a medically directed multidisciplinary program providing physical, emotional, and spiritual care to the terminally ill as inpatients and in their homes. Bell is an ordained minister with experience in death education, community programming, administration, and hospital chaplaincy. As past director of the Minnesota Coalition for Terminal Care, Inc., he had been active in the development of hospice programs both locally and nationally. His job description at MMC included the following:

> The Coordinator for Hospice Care is responsible to the Administrator of Special Services. During the initial year of this position, he shall be responsible for planning, organizing and implementing a hospice care program to assure the highest quality terminal care for patients and families served by MMC. The Coordinator for Hospice Care will implement a formal hospice program on either an individual or shared agency basis by October 1, 1980.

The person who chaired the Cancer Committee, a physician with the Center's Cancer Clinic, told Bell that "we are only interested in developing a hospice program for our existing patient population—we do not want to be the Mayo Clinic of the hospice movement." MMC had made no previous commitment to an integrated hospice program before hiring Bell. The Medical Center had long been serving the terminally ill through existing programs and had been sensitive to the special needs of this patient group. It also had been supportive of other hospice development in the area.

The Hospice Concept

Since the mid-1960s, much has been written about the needs of dying patients and their families. Inhibitions against discussion of death and dying in the United States have been decreasing, especially among health and human service professionals. They have come to recognize that the terminally ill and their families have special needs that had not been addressed appropriately by the existing health care system. Hospice care is a response to this problem. Although originally seen as an alternative concept for the terminally ill, by the late 1970s hospice programs were being integrated into the traditional health care system.

Hospice care focuses on pain and symptom control (palliative care); easing the physical, emotional, and spiritual discomfort of the patient; and treating the entire patient-family system rather than the individual alone. These concepts often are new to traditional acute care medicine. According to the National Hospice Organization, a group endorsed by the American Cancer Society and the American Medical Association and composed of individual hospice providers, a well-developed hospice program of care would be characterized by the following identifiable components:

1. The patient/family is the primary unit of care.
2. The emphasis is on symptom control rather than cure.
3. There is overall medical direction in the program.
4. The home care, inpatient, and bereavement services are coordinated.
5. The services are provided by an interdisciplinary core team that includes physician, nurse, social worker, patient care coordinator, volunteer director, and chaplain.
6. There is 24-hour-per-day, 7-day-per-week coverage with emphasis on the availability of nursing skills.
7. The program uses volunteers as an integral part of the hospice team.
8. The care of the family extends through the bereavement period.

Hospice programs are organized and administered through different delivery modes across the country (Exhibit 11-2). While no approach has been more successful than others, the hospital-based alternative is the most prevalent. All hospice programs based on hospitals or nursing homes have worked toward developing a coordinated home care component; conversely, those based on home care have sought a coordinated inpatient component. While most hospice patients are suffering from cancer, any individual with a degenerative disease and a terminal prognosis of six months or less is admitted to most programs. Age generally is not a criterion for admission, although some programs do not accept children.

The National Hospice Organization (NHO), in Washington, D.C., has been the vanguard for the hospice movement. In the fall of 1979, it approved the sixth and final draft of "Criteria and Standards for Hospice." The standards basically call for the development of programs with the components just listed. While the National Hospice Organization as of October 1979 had not been given any legal accrediting powers, it was expected that its criteria and standards would be adopted by third party payers and regulatory agencies. The growth of hospice programs in the

Exhibit 11-2 Hospice Service Delivery Modes

1. *Free Standing* (Independent)

   A separate facility with all beds and staff assigned to providing care to dying patients. It is an autonomous economic entity governed by its own management and board.

2. *Hospital Based*

   a. An acute care hospital with a centralized hospice unit: a separate unit within a general hospital with the staff and beds designated for providing care for the dying.
   b. An acute care hospital with a hospice "floating team" that carries on a consulting and supporting program of care for dying patients and staff throughout the institution.

3. *Hospital/Medical Center Affiliated Free Standing*

   A separate facility with all beds and staff assigned to providing care to dying patients. The facility is located adjacent to a hospital or medical center or is in the community but is owned by the hospital or medical center.

4. *Home Care*

   A program that provides and/or coordinates hospice care in the home but does not own or operate a designated inpatient hospice unit.

5. *Extended Care Facility or Nursing Home*

   A nursing home or extended care facility that has converted beds or established a separate unit for hospice care.

Minneapolis-St. Paul area and in the United States is shown in Table 11-1. Recognizing this increase, the NHO's objectives for 1979 were to:

1. define a common data collection base to be used to demonstrate definitive national trends in the care of the terminally ill and their families
2. design a policy to be considered by legislators and governmental agencies for provision of care for the terminally ill and their families
3. develop standards and procedures for giving accreditations to hospice organizations
4. provide opportunities for training through workshops, seminars, and other similar programs

The Minneapolis Medical Center

The Minneapolis Medical Center consists of more than 800 acute care medical/surgical beds, a 100-bed children's hospital and clinic, a physical rehabilitation center, educational facilities, and various outpatient health programs and clinics. The center has a comprehensive cancer program with inpatient beds, a clinic, modern therapies, and a specially trained staff. Two-thirds of the metropolitan region's certified cancer specialists are related to the program in some way.

The Environment

The MMC operates in a highly competitive environment. The Minneapolis-St. Paul area includes 37 general acute care hospitals and medical centers, three specialty centers, and 157 long-term care facilities. The

Table 11-1 Growth of Hospice Programs, 1974–80

Year	St. Paul/Minneapolis	State of Minnesota	U.S. and Canada
1974	0	0	1
1975	0	0	3
1976	0	0	5
1977	1	1	22[1]
1978	3	4	80[1]
1979	11	13	140[1]
1980	12[2]	14[2]	200 plus[1]

[1] These are estimations that include hospices in late planning stages as well as those actually giving care.

[2] These include the proposed hospice program of Minneapolis Medical Center to be implemented in the fall of 1980.

administration of the MMC defines its service area primarily as two counties (Figure 11-1). Ninety percent of its patients come from Minneapolis and the western portion of the metropolitan area. The map shows the other hospitals in the area with hospice programs. The services they offer are listed in Table 11-2. According to the Minnesota Coalition for Terminal Care, Inc., 17 other health care organizations in the area have expressed interest in delivering some form of hospice care—ten other hospitals, four nursing homes, and three home care agencies.

Regulatory Pressures

The occupancy rates at area hospitals have been decreasing over the last ten years (Figure 11-2) even though population has been increasing and was expected to grow further (Figure 11-3). This has caused an overbedded situation in the area, with hospitals looking for new growth opportunities. The Metropolitan Health Board, the region's Health Systems Agency (HSA) in charge of certificate of need and planning for regional health services, issued a moratorium on the licensing of all new hospital construction until beds are reduced by 1,000 in the area. Occupancy rates at the MMC had been running at 75 to 85 percent of capacity—above the regional average for general hospitals.

The MMC's Patient Population

The population served by the MMC is fairly diverse but a majority of patients tend to be middle-class, white, and professional. The population in the region overall was more than 2 million and increasing. The population density of the Minneapolis communities surrounding the MMC was expected to increase as people moved back to the city because of the energy situation.

Table 11-3 shows that cancer accounted for 18.6 percent of the deaths in the area between 1965 and 1975. Records at the MMC showed that 805 new cases of cancer were diagnosed at the Center in 1977, 846 in 1978, and 880 expected in 1979. This reflects increased cancer rates and better detection techniques.

HMOs: Home Care and Long-Term Care

Other prevalent actors in the area's health care environment include seven health maintenance organizations (HMOs). These prepaid health programs contracted with area hospitals and accounted for 13 percent of the health insurance market in the area, well above national averages. The enrollment in HMOs overall had been increasing 27 percent per year since

Figure 11-1 Service Area of the MMC

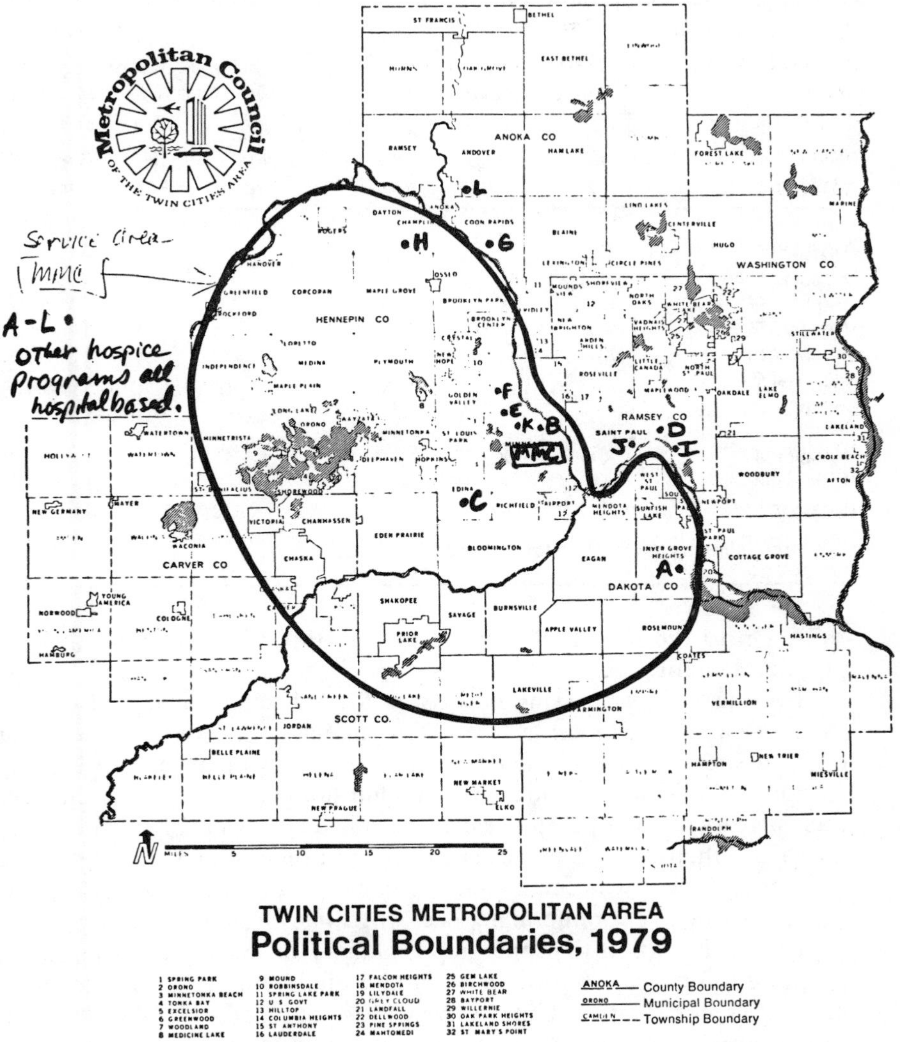

TWIN CITIES METROPOLITAN AREA
Political Boundaries, 1979

1 SPRING PARK	9 MOUND	17 FALCON HEIGHTS	25 GEM LAKE
2 ORONO	10 ROBBINSDALE	18 MENDOTA	26 BIRCHWOOD
3 MINNETONKA BEACH	11 SPRING LAKE PARK	19 LILYDALE	27 WHITE BEAR
4 TONKA BAY	12 U S GOVT	20 GREY CLOUD	28 BAYPORT
5 EXCELSIOR	13 HILLTOP	21 LANDFALL	29 WILLERNIE
6 GREENWOOD	14 COLUMBIA HEIGHTS	22 DELLWOOD	30 OAK PARK HEIGHTS
7 WOODLAND	15 ST ANTHONY	23 PINE SPRINGS	31 LAKELAND SHORES
8 MEDICINE LAKE	16 LAUDERDALE	24 MAHTOMEDI	32 ST MARY S POINT

ANOKA ____ County Boundary
ORONO ____ Municipal Boundary
CAMDEN -‒-‒ Township Boundary

The letters A through L denote other hospice programs, all of them hospital based.
Source: Metropolitan Council of the Twin Cities Area.

Table 11-2 St. Paul/Minneapolis Hospice Programs: Stage of Development, Fall 1979

Hospice	Hospice Services (Operational)			Planned Hospice Services (Nonoperational)		
	24-Hour Home Care	Backup Beds	Bereave- ment	24-Hour Home Care	Backup Beds	Bereave- ment
Hospital A	X	X				X
Hospital B	X		X	X		
Hospital C	X		X			
Hospital D	X	X	X			
Hospital E	X		X			
Hospital F	X		X			
Hospital G	X		X			
Hospital H	X		X		X	
Hospital I	X		X		X	
Hospital J	X	X	X			
Hospital K	X	X	X			
Hospital L	X		X			

Source: Minnesota Coalition for Terminal Care, Inc.

1971. Up to the fall of 1979, none of the HMOs had offered a hospice program benefit.

There also was a growing movement toward more home care services in the area. The Minnesota State Department of Health called for additional home care services and reimbursement for them in a 1979 study. Although the MMC did not have an adult home care program, the Children's Hospital had operated a special service for terminally ill youngsters that aided their parents in caring for them in their homes.

Although there were many nursing homes in the area, their occupancy rates generally were quite high. The MMC had been in discussion with a nonprofit foundation that operated a number of nursing homes and was planning to open a new one in an old hospital about two miles from the medical center campus. Until it decided to hire Bell, the MMC had not had any plans to provide long-term care. In addition to the hospice programs already mentioned, the Minnesota Coalition for Terminal Care had identified another 50 health and social service agencies in the area that offered some sort of specialized services to the terminally ill and their families.

Figure 11-2 Hospital Use Rates for Medical/Surgical and Pediatrics Services, 1970–1978

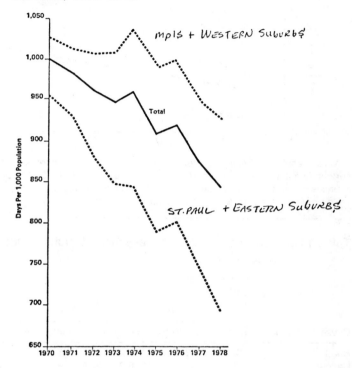

Note: The decline in use rates has resulted in an oversupply of acute care hospital beds. At 80 percent occupancy, there was an excess of approximately 2,000 licensed beds in 1978. If the 1978 use rate (1,090 days per 1,000 population) continued, as population increased, there still would be an excess of 1,830 acute care beds in 1980 and 962 in 1990, at 80 percent occupancy.

Source: Minneapolis-St. Paul Metropolitan Health Board.

Figure 11-3 Population 1950–2000, St. Paul/Minneapolis Metropolitan Area

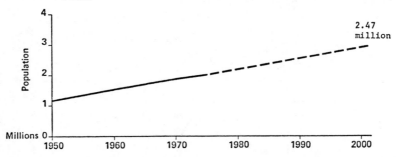

Note: Despite a diminished growth rate in the St. Paul/Minneapolis metropolitan area, surrounding counties have experienced rapid growth since 1970. The population in these counties depends to a great extent on the seven-county area for employment and services.
Source: U.S. Census, Metropolitan Council Forecasts.

Table 11-3 Age-Specific and Cause-Specific Deaths in Metropolitan Area, 1965–1975

Cause of Death	Percent of Deaths All Ages	0–4 No.	0–4 Rank	0–4 Rate	5–14 No.	5–14 Rank	5–14 Rate	15–24 No.	15–24 Rank	15–24 Rate
Heart	37.2	43	7	2.2	24	5	0.5	57	6	1.5
Cancer	18.6	133	5	6.9	267	2	6.0	276	3	7.4
Cerebro	12.2	23	9	1.2	16	7	0.4	27	7*	0.7
Accidental	5.7	479	3	24.9	673	1	15.2	1,945	1	52.1
Flu & Pneu.	3.2	266	4	13.8	37	4	0.8	27	8*	0.7
Arterio	1.8	0		0.0	1		0.1	0		0.0
Diabetes	1.7	3		0.2	9	9	0.2	15	9	0.4
Suicide	1.3	0		—	8	10	0.2	364	2	9.7
Bronchitis/ Asthma/ Emphysema	1.5	24	8	1.3	11	8	0.2	7		0.2
Perinatal	2.3	3,575	1	185.7	1		0.1	0		—
Cirrhosis	1.4	3		0.2	5		0.1	8	10	0.2
Cong. Anom.	1.1	1,307	2	67.9	117	3	2.6	70	5	1.9
Peptic Ulcer	.4	4		0.2	0		0.0	5		0.1
Homicide	.5	22	10	1.1	22	6	0.5	208	4	5.6
Hernia/ Intestine	.4	61	6	3.2	3		0.1	5		0.1
Hypertension	.4	1		—	0		0.0	1		0.1
Other	10.3	1,187		61.7	255		5.8	463		12.4
Total	100.0	7,131		369.3	1,449		32.8	3,478		93.1

Table 11-3 continued

Cause of Death	Percent of Deaths All Ages	25–44			45–64			65 +		
		No.	Rank	Rate	No.	Rank	Rate	No.	Rank	Rate
Heart	37.2	1,299	3	25.5	12,700	1	349.8	43,212	1	2,399.1
Cancer	18.6	1,459	2	28.6	9,297	2	256.1	17,295	2	960.2
Cerebro	12.2	324	5	6.3	2,125	3	58.5	16,278	3	903.8
Accidental	5.7	1,689	1	33.1	1,718	4	47.3	2,338	6	129.8
Flu & Pneu.	3.2	108	9	2.1	607	7	16.7	3,835	4	212.9
Arterio	1.8	7		0.1	88		2.4	2,617	5	145.3
Diabetes	1.7	159	8	3.1	481	9	13.2	1,922	7	106.7
Suicide	1.3	693	4	13.6	708	6	19.5	280		15.5
Bronchitis/ Asthma/ Emphysema	1.5	38		0.7	486	8	13.4	1,683	8	93.4
Perinatal	2.3	0		—	0		—	0		—
Cirrhosis	1.4	267	7	5.2	1,303	5	35.9	605	9	33.6
Cong. Anom.	1.1	87	10	1.7	77		2.1	65		3.6
Peptic Ulcer	.4	28		0.5	180	10	5.0	429		23.8
Homicide	.5	280	6	5.5	117		3.2	37		2.1
Hernia/ Intestine	.4	11		0.2	74		2.0	464		25.8
Hypertension	.4	12		0.2	89		2.5	534	10	29.5
Other	10.3	1,100		21.6	3,540		97.5	9,392		521.4
Total	100.0	7,561		148.1	33,590		925.1	100,985		5,606.7

* Tied for 7th and 8th places.
Source: Metropolitan Health Board.

Bell's Present Options

After a month on the job, Bell realized that planning a hospice program at the MMC would be even more challenging than he had anticipated. The center's Cancer Committee, representing administration, nursing, and physicians, had instructed him to examine different modes of organizing a hospice, specifically the following alternatives that the MMC had available:

1. the use of existing hospital beds at the MMC
2. the conversion of an existing house on the MMC campus
3. the designation of beds at an affiliated off-campus nursing home
4. the designation of beds through other area nursing homes
5. the utilization of other beds at a hospice program(s) in another hospital(s) through a shared service agreement

6. the development of a hospital-based home care service vs. contracting with existing home care services in the area

Being active in local hospice development, Bell had been in close contact with the directors of other programs in the area. He felt strongly that a hospice should be community-based and noncompetitive and that potential competitive problems could be avoided. He had not ruled out any of the alternatives suggested by the Cancer Committee. As he began examining each one and planning a program, he was most concerned about the following issues.

Acceptance and Understanding of Hospice

Although the Cancer Committee was supportive of hospice, Bell was uncertain as to how physicians in general would view such a new program at the MMC. One cancer specialist in the area had written in an editorial in a national medical journal that, "the use of the word terminal in describing patients should be limited to morticians who make the funeral arrangements and to clergymen when they deliver the eulogy." Bell knew that the general public often was ill-informed about hospices and held many misconceptions about what they actually were. He also had not had an opportunity to survey the MMC staff on the subject. He wondered how its members would deal with working with a concentrated group of terminally ill patients if a unit were formed at the center. Some area hospice programs had had difficulty maintaining nursing staffs, as evidenced by advertising for full-time staff in the newsletter of the Minnesota Coalition for Terminal Care.

Reimbursement for Hospice Services

By late 1979, it was unclear where reimbursement would come from for hospice services. Bell had been told by the MMC administrator of special services to "pursue all efforts to maximize reimbursement using all available mechanisms." Although hospice care generally was considered less expensive than other alternatives, reliable comparative data had been collected only recently. He was aware of one favorable cost analysis study done at the Kaiser Permanente Medical Center in California. Its summary cost data on patients before and after implementation of a hospice program are shown in Table 11-4. No new state or federal legislation regarding reimbursement for hospice service was expected in 1980. Third party payers were examining hospice care and Bell had scheduled a meeting with the regional Blue Cross and Blue Shield representatives who were looking at how they could make reimbursements for such service.

Table 11-4 Kaiser Permanente Cost Analysis Study

Cost Data for Patients Who Died in Prehospice Program Group (April–September, 1977)
N = 45 vs. Posthospice Program Group (April–September, 1978) N = 62

	Cost Per Patient			Cost Per Diem		
	Pre- hospice	Post- hospice	% Change	Pre- hospice	Post- hospice	% Change
Inpatient						
Basic Care	$2,424	$2,688	+11	$146	$173*	+18
Physician	453	388	−14	27	25	−7
Laboratory	1,073	238	−78	65	15	−77
Radiology	96	72	−25	6	5	−17
Nuclear Medicine	41	12	−71	2	1	−50
Operating Room	321	187	−42	19	12	−37
Other	16	22	—	1	1	—
Totals	4,424	3,607	−18	266	232	−13

Source: Reprinted from *Hospice Pilot Project Report* by permission of Kaiser Permanente Medical Center, Haywood, Calif., © 1979, p. 154.

The federal government had just announced that it would reimburse 26 hospice programs, including one in St. Paul, for two years on a pilot study basis through waiver of certain Medicare and Medicaid regulations. This study was to begin in March 1980, so no change in Medicare or Medicaid reimbursement was expected until the project was completed and evaluated. Bell had not been given any proposed budget figures for the hospice program to be implemented in October 1980. The administrator of special services asked him to turn in proposed figures to corporate planning, as the budgetary planning cycle for 1981 was to begin in six weeks.

Criteria and Standards of Care

Thus far the area HSA had not attempted to regulate the development of hospice programs nor had any formal criteria and standards been developed beyond those proposed by the National Hospice Organization. There was some concern that there were too many hospices in the region and that some programs were not meeting the goals laid out by the NHO. Bell was not aware of any adverse feedback from patients or families about the hospice care at other hospitals.

The Actual Need for Hospice Services at the MMC

After becoming familiar with the services and staff at the MMC, Bell had become convinced that the patients could benefit from an integrated hospice program. While no data had been collected at the MMC, opinion surveys by the Minnesota Coalition for Terminal Care and other hospice programs in the area documented the dissatisfaction of families and health professionals with how the terminally ill had been cared for in the past.

The medical center did keep an updated computerized cancer tumor registry on all cancer patients treated there. Bell was informed that the registry would have information on all cancer-related deaths since January 1978, including data on place of death, cause of death, diagnosis prior to death, place of residence, last stay in the hospital, and patient's age, sex, and race. He used this registry to obtain the initial data shown in Table 11-5. He felt this and other information in the system could give him an idea on how many patients a new hospice program might serve.

Within two weeks, Bell was to present the administrator of special services with a plan of action that would culminate in a program by October 1, 1980. As he began this task, he thought about two hospices elsewhere in the country that recently had discontinued operations because of inadequate numbers of patients.

OVERVIEW OF CASE 21

Issues to Consider

1. What alternatives are available to Bell?
2. What additional data are necessary in evaluating the alternatives?
3. What are the target markets and key publics that Bell must examine?

Discussion

1. Available Alternatives

There are several options for the establishment of a hospice program by the MMC. It must be determined whether the center wants to include pediatric clients in its hospice program, to provide a total hospice service (i.e., home care, backup beds, bereavement) or a partial one; and which of the following alternatives will best meet client needs:

a. utilization of existing MMC hospital beds
b. use of nursing home locations
c. home care services only or in addition to hospital or nursing home facilities

The first decision Bell must make is how the Cancer Committee's request can best be implemented. There are two choices. The first is a totally

Table 11-5 Minneapolis Medical Center Tumor Registry Data
(Number of cancer patients treated at the MMC who died during study period June 1, 1978–May 31, 1979: N = 474)

Location of Death: N = 474	Number	Percent
MMC	248	53
Unknown	106	22
Elsewhere	81	17
Other hospitals in Minnesota	39	8

Place of Residence: N = 474	Number	Percent
Minneapolis	185	39
Minneapolis suburbs	104	21
St. Paul	14	3
Others in metropolitan area	59	12
Outstate Minnesota	80	17
Other states	36	8

Deaths at MMC (N = 248) Place of Residence	Number	Percent
Minneapolis	118	48
Minneapolis suburbs	57	18
St. Paul & suburbs	5	2
Others in metropolitan area	29	12
Outside metropolitan area	49	20

integrated program that would involve modifying the present structure of care for the terminally ill to include components that the MMC does not provide. The MMC could offer some of these on campus and contract others out, e.g., home care, until demand is great enough to warrant a separate program.

The second alternative is to add an entirely separate program of hospice care to the current services. This would involve such factors as location, staff, certification, and attracting a separate market segment to use these services as opposed to the package deal offered by the first choice.

The decision can be made only after Bell has researched the benefits and problems involved in each choice thoroughly. He should solicit ideas from the Cancer Committee members, the MMC medical and administrative staffs, and patients who would or could use this type of service.

2. Additional Data

Bell has considerable data to use in analyzing the alternatives. However, additional information will be useful. Although the service area is defined geographically, what other stratification factors would be useful in subdividing this rather large, amorphous market, e.g., age, income, present source of medical care (HMO, private M.D., none)? After segmenting the catchment area into various markets, Bell must determine the actual and potential users of the proposed program. These segments then can be subdivided further either demographically or psychographically into several more or less homogeneous groups. Each group may be considered a target market for which a unique marketing approach would be developed.

In addition to defining and understanding potential users, it is necessary also to define and understand potential competitors. Analysis of consumers' behavior must consider where they go now, what this facility offers, the degree of satisfaction, and loyalty to their present source of care. In addition, input regarding competitors' fees, hours, services, etc., would enable Bell to define his program's position in the marketplace of care for terminally ill patients. This also would assist him in determining whether the MMC catchment area needs hospice care as a separate entity at this time.

To help develop a successful plan for hospice care, Bell should communicate with the two hospices mentioned that discontinued their services. Learning from another's experience can be a valuable tool in avoiding those same mistakes.

A budget for this program must be developed. Bell, in addition to determining costs to the MMC and proposing fees to be charged, should investigate the source of funds for other hospice programs. Before his meeting with Blue Cross and Blue Shield, he should become familiar with operation of other programs, including the types of reimbursement systems.

A survey should be conducted as to how patients are referred to, or choose, a particular program. Each of the avenues deemed to be important sources of information and/or referral needs to be investigated and a promotion plan developed to introduce the new program or the new approach to care for the terminally ill and the range of services offered.

3. Target Markets

At least four important target markets exist: (1) terminally ill MMC clients, (2) physicians, (3) MMC staff, and (4) the general public. Data must be obtained concerning their image, understanding, and desires as they relate to a hospice program. These data then must be heeded in setting objectives for a new hospice and in determining services to be offered, price, place, and types of promotion. Marketing research is only the first step in the overall process but it is an indispensable one.

The only way to define the needs of the potential MMC patient population is to ask for feedback. Terminally ill patients and/or their families could be given questionnaires or be interviewed concerning their desires and needs. This can be done tactfully if those questioned understand that the purpose of the project is to better serve them, their loved ones, and others in similar circumstances. The data will greatly facilitate decisions as to the type and scope of hospice services to offer to best meet client needs. In other words, more accurate and specific objectives can be drawn up.

In segmenting the market further, physicians comprise a second target population about which something must be known. Without physician support in the form of referrals, the new hospice program could be doomed. Physicians thus should be questioned to ascertain what percentage of them knows what a hospice is, what in their view makes up a quality hospice, how many patients they would refer to the MMC's hospice, and their impression or image of hospices in general. If physicians' image and support is favorable, it should be reinforced. If their reaction is negative, promotional activity will be necessary.

The same holds true for a third key public, the MMC staff. Bell is concerned about possible reactions to working with terminally ill patients. Unless the staff needs are met, high personnel turnover will result, thus compromising the continuity of care and stable staff-patient relationships that are so important in a hospice situation. If there is a strong negative reaction from the staff members, it is possible that no amount of education and promotion will change their feelings and a separate staff and/or facility will be required. After all, meeting the needs of the terminally ill takes a unique person with specific qualities. A hospice program without the right kind of staff could be disastrous. Therefore, staff members must be asked about their needs and perceptions via questionnaires or interviews.

Another important group, the general public, appears to be ill informed and to have many misconceptions about hospices. Issuing questionnaires or conducting a telephone survey of such a large population, even if randomized, could be time consuming and expensive, yet this support might be very important since the source of reimbursement for the hospice is unclear. Donations from the general public might prove to be vital at least initially until Medicare, Medicaid, and private third party payers change their policies to include hospices. Focus groups might be a useful tool in assessing the general public's image of hospices.

CASE 22. COMMUNITY HEALTH PLAN: MARKETING FOR AN HMO

The Community Health Plan, Inc., known as the CHP, was Rhode Island's first nonprofit health maintenance organization (HMO), established in June 1971. With the support and assistance of local organized labor, the CHP became the first viable alternative to sometimes costly and piecemeal medical coverage and services. For the first time in Rhode Island, families were offered the opportunity to obtain total care at a reasonable cost under one roof.

Although the CHP had been widely respected in its two years of service to the community, the same problems experienced by other HMOs presented themselves in this setting. Group practice remained a fairly new and innovative concept about which some individuals remained skeptical, given long-standing relationships with private physicians. The newness of the organization also presented questions at first concerning its stability as compared to older, more established methods of health care delivery and insurance.

The CHP started with 1,200 members (subscribers and their families), although the opening enrollment had been forecast at 6,000. In 1973, the organization had 12,000 subscribers who had been offered the CHP plan on a dual choice basis through their particular group setting, usually at their place of employment. The CHP marketing team was responsible for tapping the available group resources and arranging for dual choices to be offered.

Because of insufficient enrollment, the CHP found it necessary to obtain large loans from the Prudential Insurance Company. The organization was near its operational break-even point, estimated at 16,000 members. However, at that point it would not be retiring its debt or setting money aside for expansion or replacement of capital equipment.

The CHP had experienced problems administratively. The fourth director was Philip Nelson, who was brought in by Prudential in an effort to strengthen the organization and ensure its success. As it entered its third year of operation, Nelson intended to refine both services and operations. He hoped to expand it to include new markets, additional medical capabilities, and larger and more numerous treatment facilities.

One of Nelson's first tasks as director was to evaluate the CHP's marketing. He requested a copy of the association's 1973 marketing plan, which had been prepared by Ralph Wilbur, director of marketing. Nelson also reviewed CHP's past marketing strategies and decisional inputs as a guide for future marketing activities.

The Basic HMO Model

The term HMO has been used to designate a variety of health care delivery systems. The most commonly accepted definition is that of a medical care delivery system that accepts responsibility for the organization, financing, and delivery of health care services for a defined population. The HMO is characterized by the combination of a financing mechanism—prepayment—and a particular mode of delivery—group practice—by means of a managerial-administrative organization responsible for ensuring the availability of health services for a subscriber population.

The principles of HMOs' operations may be divided into six primary characteristics:

1. Responsibility of organizing and delivering health services: the HMO is not merely a financing mechanism but is concerned with obtaining, through contracts with providers, an assured source of supply of health services for its members.
2. Prepayment: costs of the organization are met through fixed periodic payments from subscribers. Many plans, however, supplement prepayment income with copayments charged at the time treatment is incurred, e.g., a $2 charge for an office call.
3. Group practice: physicians are organized into multispecialty groups of sufficient size to maintain facilities that are capable of providing comprehensive, continuous care. In the early stages, a developing HMO may include only primary care physicians and may depend on referrals to outside specialists for services beyond its capabilities.
4. Comprehensive benefits: although "comprehensiveness" varies, most plans offer a complete range of medical services, including some forms of preventive care.
5. Compensation of physicians: the physicians usually are compensated through the capitation principle (the payment of an amount of money equal to a fixed per capita sum for each subscriber multiplied by the number of subscribers enrolled). In addition, most physician groups participate in any savings generated through effective management of the plan.
6. Voluntary enrollment: most HMOs enroll through a dual choice mechanism under which employees may choose between an indemnity plan or the HMO.

Group practice prepayment was initiated in the United States in a small clinic in Elk City, Okla., in 1932 and first implemented on a large scale by the Kaiser Foundation Health Plan on the West Coast. Since then, plans have been organized by diverse groups such as consumers at Puget Sound, a medical school which is part of the Harvard Community Health Plan, and an insurance company in Columbia, Md.—and in equally diverse forms. In 1970, 75 HMOs provided health care for more than eight million persons nationally. The data derived from those participants indicate that HMOs have been able to supply health care for substantially less dollar outlay than has the predominant fee-for-service system.

The Community Health Plan

The CHP embraced all of the concepts that made up the HMO definition—prepayment, group practice, and the organizational responsibility for ensuring the availability of health services for the defined population.

The prepaid premium covered all benefits outlined in the CHP contract and precluded any additional expense to the subscriber except for items excluded under that agreement. By and large, it could be said that all routine medical expenses were covered by the prepayment mechanism, as were most unexpected major medical eventualities, including surgery, hospitalizations, specialty consultations required by CHP physicians, and so forth.

Its marketing plan involved the four basic elements of this field: product, promotion, price, and place—the four Ps, as follows.

Product

A principal marketing advantage of prepaid group practice programs over traditional health insurance is a comprehensive benefit package. Such programs also claim the potential to deliver broader benefits at a lower cost than similar benefits under a fee-for-service plan.

In designing an HMO benefit package, primary emphasis is given to elements considered essential to provide flexibility for the medical group treating patients. Any additions to this package must take into account the attractiveness of benefits to potential subscribers, their cost-effectiveness, and the nature and price of competitive benefits in the community. Although most programs include copayments and deductibles, the CHP had none except for house calls. The CHP benefit package was described in a brochure distributed to prospective members. A copy of part of this brochure is shown in Exhibit 11-3.

Promotion

A substantial part of the work of an HMO involves promotion. For example, the community must be educated about prepaid group practice,

Exhibit 11-3 Sample Page from HMO Benefit Package

MEDICAL, SURGICAL AND HOSPITAL SERVICES

IN THE COMMUNITY HEALTH CENTER	Visits to Doctor's office	No Charge
	Laboratory Tests-X ray- Physical Therapy	"
	Casts and Dressings	"
	Injections-Allergy Injections	"
IN THE HOSPITAL	Services of Physicians and Surgeons and Other Health Personnel - Including Operations	"
	Room and Board - General Nursing - use of Operating Room - Anesthesia	"
	X-ray and Laboratory Examinations -X-ray Therapy Dressings - Casts - Blood Transfusions If Blood is Replaced	" "
AMBULANCE SERVICE		Provided Without Charge If Authorized by CHP Personnel
IN YOUR HOME	House Calls by CHP Physicians	$5 for first for each Acute Illness No charge after first visit for the Same Illness. House calls will be made at the judgement of a CHP Physian.
MATERNITY CARE	Full Physician's Services Including Prenatal Care	No Charge
	Hospital Care - Full Hospital Care is provided to a member after 180 days continuous family membership in CHP - or when continued combined membership in an alternate plan and CHP totals 180 days of family coverage.	"

Source: By permission of Rhode Island Community Health Program, Inc., © 1971.

management and union leadership must be sold on the idea of dual choice for the firm's employees, individuals must be enrolled in the program.

The marketing department at the CHP consisted of four employees. Wilbur was the director, with previous experience in marketing but not in the health field. The other three persons had no previous experience in marketing. These four called on employees and employers in an effort to sell the concept of prepaid group practice.

Prospective subscribers appeared to respond best to three sales themes: (1) comprehensive services are delivered at one place; (2) services are completely prepaid; and (3) high-quality medical care is obtained.

In addition to personal selling efforts, the CHP twice used newspaper advertising. Physicians then were bound by professional codes of conduct that considered it unethical to solicit patients directly or indirectly. Thus, any promotion must be handled delicately so that no charges of unethical conduct can arise. In addition, HMOs had been subjected to charges of socialized medicine and had suffered from the stigma associated with such contentions. For these reasons, prepaid group practice programs generally were conservative in advertising and promoting. Some groups did not aggressively seek out new business but relied on their reputations to attract new accounts. However, for new prepaid programs in their infancy there was pressure to meet enrollment quotas and educate the citizenry; thus, promotion was sometimes more aggressive.

In November 1972, the CHP ran a newspaper advertisement (Exhibit 11-4). As a result, the Rhode Island Medical Society lodged a complaint against the CHP over its merchandising tactics.

Price

A 1964 study compared out-of-pocket costs in a prepaid group practice with two traditional health insurance plans. It found that the prepaid program premium covered 76 percent of costs of physician services, prescription drugs, and hospitalization while the other programs covered 55 percent and 59 percent, respectively. Thus, price could be a significant marketing advantage in terms of out-of-pocket costs of prepaid programs.

Although copayments are a feature of most prepaid plans, the CHP had only one. A reason for their use is that prepaid premiums can be set more competitively. Many programs included small charges for office visits ($1 to $3). With such an approach, Nelson believed the CHP could reduce its price below its major competitor, which in 1973 wrote about 85 percent of the health insurance in the state.

The CHP's primary competitor offered a low-option benefit package that fitted the needs of a particular group of employees in the state, namely, low-pay, low-fringe-benefit industries such as jewelry and textiles. The competitor's plan paid for approximately 60 percent of health care expenses but cost substantially less than CHP's only plan, a high-option benefit package.

Another variable influenced by competition concerned the number of price steps. Both the major competitor and the CHP had two price steps—one rate for a single person and another for families, regardless of size. However, Nelson had considered adding another price step so the rates would be categorized three ways—for one person, two, and three or more. The result if implemented would be to skew CHP's membership more to one- and two-person enrollees since their rates would be lower. However, large families would have a greater incentive to subscribe to the competitor's plan because their rate would increase with the CHP. Although Nelson was considering such a move, he was unsure what ramifications this might have on employer acceptance, membership size, the CHP's break-even point, or competitive reaction.

Exhibit 11-4 Advertisement

ATTENTION FEDERAL AND STATE EMPLOYEES AND OTHER EMPLOYEE GROUPS: WITH THE CHP PLAN YOU RECEIVE TOTAL FAMILY HEALTH CARE

Yes, emergency medical care and advice is available to you 24 hours a day, 365 days a year, under the Comprehensive Health Care Plan provided by CHP.

There is no other plan to match CHP. Besides providing full inhospital coverage for a semiprivate room, other hospital service charges and all surgical and medical charges, the plan has many unique features not generally offered by other plans such as:

— Full coverage for all visits to your CHP physician or other specialists to whom you may be referred by your CHP doctor—whether for treatment, advice, diagnosis or just a check-up.

— Full coverage for all visits to CHP pediatricians at the CHP family health care center, including well-baby care, inoculations and immunizations.

— Complete maternity care, including prenatal, delivery and postnatal care by your CHP obstetrician, at no charge to you.

— Eye examinations and prescriptions for glasses from your CHP vision center.

November 15–30 is open enrollment period for federal and state employees and their families. (It's always open enrollment for other groups of employees.)

Whether you live in Rhode Island or Southeastern Massachusetts, you owe it to yourself and your family to take advantage of this once-a-year opportunity to join CHP for complete personal and family care. Obtain CHP literature and application forms from your payroll clerk or by calling CHP. Visit the new Health Care Center, Plenty of free Parking.

OPEN HOUSE
TODAY 1 to 4 p.m.
TOMORROW EVENING 7 to 9 p.m.
COMMUNITY HEALTH PLAN
North Providence, R.I.
A Nonprofit Organization

Place

The CHP was located adjacent to a medium-size hospital in North Providence, one of the most heavily populated areas of the state. It was convenient to the main traffic arteries in the northern part of the state.

Nelson estimated that the CHP would exhaust the capacity of the present building when it reached 16,000 enrollees, so thought must be given to expanded facilities and their location.

One barrier to greater enrollment was the distance some members had to travel to reach the facility. Studies of other HMO programs indicated that distances of 10 miles or more from the facility significantly retarded membership and utilization by members. However, because the CHP lacked precise knowledge of the geographic distribution of its membership, Nelson was uncertain of the extent to which this could be a problem.

If the CHP were to open additional locations, a number of areas in the state might be considered. Figure 11-4 presents a map of the state and population data. Two appealing locations to Nelson were Warwick and South Kingston. Warwick's population had expanded rapidly. The city offered a central location in the state and it featured Rhode Island's two major regional shopping centers. The other area was near the state university, in South Kingston, which had a student and employee population of more than 15,000. In fact, preliminary negotiations had been undertaken in the past on the possibility of the CHP's assuming a major role in the student health service.

Soon after Nelson had reviewed these aspects of the CHP's marketing situation, Wilbur submitted the proposed marketing plan for 1973 (Exhibit 11-5), which indicated what marketing directions were planned for the coming year.

OVERVIEW OF CASE 22

Issues to Consider

1. What would be the reaction to Wilbur's proposed marketing program if the reader were Nelson?
2. How might the plan be improved?
3. What are the unique features of this organization that influence marketing decisions?
4. What recommendations should be made for CHP's marketing strategy?

Figure 11-4 Rhode Island Population by Counties & Select Cities

	Population Census	
	1960	1970
Kent County	112,619	142,382
Warwick	68,504	83,694
Other Areas	44,115	58,688
Bristol County	37,146	45,937
Newport County	81,405	94,220
Newport	47,049	34,231
Other Areas	34,356	59,989
Washington County	59,640	85,706
South Kingston	11,942	16,913
Other Areas	47,698	68,793
Providence County	568,778	581,470
North Providence	18,220	24,337
East Providence	41,955	48,207
Pawtucket	81,001	76,984
Providence	207,498	179,116
Woonsocket	47,080	46,820
Other Areas	173,024	206,006
State	858,488	949,723

Source: Abstracted from U.S. Census (1970).

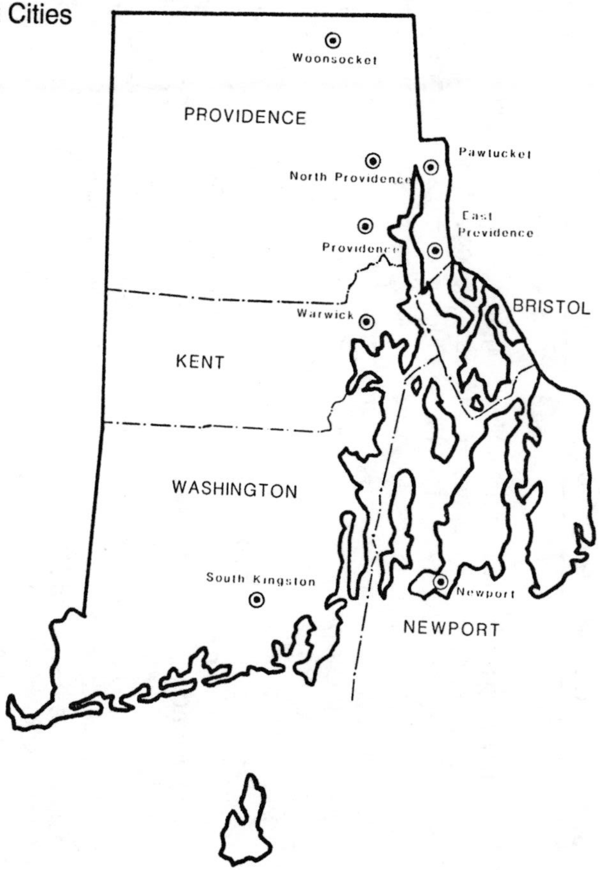

Exhibit 11-5 1973 Marketing Program for Community Health Plan

---

Preface

The following recommended marketing program is based on the premise that the prepaid, group practice health care concept offered by the Rhode Island Community Health Plan is a highly marketable program. This is not to say that it is absolutely perfect and that *no* improvements could be made in the plan. Slight improvements may be made.

We face certain problems . . . some of which come under the category of demographics. Our market is unlimited by age. Every employed individual and adult family member with or without children is a prospective enrollee. However, at our present stage of growth and development, with one Health Care Center located in North Providence, CHP is somewhat limited geographically. While we are located almost in the heart of the Providence metropolitan area and the extension of Route 295 will place us in close proximity to a major expressway, our present facility is still far removed from southern areas of the State, both on the east and west sides of Narragansett Bay. Obviously, the answer is the future establishment of a family health care facility somewhere south of Warwick, which is the fastest growing city in the State. With this as a future goal, we still have the advantage of being located in an area with the greatest mass concentration of population in Rhode Island. Even a modest share of enrollees out of the potential in our present location could flood the CHP Center.

Based on a successful marketing program, the initial CHP planning grant projected an enrollment of 17,500 persons by June 1973, and 20,000 by June 1974. If these enrollments are attained, it leads to immediate consideration of a larger facility in the metropolitan area and/ or a second facility in southern Rhode Island, plus expansion of the medical staff. We call your attention to goals and objectives later in this presentation.

A problem we will always face under our present concept is the disruption of previously established doctor-patient relationships. This is a particularly difficult problem with a segment of the female population. We see no simple solution of this problem. The Marketing Department's job will be to "sell" the CHP concept, the high degree of competence, experience and professionalism and ongoing availability and accessibility of our staff physicians as well as the importance of containment of the cost of health care.

In presenting a marketing "game plan," it is necessary to discuss some basic marketing techniques:

Exhibit 11-5 continued

1. It is absolutely essential that the general public be totally aware of and familiarized with the existence of the product or service (Community Health Plan). We have made great strides in this direction during the past two months. However, *much* remains to be done. To coin a very hackneyed expression, CHP must become a "household word."

2. After CHP is known to the mass public, we must educate the people to accept the CHP concept of prepaid, group practice health care . . . the total health care . . . the preventive health care available under the plan.

3. Finally, we must break down old associations, market the acceptability of the CHP plan and *MOTIVATE* the individual to enroll. Once he is enrolled, we must provide the highest quality of health care, thereby creating satisfied customers, each of whom in a sense becomes a member of our Marketing Department, spreading the word of his satisfaction and the CHP concept. Once we have acquisition, we must have a very concentrated effort in retention . . . and this objective must permeate the entire CHP staff in their dealings with our membership. This is an extremely important area of the CHP marketing program . . . the constant liaison with the employer contacts and union representatives. It is through them that we gain the entree to the employee groups and the growth of our membership. This requires constant telephone and personal contact, *especially personal contact*, with visual presentations and/or visits to the CHP Family Health Care Center. Through good advertising and public relations, we hope to gain total public awareness of the CHP plan and the entree to management and unions.

How do we accomplish these objectives? Without high public mass media exposure, success will be slow in coming. It is essential that we establish a firm advertising and public relations budget. This can be formulated by setting an enrollment goal and a cost of acquisition for each individual enrollee. During the Blue Cross–Blue Shield Open Enrollment period in October 1972, we have learned that its cost of acquisition was $5.00 per enrollee.[1] Figuring our cost of acquisition at $2.50 and now projecting a total membership of 25,000 by December 31, 1973, or an increase of approximately 1,000 per month, we arrive at an advertising and public relations budget of $30,000 for 1973. We propose to spend this money in the following manner:

(continues)

Exhibit 11-5 continued

Advertising and Public Relations Budget

1. Outdoor Advertising . . . A "roving," painted, high-quality 14 × 48 foot billboard. Such an illuminated billboard would be moved and the copy changed every two months or six times in a year with the board facing North on Route 95 in the downtown Providence area, South on the expressway, at the intersection of Route 146 and other choice locations. It is estimated (in fact guaranteed) that such a board delivers 18,250,000 impressions a year.

   TOTAL COST including production for year $7,800.00

2. *Providence Sunday Journal*, Business and Industry Section . . . 600-line ad once a month for 12 months. Directed toward employers and unions. Total estimated impressions . . . 4,800,000 a year.

   TOTAL COST including production for year $5,400.00

3. Balance of advertising would be spread over television, radio and other daily and weekly newspapers at selected times during the year. (Heavy concentration during November as they are federal and state reopening enrollment periods, etc.)

   TOTAL COST including production for year $10,000.00

4. Public Relations Budget for year.................................$ 2,000.00

5. Printing (new brochure, newsletter, including photography, etc.)...$ 4,400.00

6. Mimeograph machine (used) ....$ 400.00

   TOTAL 1973 Advertising and Public Relations Budget..$30,000.00

Other Activities

1. It is the Marketing Department's opinion that a new CHP general purpose brochure is needed. Generally, the brochure would be more colorful with more graphics art work to attract the eye and the reader's attention. We are securing estimates of the cost of printing.

Exhibit 11-5 continued

2. Also under way is the preparation of a CHP Newsletter to be mailed to the entire membership three or four times a year. This can be an invaluable tool in the education and retention of our membership.

3. What can we get free? In the months of November and December, 1972, CHP was highly successful in gaining a large amount of free public service and news coverage in all the media. This increased our public image and visibility enormously. Because we are a non-profit organization, we are in a better position to secure such coverage than a commercial, profit-making organization. Every effort will be made to secure free public exposure in all the mass media.

System for Follow-Up
of New and Old Marketing Group Leads

In order to guard against the possibility that any Marketing Representative might neglect the proper follow-up with a particular group at a future date, each representative should maintain a "tickler file" divided by months. At our weekly Marketing meeting, we shall continue to discuss the prospective groups with which each representative is in contact so that there is no unnecessary duplication. I do not feel it would be advantageous to establish any geographical territories to be assigned to our representatives since all of us have hundreds of contacts all over the state and established entrees with business and industry. However, we should all be aware of each other's activities in order to preclude the possibility that two of us would be pounding on different doors in the same plant at the same time.

OUR GOAL:

25,000
MEMBERS
by
December 31, 1973

Note: Blue Cross and Blue Shield spend more than $150,000 per year in advertising and public relations in the Providence area. They spent $40,000 during the open enrollment period to attract about 8,000 new members (total individuals).

Discussion

1. The Marketing Program

There appear to be several problems with Wilbur's proposed marketing plan:

a. There is a lack of a marketing audit.
b. There is no clearcut relationship to organizational goals (which are not specified).
c. There is a lack of an estimate of market potential.
d. There is an unstated assumption base for forecasts.
e. There are unspecified sources for much of the information.
f. There is vagueness in the statement of plan.
g. There is a lack of integration in the plan. It also concentrates on promotional tactics and does not answer questions of marketing strategy.

2. Plan Improvements

Wilbur's plan could be improved greatly by addressing four major problem areas:

a. The basis for the enrollment projection should be explained. Wilbur has assumed a growth rate of 1,000 members per month. Is this assumption valid? How was the figure obtained and why is the goal to increase enrollment as opposed to other methods of increasing total contribution (that is, price changes) in order to break even? The CHP's past enrollment experience has fallen short of the projected growth rate. Realistic assumptions should be stated in the plan to support monthly enrollment estimates, which should be based on stated market potential coupled with market share targets.
b. The type of enrollees desired should be specified. Wilbur should determine the following:

   • Who are they?

   • Where do they live and work?

   • What are their characteristics (demographic, organizational and life style)?

   The CHP must determine the type of target market mix it should seek, because certain groups such as large families and those of older age, if attracted in large numbers, could put a great strain on resources.

c. Recommendations should be made regarding implications of the market plan and goals. Wilbur has set an enrollment of 25,000 by December 1973. This gives a very short lead time in which new facilities must be acquired, personnel added, and so forth. Assuming that Wilbur's estimates are accurate, the projected expansion might overload the present facility and resouces since the break-even level (16,000) also is its capacity.

d. Promotional recommendations should be justified. The basis for determining the dollar per capita enrollment estimates is questionable. How was it derived? The rationale should be made clear in the plan. More importantly, the CHP should examine the expected reaction of the medical community to the use of outdoor, newspaper, television, and radio advertising. By using advertising, the CHP may be open to censure by the medical society. The CHP doctors, since they value peer acceptance, may disapprove of overt use of advertising.

3. Features of the CHP

There are several similarities between the marketing of CHP's services and of consumer products. Fundamentally, the same concepts and principles are applicable in both situations. Products must be developed, promoted, priced, and distributed. However, there are some essential differences. One is that the CHP is subject to government regulation in its rates (prices). A second concerns promotion. Promotion of professional services must rely on strictly objective, factual descriptions of the services without making claims for results or making comparative statements. Thus, promotional opportunities are more limited than for consumer goods marketers.

4. Strategy Recommendations

Recommendations for CHP's marketing strategy might include the following analysis.

Recommendations need a time frame. It seems clear that Wilbur's immediate problem is to develop a short-term marketing plan. The goal of enrollment growth probably will take high priority. In the short run, few substantive changes are possible in three of the marketing mix variables—namely, product, price, and distribution (that is, place) decisions. Therefore, one feasible short-run scenario would be to make effective use of promotional tools to encourage enrollment. Of course, in the longer run, all of the marketing mix elements should be reviewed intensively for possible modifications. For example, it seems clear that more than one location will be necessary if new market segments are to be tapped effectively in other parts of the state.

The CHP may desire to pursue a market penetration strategy as opposed to the current planned market development. Under a penetration, the CHP would focus on more intensive cultivation of its present markets with existing products. Short-run alternatives include increased efforts focused on employees of firms offering dual choice and more intensive activities directed at first subscribers from other organizations. Some recommendations also may be offered for a market development strategy in which the CHP would seek to sell its existing programs to new market segments.

Index

Note: Page number in *italic* indicates entry is to be found in an Exhibit, Figure, or Table.

D

E

About the Authors

PHILIP D. COOPER is Associate Professor of Marketing at the University of Tulsa. He has had both industrial and academic experience ranging from consumer goods corporations to health care facilities. Prior to faculty and teaching positions at the University of Virginia, Memphis State University, and the Pennsylvania State University, he served in brands management for the Hershey Foods Corporation, sales promotion for the Pillsbury Company, and sales for The Procter & Gamble Company.

Dr. Cooper has focused on the use of the marketing concept in the health care setting since 1971 and has written extensively in the area. Besides writing three books (the two most recent being this one and *Health Care Marketing: Issues and Trends*, both published by Aspen Systems Corporation), his articles have appeared in journals oriented to health care such as *Health Care Management Review*, *Hospital and Health Services Administration, Journal of Health Care Marketing, Journal of Ambulatory Care Management*, and others. He is on the editorial review boards of the *Journal of Health Care Marketing* and the *Health Care Planning and Marketing Quarterly*. Other articles on more general marketing issues by Dr. Cooper have appeared in *Business*, the *Journal of the Academy of Marketing Science, MSU Business Topics*, and many other business-oriented publications.

Dr. Cooper has worked with hospitals, health maintenance organizations, primary care centers, and hospital and nursing home corporations. He has participated in numerous seminars and workshops and has appeared as a guest speaker on health care marketing and planning for nonprofit organizations throughout the country.

LARRY M. ROBINSON is vice president, research, Nationwide Insurance Companies. He was on the faculties of Georgia State University, Antioch College, and Wright State University, then was employed by the General

Electric Company and the General Motors Corporation in manufacturing assignments. He earned a Ph.D in marketing from The Ohio State University.

Dr. Robinson has focused on marketing of hospitality, financial, and health care services and has worked in the area of customer satisfaction measurement and complaint behavior. He has coauthored two texts: *The Corporate Social Challenge* and *Marketing and Society*. With Dr. Cooper, he has coauthored *Health Care Marketing: An Annotated Bibliography*. His articles have appeared in *Journal of Marketing, Journal of Marketing Research, Journal of Consumer Affairs,* the *Journal of the Academy of Marketing Science, Business,* and the *Journal of Health Care Marketing*, where he has served as book review coeditor and is on the editorial review board.

Dr. Robinson has presented numerous seminars and workshops on the application of marketing concepts and techniques for administrators in primary care centers, hospitals, community mental health centers, and vocational rehabilitation facilities.